CHURCHILL'S POCKET
Cardiology

D0283576

Commissioning Editor: Laurence Hunter
Project Development Manager: Janice Urquhart
Project Manager: Frances Affleck
Design direction: Erik Bigland
Illustrated by: Graeme Chambers, Peter Lamb

CHURCHILL'S POCKETBOOK OF
Cardiology

Neil R. Grubb
BSc(Hons) MB ChB MRCP MD
Lecturer in Cardiology, Cardiovascular Research, University of
Edinburgh, Royal Infirmary, Edinburgh, UK

David E. Newby
BA BSc(Hons) Phd BM DM MRCP
Senior Lecturer in Cardiology, Cardiovascular Research, University of
Edinburgh, Royal Infirmary, Edinburgh, UK

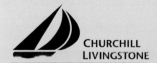

CHURCHILL LIVINGSTONE

EDINBURGH LONDON NEW YORK OXFORD PHILADELPHIA ST LOUIS
SYDNEY TORONTO 2000

CHURCHILL LIVINGSTONE
An imprint of Elsevier Limited

First published 2000

ISBN 0 443 06221 8
  Reprinted 2001, 2002, 2003, 2004

International Student Edition ISBN 0 443 06220 X
  Reprinted 2001

British Library Cataloguing in Publication Data
A catalogue record for this book is available from the British Library

Library of Congress Cataloging in Publication Data
A catalog record for this book is available from the Library of
Congress

Note
Medical knowledge is constantly changing. As new information
becomes available, changes in treatment, procedures, equipment
and the use of drugs become necessary. The authors and the
publishers have, as far as it is possible taken care to ensure that the
information given in this text is accurate and up to date. However,
readers are strongly advised to confirm that the information,
especially with regard to drug usage, complies with current
legislation and standards of practice.

**ELSEVIER
SCIENCE**
your source for books,
journals and multimedia
in the health sciences

www.elsevierhealth.com

The
publisher's
policy is to use
**paper manufactured
from sustainable forests**

Printed in China
C/05

Preface

This pocketbook serves as a guide for doctors embarking on specialist training in cardiology, and will also be useful for junior doctors who work in acute medical, cardiology and coronary care units. It is not intended to be a comprehensive text, but is written using a problem-based approach, complementing the other titles in the successful Churchill's pocketbook series.

We work in an environment of increasing dependence on the large number of high technology investigations and interventions that are available to the cardiologist. Despite this, the authors believe that there is no substitute for bedside clinical skills, and we emphasize the importance of history taking and physical examination in all sections of this guide.

The book is based on the experience of several cardiologists in training and offers concise, practical advice about assessing and managing common (and some less common!) cardiological problems. The book is divided into four broad sections. Section A provides a refresher on cardiovascular anatomy and physiology, and also covers the management of common acute cardiac emergencies. Section B deals with management of in-patients, and includes chapters on acute coronary syndromes, arrhythmias and heart failure. Section C gives advice on how to make a focused assessment of the commoner problems encountered in out-patients clinics. The *new referrals* chapter is symptom-based, since this is how patients present to the clinic. The *review clinics* chapter is diagnosis-based, and covers the common follow-up consultations (e.g. follow-up of patients with valve disease, with recent myocardial infarction, etc.). The final and largest section, Section D, covers the technical aspects of cardiology – echocardiography, cardiac catheterization and intervention, electrophysiology and pacing, and nuclear cardiology. This section provides information about indications for cardiac investigations and procedures, preprocedure checklists, hints and tips about performing procedures, and advice about dealing with their complications. It is designed to accompany practical training under expert supervision! In addition to the four main sections, we have included chapters on cardiac rehabilitation and grown-up congenital heart disease, which are often neglected in training programmes.

Neil Grubb   2000
David Newby

Acknowledgements

The authors would like to thank the following for their contributions to the manuscript: Dr Peter Currie, Consultant Cardiologist, Perth Royal Infirmary (Chapter 14, Adult congenital heart disease); Dr Omer Elhag, Staff Grade Cardiologist, Royal Infirmary, Edinburgh (contributions to Chapter 16, Electrophysiology); Dr John Reid, Consultant Radiologist, Borders General Hospital, Melrose (Chapter 19, Nuclear cardiology); Dr Ian Todd, Consultant in Rehabilitation Medicine, Astley Ainslie Hospital, Edinburgh (Chapter 15, Rehabilitation); Dr Helen Oxenham, Specialist Registrar in Cardiology, Royal Infirmary, Edinburgh (artwork, Chapter 14, Adult congenital heart disease).

We would also like to thank the following for their helpful advice and comments on the manuscript: Dr Peter Bloomfield, Consultant Cardiologist, Royal Infirmary, Edinburgh; Dr Nicholas Boon, Consultant Cardiologist, Royal Infirmary, Edinburgh; Professor Keith Fox, Consultant Cardiologist and Professor of Cardiology, Cardiovascular Unit, University of Edinburgh; Dr Nicholas Goodfield, Consultant Cardiologist, Stobhill Hospital, Glasgow; Ms Ase Irvine, Principal Pharmacist (Drug Information), Royal Infirmary, Edinburgh; Miss Jennifer Laurie, Senior Technician, Cardiology Department, Royal Infirmary, Edinburgh; Dr Hugh Miller, Consultant Cardiologist, Royal Infirmary, Edinburgh; Miss Margaret Pryde, Chief Technician, Cardiology Department, Royal Infirmary, Edinburgh; Dr Neal Uren, Consultant Cardiologist, Royal Infirmary, Edinburgh.

Contents

Abbreviations

see Chapter 17 for pacemaker codes.

A_2	aortic second heart sound
ABG	arterial blood gas
ACC	American College of Cardiology
ACEi	angiotensin-converting enzyme (inhibitor)
AF	atrial fibrillation
AHA	American Heart Association
AICD	automatic implantable cardioverter/defibrillator
AMI	acute myocardial infarction
ANF	antinuclear factor
AP	antero-posterior
aPTT	activated partial thromboplastin time
ARP	atrial refractory period
ASD	atrial septal defect
ASH	asymmetrical septal hypertrophy
ASO	antistreptolysin O
AST	aspartate transaminase
AV	atrioventricular
AVNRT	atrioventricular nodal re-entry tachycardia
AVR	aortic valve replacement
AXR	abdominal X-ray
BCS	British Cardiac Society
BCIS	British Cardiac Intervention Society
BD	twice daily
BP	blood pressure
BPEG	British Pacing and Electrophysiology Group
bpm	beats per minute
BSA	body surface area

CABG	coronary artery bypass graft
CAD	coronary artery disease
CCS	Canadian Cardiovascular Society (functional class)
CFM	colour flow mapping
CHB	complete heart block
CK	creatine kinase
CK-MB	creatine kinase MB isoform
COA(P)D	chronic obstructive airways (pulmonary) disease
CRP	C-reactive protein
CS	coronary sinus
CSM	carotid sinus massage
CT	computerized tomography
CVP	central venous pressure
C_x	circumflex coronary artery
CXR	chest X-ray
D_1, D_2	first and second diagonal branches (of LAD)
DVT	deep vein thrombosis
DCA	directional coronary atherectomy
DFP	diastolic filling period
DIC	disseminated intravascular coagulation
DVT	deep venous thrombosis
EAT	ectopic atrial tachycardia
ECG	electrocardiogram
EDM	early diastolic murmur
EEG	electroencephalogram
EF	ejection fraction

EMD	electromechanical dissociation		**ISA**	intrinsic sympathomimetic activity
EMG	electromyogram		**IV**	intravenous
EP(S)	electrophysiology/ electrophysiological study		**IVC**	inferior vena cava
			IVI	intravenous infusion
ESC	European Society of Cardiology		I_x	investigations
ESM	ejection systolic murmur		**JVP**	jugular venous pressure
ESR	erythrocyte sedimentation rate			
			LA	left atrium
ETT	exercise tolerance test		**LAD**	left anterior descending coronary artery
F	French (diameter of catheter)		**LAO**	left anterior oblique
			LBBB	left bundle branch block
FBC	full blood count		**LDH**	lactate dehydrogenase
FEV_1	forced expiratory volume in one second		**LDL**	low density lipoprotein
			LFT	liver function tests
FOB	faecal occult blood		**LSE**	left sternal edge
FVC	forced vital capacity		**LVEDP**	left ventricular end-diastolic pressure
GKI	glucose-potassium-insulin infusion		**LVEDV**	left ventricular end-diastolic volume
GTN	glyceryl trinitrate		**LVEF**	left ventricular ejection fraction
GUCH	grown-up congenital heart disease		**LVESV**	left ventricular end-systolic volume
HAD	hospital anxiety and depression questionnaire		**LVF**	left ventricular failure
			LVH	left ventricular hypertrophy
HCSS	hypersensitive carotid sinus syndrome		**LVIDD**	left ventricular internal diastolic dimension
HDL	high density lipoprotein		**LVISD**	left ventricular internal systolic dimension
HGV	heavy goods vehicle			
H(O)CM	hypertrophic (obstructive) cardiomyopathy		**LVOT**	left ventricular outflow tract
HRA	high right atrium		**LVSW(I)**	left ventricular stroke work (index)
HR	heart rate			
HRT	hormone replacement therapy		**MDM**	mid-diastolic murmur
			MI	myocardial infarction
H_x	history		**MIC**	minimum inhibitory concentration
IABP	intra-aortic balloon pump			
IHD	ischaemic heart disease		**MRI**	magnetic resonance imaging
IM	intramuscular		**MV**	mitral valve
INR	international normalized ratio			

MVA	mitral valve area	**PTCA**	percutaneous transluminal coronary angioplasty
MVR	mitral valve replacement	**PV**	pulmonary valve
NASPE	North American Society for Pacing and Electrophysiology	**PVARP**	post-ventricular atrial refractory period
NO	nitric oxide	**PVR(I)**	pulmonary vascular resistance (index)
NSAID	non-steroidal anti-inflammatory drug	**QID**	four times daily
NYHA	New York Heart Association (functional class)	**RA**	right atrium
nQMI	non-Q wave myocardial infarction	**RAO**	right anterior oblique
		RBBB	right bundle branch block
OD	once daily	**RCA**	right coronary artery
OM_1, OM_2	first and second obtuse marginal branches (of circumflex)	**RF**	radiofrequency
		RIMA	right internal mammary artery
PA	pulmonary artery	**RV**	right ventricle
P_2	pulmonary second heart sound	**RVEDP**	right ventricular end-diastolic pressure
pCO_2	partial pressure of carbon dioxide	**RVH**	right ventricular hypertrophy
PCTA	percutaneous transluminal coronary angioplasty	**RVOT**	right ventricular outflow tract
PCWP	pulmonary capillary wedge pressure	**RVSW(I)**	right ventricular stroke work (index)
PDA	patent ductus arteriosus	**R_x**	treatment
PE	pulmonary embolism	**S_1, S_2, etc.**	first heart sound, second heart sound, etc.
PFTs	pulmonary function tests	**SACT**	sino-atrial conduction time
PI	pulmonary incompetence	**SBE**	subacute bacterial endocarditis
PJRT	permanent junctional reciprocating tachycardia	**SC**	subcutaneous
PMR	percutaneous myocardial revascularization	**SEP**	systolic ejection period
		SNRT	sinus node recovery time
pO_2	partial pressure of oxygen	**SPECT**	single position emission computed tomography
PPM	permanent pacemaker	**SVC**	superior vena cava
PS	pulmonary stenosis	**SV(I)**	stroke volume (index)
PSA	pacing system analyser	**SVG**	saphenous vein graft
PSM	pan-systolic murmur	**SVR(I)**	systemic vascular resistance (index)
PSV	public services vehicle		

SVT	supraventricular tachycardia		**TV**	tricuspid valve
			T$_x$	treatment
TB	tuberculosis		**U&Es**	serum urea and electrolytes
TGA	transposition of the great arteries			
TGV	transposition of the great vessels		**VF**	ventricular fibrillation
			VLDL	very low density lipoprotein
TI	tricuspid incompetence			
TID	thrice daily		**VPB**	ventricular premature beat
TMR	transmyocardial laser revascularization		**VSD**	ventricular septal defect
TOE	transoesophageal echocardiogram		**VT**	ventricular tachycardia
TnT, TnI	troponin T, troponin I		**WCC**	white cell count
tPA	tissue plasminogen activator		**WHO**	World Health Organization
TS	tricuspid stenosis		**WPW**	Wolff–Parkinson–White syndrome
TTE	transthoracic echocardiogram			

TRAINEE'S SURVIVAL GUIDE

CHAPTER 1

REFRESHER COURSE IN BASIC CARDIOLOGY

THE CARDIOVASCULAR HISTORY

BACK TO BASICS

An accurate clinical history is the most valuable diagnostic test available to the cardiologist. A good attempt at a diagnosis can be made in most cases from the history alone; examination and tests most often serve to confirm what was suspected from the history in the first place. You should be skilled at history taking already and this section is designed to serve as a 'memory jogger' for doctors working in a cardiac unit for the first time.

COMMON PRESENTING COMPLAINTS

Chest discomfort

This is the most common symptom you will assess. Although many patients with ischaemia have typical, constricting central pain, often radiating to the left arm or neck, many do not have a 'full house' of symptoms. In patients with chronic angina it helps to ask if the current symptom resembles their normal angina. Remember, angina can present with epigastric or shoulder discomfort, isolated arm or jaw discomfort, back pain, or without discomfort at all. In patients with atypical symptoms look for typical precipitants (effort, emotion), relieving factors (rest, sublingual nitrate) and associated symptoms (breathlessness, autonomic features, e.g. sweating, nausea, vomiting, pallor), and look for supportive evidence from the ECG and cardiac enzymes. Most importantly, keep an open mind: you can't rely totally on the patient's description. Don't forget that 'heartburn' is one of the commonest symptoms of an inferior infarct!

Breathlessness

Causes to remember are pulmonary oedema, arrhythmia, chronic low-output state, ischaemic left ventricular dysfunction, systemic acidosis and occasionally β-blockade/bronchospasm. Don't forget, patients are prone to pulmonary embolism, hospital-acquired pneumonia and anxiety. Ask about precipitants (effort, lying flat), relieving factors (rest, glyceryl trinitrate (GTN), sitting up) and associated symptoms (chest discomfort, palpitation) to try and differentiate the causes.

When assessing symptom severity, it is helpful to use one of the symptom rating scales given in Table 1.1 and to document functional ability in the case records (e.g. under diagnosis list: **CCS class III angina**, or **NYHA class II cardiac failure**).

Palpitation

This means different things to different patients. Some are unusually aware of their normal rhythm; in other cases a 'flutter' may signify anxiety. A good description helps diagnose the underlying problem. Is the onset sudden? (Gradual onset and resolution suggests sinus tachycardia.) Is the rhythm fast, slow, forceful, regular or irregular? Pauses and thumps often indicate extrasystoles. Ask the patient to tap out the rhythm. Look for precipitants: palpitation brought on by effort or an anginal episode may signify ventricular arrhythmia. Alcohol may induce atrial flutter or fibrillation. Atrial arrhythmias rarely cause syncope unless very fast or in patients with severe myocardial or valvular disease.

TABLE 1.1 Grading symptoms of disability due to heart disease

New York Heart Association (NYHA) Functional Classification (applies to fatigue, dyspnoea or angina)

Class I No limitations during ordinary activity

Class II Slight limitation during ordinary activity, e.g. mild or occasional angina/dyspnoea

Class III Marked limitation of normal activities without symptoms at rest

Class IV Unable to undertake physical activity without symptoms; symptoms may be present at rest

Canadian Cardiovascular Society (CCS) Functional classification (applies to angina only)

Class I No angina with ordinary activity. Angina with strenuous, rapid or prolonged exertion

Class II Slight limitation of ordinary activity; angina when walking up stairs briskly, or walking on a cold or windy day

Class III Marked limitation: angina when walking at normal pace up flight of stairs, or walking 1–2 blocks distance

Class IV Angina on minimal exertion or at rest

Dizziness

This non-specific symptom is common in cardiac patients. Make sure the patient does not mean rotational vertigo. Common causes are vasodilator drugs (most antianginal medications can cause dizziness), diuretics (volume depletion) or a low cardiac output state; these cause postural hypotension. Ask about associated symptoms (flushing, palpitation or syncope can suggest an arrhythmia, or vasovagal syndrome). Dizziness may also reflect carotid, vertebrobasilar or cerebrovascular disease. In the elderly dizziness is often multifactorial – a combination of heart disease, medication, impaired autoregulatory reflexes and sometimes cerebrovascular disease.

Blackouts

Blackouts must be meticulously assessed as they can reflect serious cardiac disease. Exertional syncope suggests aortic stenosis, outflow obstruction or exercise-induced arrhythmia. Precipitation by prolonged standing, emotion, noxious stimuli, cough or micturition suggests vasovagal syncope, especially if there is premonitory dizziness or flushing (see Chapters 11 and 13).

PREVIOUS MEDICAL HISTORY

The next person to read the case notes will thank you for good, chronological documentation of previous cardiac problems, with attention to the following points.

'Heart attacks'

Don't believe the patient who tells you they've had 10 heart attacks! Some 'notch up' any admission with chest pain as a heart attack. Check the notes.

Angina

For patients who have this diagnosis:

- **question it!** Check the history is consistent with angina. Is there objective evidence of ischaemia from stress testing? It is difficult to shake off a label once it has been applied, so keep an open mind
- log a good description of what the patient's angina symptoms are
- look out previous angiogram reports (a two-line summary in the notes is helpful) and percutaneous interventions
- log peripheral vascular problems (important during angiography)
- log varicose veins, if present (important for a cardiac surgeon to know).

Cardiac surgery

'Previous CABG' or 'valve replacement' is inadequate.

- For CABG, document how many grafts, types of graft (vein, internal mammary, radial artery) and to which vessels. This makes life much easier when interpreting stress tests or planning angiography.
- For valve patients, document valve model, size and position. Different valve types and sizes have different properties which become important when assessing echo and cardiac catheterization measurements. Document if concomitant CABG done.

Coronary risk factor profile

Keep this up to date in the notes:

- total cholesterol, HDL cholesterol and triglycerides (within past 6 months)
- smoking status (include past smoking history – 'non-smoker' is not the same as 'ex 60-a-day smoker for 30 years, gave up last week'!)
- diabetes mellitus (check: blood glucose levels are often filed and overlooked)
- blood pressure (include past history of hypertension and current BP)
- family history (only really relevant in first-degree relatives under the age of 60).

Valve patients

Don't forget:

- history of rheumatic fever or scarlet fever?
- previous interventions (valvotomies, valvuloplasties).

MEDICATION

Cardiac patients are victims of polypharmacy! Encourage patients to carry a list with them. Record drug type and, for sustained-release preparations, brand. Check dosing frequency and duration of treatment. **Is the drug really needed?** Sometimes patients are continued on antianginal treatment which they have found completely ineffective. Note true allergies (i.e. urticaria, rash, bronchospasm, anaphylactic reaction) and intolerances (because of side effects). Patients may have side effects and not associate them with their medication, so ask specifically (e.g. impotence and β-blockers; cough and ACE inhibitors; oedema and calcium channel blockers).

PSYCHOSOCIAL ASPECTS

Work

Ask about patients' employment: what their job involves. Is there a significant physical component? Psychological stress? Some occupations have specific regulations for employees with heart disease, e.g. heavy-goods and public-service vehicle drivers, and pilots.

Home

For older patients, cardiac symptoms seriously affect independence. Housing may be unsuitable because of stairs, or distance to shops etc. Rehousing or social services input may be needed in these cases. Also ask about dependants: your patient with NYHA class III angina might be struggling to care for a housebound spouse or parent!

Alcohol

Although there is some evidence for the benefit of a glass of red wine a day, alcohol often spells trouble for cardiac patients. If you are suspicious about consumption, try to corroborate alcohol history through a relative. Although alcohol is not a direct coronary risk factor, abuse is associated with hypertension, dilated cardiomyopathy and atrial fibrillation.

Psychological problems

Chronic anxiety and depression affect up to 50% of patients with ischaemic heart disease. Depression after myocardial infarction is associated with premature death. Fear of death, illness or dependency is a common symptom and patients may feel out of control. Ask specifically about these symptoms: fears sometimes arise from misconceptions about or lack of understanding of the condition. The Hospital Anxiety and Depression (HAD) questionnaire can be used to screen for these symptoms. Several specific cardiac screening questionnaires have also been devised:

- Heart Patients Psychological Questionnaire
- Cardiac Threat Questionnaire
- Cardiac Depression Scale.

CARDIOVASCULAR EXAMINATION

BACK TO BASICS

As with history taking, by this stage you should be competent at examining patients. In the assessment of any patient admitted to hospital and any new patient attending the hospital clinic, a full systematic physical examination is mandatory. However, in review clinic and during ward rounds and interdepartmental consults, you need of necessity to be focused and concise in your examination because of the demands on your time. This chapter concentrates on cardiovascular examination and also serves as a 'memory jogger'. A detailed text which covers all the systems is *Macleod's Clinical Examination* (Churchill Livingstone 1995).

GENERAL INSPECTION

When you take the history, take a mental step back and ask yourself 'does he/she *look* unwell?'. This is the most important 'knack' to learn in examination. Does the patient look frightened? Pale, grey, sweaty? Some doctors (and more so nurses) have an uncanny talent for spotting patients who say they are well but who are heading towards cardiogenic shock or heart failure, or even cardiac arrest. Check systematically for the following:

- Demeanour   (anxious, alert, orientated, confused?)
- Colour
  - pallor   (suggests poor perfusion or anaemia)
  - central cyanosis   (low O_2 saturation due to pulmonary oedema, pulmonary embolism, infection, lung disease or cyanotic congenital heart disease)
  - peripheral cyanosis   ($\downarrow$ perfusion; vasoconstriction or low output)
  - jaundice   (hepatic congestion, haemolysis, drug-induced)
  - plethora   (polycythaemia, vasodilatation)
  - malar flush   (mitral stenosis, chronic low-output state)
- Build
  - obesity   (check height and weight, calculate BMI
  - cachexia   (common in chronic cardiac failure)
  - Marfanoid   (risk of aortic valve disease, aortic dissection)

dysmorphic

hypertelorism (wide-set eyes)	→	pulmonary stenosis
elfin facies (receding jaw, flared nostrils, pointed ears)	→	supravalvar aortic stenosis
Down syndrome (trisomy 21); (flat profile, small nose, low-set ears, simian crease)	→	endocardial cushion defects.

HANDS AND FACE

These are normally inspected while you are checking the pulse and respiratory rate. Specific areas for attention are detailed below:

- Temperature (tells you about peripheral perfusion)
- Sweating (pyrexia or sympathetic activation)
- Digital clubbing (cyanotic congenital heart disease, infective endocarditis [late sign])
- Cutaneous features of endocarditis
  petechiae
  splinter haemorrhages (linear haemorrhages in nailbeds – vasculitic)
  Osler's nodes (small, purplish nodules on pulps of fingers and toes, sometimes in palms and soles)
  Janeway lesions (raised, non-tender, haemorrhagic lesions in palms and soles)
- Xanthomata (yellowish deposits of lipid in tendons, skin and soft tissues)
  tendon xanthomata (commonly Achilles tendon, extensor digitorum) [association: type II hyperlipidaemia]
  palmar xanthomata (skin creases of palms and soles) [association: type III hyperlipidaemia]
  xanthelasma (skin of eyelids, often upper) [can occur in absence of hyperlipidaemia]
- Teeth (poor dentition increases risk of endocarditis)
- Eyes
  corneal arcus (hyperlipidaemia; also occurs with age)
  hypertensive retinopathy
  - grade I arterial tortuosity, change in calibre giving 'silver wiring' appearance
  - grade II arteriovenous nipping; right-angle arteriovenous crossing (arterial smooth muscle hypertrophy)
  - grade III flame-shaped haemorrhages, hard and soft exudates (often in accelerated hypertension)
  - grade IV papilloedema (sign of cerebral oedema)
  diabetic retinopathy
  - background microaneurysms, blot and dot haemorrhages, hard exudates (lipid deposition in retina)

proliferative soft exudates, flame haemorrhages, new vessel
formation

Roth spots (retinal haemorrhage with central white spot due
to retinal vasculitis – occurs in endocarditis).

THE ARTERIAL SYSTEM

Examination of the arterial system gives information about the patency of the
arteries and also about the function of the heart.

The pulses

- Check rate, rhythm and for apical–radial deficit (atrial fibrillation)
- Radio–radial delay (aortic dissection)
- Pulse volume/character (use brachial or carotid pulse to assess)

  low volume (low output, hypovolaemia, arterial insufficiency)

  high volume (high-output state [pyrexia, vasodilatation, aortic
  regurgitation])

  pulsus alternans (alternating low- and high-volume beats which
  occur during bigeminy and in severe LVF)

  pulsus paradoxus (inspiratory decrease in pulse volume (see Blood
  pressure, below))

  pulsus bisferiens (double systolic peak, associated with aortic
  regurgitation and sometimes HOCM)

  collapsing pulse (check pulse character with arm raised above
  head; rapid 'downstroke' in severe aortic
  regurgitation)

  slow rising pulse (delayed 'upstroke' of pulse in severe aortic
  stenosis)

  jerky pulse (rapid 'upstroke' followed by rapid decline
  caused by outflow obstruction in HOCM)

- Peripheral pulses

  These are checked for signs of aortic disease and as a test of peripheral
  arterial patency

  femoral pulse (check volume, radiofemoral delay [aortic
  coarctation], bruits, Duroziez's sign [diastolic bruit
  when artery compressed])

  popliteal (check with knee slightly flexed; located deep, in
  middle of popliteal fossa)

  dorsalis pedis (lateral to extensor hallucis tendon)

  posterior tibial (behind medial malleolus).

Blood pressure

- *Check BP in both arms* if aortic coarctation or dissection suspected.
- *Pulsus paradoxus* is an exaggerated inspiratory fall in BP. Check systolic BP
in inspiration and expiration by letting cuff pressure fall by 2 mmHg per

heartbeat. A difference >10 mmHg signifies pulsus paradoxus. Occurs in cardiac tamponade and severe airway obstruction.

● *Compare supine upper and lower limb BP* in patients with aortic coarctation, to estimate pressure gradient.

Key points on checking blood pressure

● Have the patient in a relaxed and comfortable position.
● Use cuff size appropriate to the upper arm diameter.
● **Do not** check blood pressure through clothing.
● Palpate rather than listen as you inflate the cuff to avoid the 'auscultatory gap'.
● Check BP with arm resting at level of heart.
● If using mercury sphygmomanometer, have it at eye level and at level of patient's chest.
● Use Korotkov phase V for diastolic BP (i.e. complete disappearance of sounds).
● Recheck BP after 5 minutes' rest if result abnormally high.

THE JUGULAR VENOUS PULSE (JVP)

The JVP gives an index of right atrial pressure, which is elevated in cardiac failure and fluid overload. In addition, the JVP waveform gives an index of cardiac function (see Fig. 1.1). Ensure patient is reclined to 45°. Time against contralateral carotid pulse.

Abnormalities of the JVP

● Large a-wave   right ventricular hypertrophy (↓ compliance), tricuspid stenosis
● Cannon waves   [atrial contraction against closed tricuspid valve] junctional rhythm with retrograde atrial activation complete heart block (irregular cannon waves)

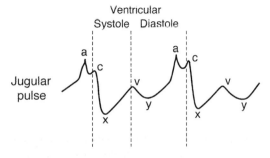

Fig. 1.1 Waveform of jugular venous pulse. (From *McLeod's clinical examination*, with permission.)

- Large v-wave — tricuspid regurgitation
- Rapid y descent — any condition with myocardial dysfunction and ↑ CVP ASD, constrictive pericarditis
- Kussmaul's sign — rise of JVP on inspiration (constrictive pericarditis, tamponade)
- Fixed, raised JVP without waveform — SVC obstruction.

Elements of the JVP

- a-wave — Rise in JVP due to RA contraction
- c-wave — Transmitted carotid impulse at onset of systole
- v-wave — Rise in RA pressure due to filling against closed tricuspid valve in systole
- x descent — RA relaxation followed by descent of tricuspid ring in systole
- y descent — Pressure drop as tricuspid valve opens at start of diastole

---

THE PRECORDIUM

Inspection

- Scars (sternotomy, valvotomy [in rib line, lower left chest] thoracotomy)
- Deformity (pectus excavatum, kyphoscoliosis – Marfan syndrome)
- Pulsations (see 'heaves' below)
- Gynaecomastia (digoxin, spironolactone).

Palpation

Apex position, character

- Absent impulse (emphysema, obesity, pericardial effusion, dextrocardia)
- Forceful impulse (LVH)
- 'Tapping' impulse (mitral stenosis)
- Dyskinetic impulse (due to paradoxical ventricular wall movement in systole, e.g. anterior MI).

Heaves and thrills

- Parasternal heave due to RV dilatation or hypertrophy – most often seen in mitral valve disease and cor pulmonale
- Thrills.

Percussion

Percussion of cardiac dullness is not clinically very useful: the CXR gives a better idea of heart size. Still, check for pleural effusions; upper chest dullness can occur with aortic aneurysm.

Auscultation

This acquired skill is one of the keys to diagnosis in cardiology. The best way to learn is to see plenty of examples of the common added sounds and murmurs, as you will do in review clinics.

Auscultation technique

- Time heart sounds and murmurs against the carotid pulse.
- The **bell** is best for low-pitched sounds, **diaphragm** for high-pitched sounds.
- Listen in turn over the apex (diaphragm *and* bell), upper and lower left and right sternal borders, under the clavicles, over carotids and in axilla (diaphragm ± bell).
- Listen at apex, with patient rolled to left side (mitral stenotic murmur).
- Listen at lower left sternal border, with patient sitting forward, in expiration (aortic incompetence murmur).
- Listen **individually** to the S_1 and S_2:
    Is either sound loud?
    Is there splitting?
    Does splitting increase or decrease with inspiration?
- Listen for added sounds; note their timing relative to S_1 and S_2.
- Listen for murmurs:
    Systolic or diastolic?
    Which part of systole/diastole (pan-, early, mid, late)?
    Quality of murmur (harsh, soft, low/high-pitched)?
- Listen for prosthetic sounds.

Heart sounds

The heart sounds themselves are often overlooked as murmurs are sought. They give useful additional clues to underlying pathology.

- Loud S_1 high-output states
                mitral stenosis (corresponds with 'tapping' apex)
- Split S_1 RBBB (wide splitting)
                Ebstein's anomaly
- Loud S_2 pulmonary hypertension (loud P_2)
                systemic hypertension (loud A_2)
                high-output states
- Split S_2 (A_2P_2)   *physiological* (normal on inspiration, especially in young)
                delayed pulmonary valve closure (RBBB)
                prolonged RV systole (massive pulmonary embolism, pulmonary hypertension, pulmonary stenosis, ASD)
                early aortic valve closure (mitral regurgitation, VSD)
- Reverse split   *delayed aortic valve closure* (LBBB, RV paced rhythm)

S_2 (P_2A_2)	*prolonged LV systole* (LVOT obstruction, aortic stenosis, hypertension)
	patent ductus arteriosus
	early pulmonary valve closure (WPW syndrome type B)
● Fixed split S_2	*inspiration has same effect on left and right heart output* (medium-sized or large ASD).

Added sounds

● A **third heart sound** (S_3) is due to rapid ventricular filling (e.g. in left ventricular failure). It occurs shortly after the S_2 and is usually low-pitched. It can occur in athletic individuals with slow resting HR.

● A **fourth heart sound** (S_4) is due to atrial systole against a poorly compliant ventricle (e.g. LVH, hypertension). It occurs just before S_1.

● An **ejection click** is high-pitched and closely follows S_1. It occurs in congenitally bicuspid aortic valve/aortic stenosis, valvular pulmonary stenosis and idiopathic dilatation of the pulmonary artery.

● A **midsystolic click** is due to mitral valve prolapse.

● An **opening snap** is high-pitched, occurs after S_2 and occurs as a stenotic mitral valve opens. In severe mitral stenosis the opening snap may be absent owing to immobility of the leaflets.

● **Prosthetic sounds** – mechanical prostheses should have both an opening and a closing sound. Absent prosthetic sounds may be a sign of valve dysfunction (e.g. thrombosis, pannus encroachment on valve, or (rarely) valve disintegration (patient is critically compromised; the best documented case is of strut fracture and disc embolism in specific Bjork–Shiley concavoconvex (CC) valves in the mitral position).

Murmurs

● Ejection (mid) systolic murmur

aortic stenosis	(radiates to aortic area/carotids)
aortic valve calcification	(similar radiation; often not carotids)
pulmonary stenosis	(radiates posteriorly and to pulmonary area)

TABLE 1.2 Grading system for cardiac murmurs	
Grade I	Just audible in quiet room, with patient holding breath
Grade II	Quiet
Grade III	Easy to hear, no accompanying thrill
Grade IV	Loud, with thrill
Grade V	Very loud, with thrill
Grade VI	Audible without stethoscope

ASD with left to right shunt   (increased flow into dilated PA)

'innocent' flow murmur   (anaemia, thyrotoxicosis, pyrexia, pregnancy)

- Pansystolic (holosystolic) murmur (S_2 may be obscured)

  mitral regurgitation   (often radiates to axilla)

  tricuspid regurgitation   (louder on inspiration)

  VSD   (harsh, can radiate to right sternal border)

  PDA   (component of 'continuous murmur')

- Early systolic murmur

  severe mitral regurgitation   (ejection ends before S_2)

- Late systolic murmur

  mitral valve prolapse   (midsystolic click may precede murmur)

- Early diastolic murmur

  aortic regurgitation   (may radiate to right sternal border*)

  pulmonary regurgitation   (in pulmonary hypertension, loud S_2 then EDM – Graham Steell murmur)

  (* the EDM of acute severe aortic regurgitation is short and medium pitched, as the LV is small and non-compliant. The EDM of chronic aortic regurgitation is prolonged and high-pitched.)

- Mid-diastolic murmur

  mitral stenosis   (low-pitched; in sinus rhythm, louder late in diastole (presystolic accentuation))

  tricuspid stenosis   (louder on inspiration; lower left sternal border)

  severe mitral regurgitation   (due to increased forward flow)

  aortic regurgitation   (aortic regurgitant jet hits anterior mitral leaflet, $\rightarrow$ vibration ± functional mitral stenosis (Austin Flint murmur))

  pulmonary regurgitation   (with normal PA pressure)

- Late diastolic (presystolic) murmur

  mitral stenosis in sinus rhythm   (see above)

  tricuspid stenosis in sinus rhythm.

FINAL POINTS

- **The abdomen.** Check for pulsatile hepatomegaly (right heart failure with tricuspid incompetence), ascites, splenomegaly (endocarditis) and renal bruits (renal artery stenosis – hypertension).
- **Oedema.** Check for ankle and sacral oedema. Note whether it is pitting or non-pitting, signs of chronic oedema (haemosiderin pigmentation).
- **Lower limbs.** Check pulses and for capillary refill (peripheral perfusion), venous or arterial ulcers, varicose veins.
- For examination during vagal manoeuvres and carotid sinus massage, see Chapter 11.

Warning: Check for varicose veins in patients you consider for coronary artery bypass surgery. Don't let the surgeon find them first at the operation!

CARDIAC ANATOMY

GENERAL STRUCTURE

TABLE 1.3 Normal reference values for the cardiac chambers

Chamber diameter	Men (mm)	Women (mm)
Left atrium	30–45	27–40
LV end-diastolic diameter	43–59	40–52
LV end-systolic diameter	26–40	23–35
Posterior wall (diastole)	6–12	5–11
Interventricular septum (diastole)	6–13	5–12

VASCULAR ANATOMY

The anatomy of the epicardial vessels is shown in Figure 1.3. More detail on coronary anatomy is given in Chapter 18 (angiography).

TABLE 1.4 Normal reference diameters for the aorta

Aortic site	Range (mm)
Aortic annulus	17–25
Sinuses	22–36
Arch	14–29
Abdominal	10–22

CARDIAC PHYSIOLOGY

HAEMODYNAMICS

Cardiac ouput is the product of the stroke volume and heart rate and is normally around $5\,l\,min^{-1}$ at rest. Although it is easy to think of cardiac output as being determined solely by cardiac contractility, systemic vascular resistance (SVR) is equally important in determining cardiac output. SVR and

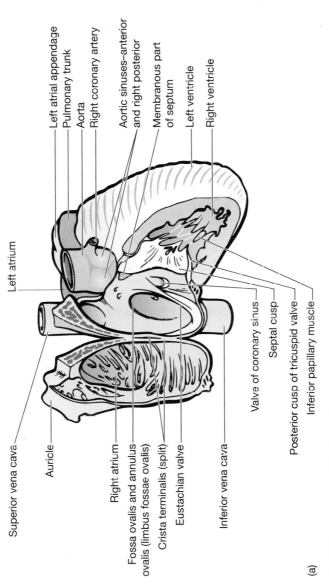

Fig. 1.2 Internal anatomy of the left and right heart.

(a)

Left atrial appendage
Pulmonary trunk
Aorta
Right coronary artery
Aortic sinuses–anterior and right posterior
Membranous part of septum
Left ventricle
Right ventricle

Left atrium

Superior vena cava

Auricle

Right atrium
Fossa ovalis and annulus ovalis (limbus fossae ovalis)
Crista terminalis (split)
Eustachian valve

Inferior vena cava

Valve of coronary sinus
Septal cusp
Posterior cusp of tricuspid valve
Inferior papillary muscle

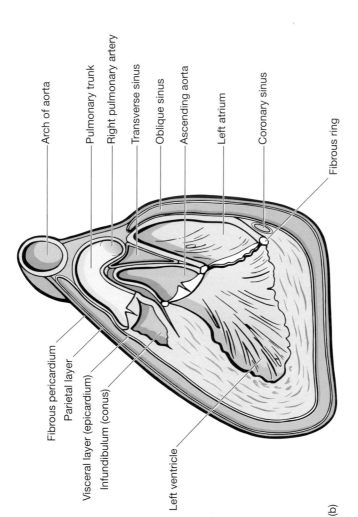

Arch of aorta

Pulmonary trunk

Right pulmonary artery

Transverse sinus

Oblique sinus

Ascending aorta

Left atrium

Coronary sinus

Fibrous ring

Fibrous pericardium

Parietal layer

Visceral layer (epicardium)

Infundibulum (conus)

Left ventricle

(b)

Fig. 1.2 (cont'd)

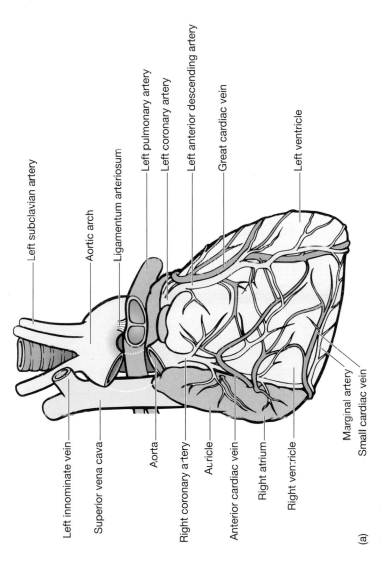

Fig. 1.3 Valvular and vascular anatomy of the heart.

(a)

Left innominate vein

Superior vena cava

Aorta

Right coronary artery

Auricle

Anterior cardiac vein

Right atrium

Right ventricle

Marginal artery

Small cardiac vein

Left subclavian artery

Aortic arch

Ligamentum arteriosum

Left pulmonary artery

Left coronary artery

Left anterior descending artery

Great cardiac vein

Left ventricle

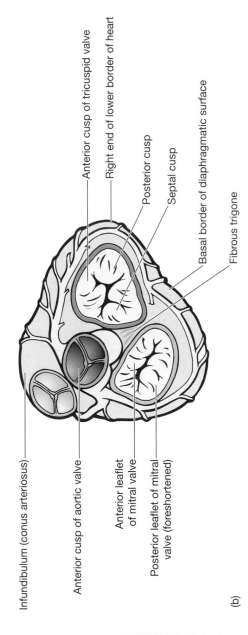

(b)

Fig. 1.3 *(cont'd)*

cardiac contractility determine cardiac output in a manner analogous to Ohm's law ($V = IR$):

$$\text{Current (I)} = \frac{\text{Voltage (V)}}{\text{Resistance (R)}}$$

Systemic vascular resistance

$$\text{Cardiac output} = \frac{\text{Mean aortic pressure} - \text{Mean right atrial pressure}}{\text{Systemic vascular resistance (SVR)}}$$

So, to calculate systemic vascular resistance accurately, you need to know:

- Mean aortic pressure (from BP measurement)
- Mean right atrial pressure (from central venous line, right heart catheter, or estimated from JVP)
- Cardiac output (from thermodilution catheter, Fick principle (see Chapter 18) or echo (less accurate).

Right heart (Swan–Ganz) catheterization is required for an accurate estimation of SVR. When right atrial pressure is unknown this term is dropped and the equation can be simplified:

$$\text{Cardiac output} \cong \frac{\text{Mean aortic pressure}}{\text{'Total peripheral resistance'}}$$

Pulmonary vascular resistance

For the pulmonary circulation, the same principle is used:

$$\text{Cardiac output} = \frac{\text{Mean PA pressure} - \text{Mean left atrial pressure}}{\text{Pulmonary vascular resistance (PVR)}}$$

To calculate pulmonary vascular resistance accurately, you need to know:

- Mean PA pressure (from right heart catheter)
- Mean left atrial pressure (inferred from pulmonary capillary 'wedge' pressure – right heart catheter)
- Cardiac output (as for SVR calculation above).

Right heart (Swan–Ganz) catheterization is also required for an accurate estimation of PVR.

Tip:
- SVR and PVR are expressed in dyne.s cm^{-5}, or Wood units ($mmHg/l\,min^{-1}$).
- Wood units are easier to calculate from pressure and cardiac output data.
- 80 dyne.s $cm^{-5} \cong 1$ Wood unit.

Most of the resistance to systemic and pulmonary blood flow is mediated by small arterioles (resistance vessels), with only a small contribution from the larger conduit arteries.

Over 75% of normal circulating blood volume is contained within the venous system and capacitance vessels. The latter can accommodate a large reservoir of blood and virtually the entire volume of any infused blood or fluid will initially be accommodated in the capacitance vessels.

The organs of the systemic circulation are arranged in parallel circuits so, as the demands of any one vascular bed increase, there is a relative reduction in blood flow elsewhere. This may be compensated for by an increase in cardiac output. For example, blood flow is diverted from the splanchnic circulation to skeletal muscle during exercise; the reverse occurs after a large meal. Regional blood flow is regulated by local, humoral and neural factors.

Coronary perfusion

Coronary blood flow occurs predominantly in diastole. Coronary perfusion pressure is determined by the pressure gradient across the coronary vascular bed:

TABLE 1.5 Normal ranges of haemodynamic parameters (see inside cover)

Parameter	Range	Units
Heart rate	60–100	bpm
Right atrial pressure	0–7	mmHg
Left atrial pressure	4–12	mmHg
Left ventricular pressure	90–140/5–12	mmHg
Right ventricular pressure	15–30/0–8	mmHg
Systemic arterial pressure	90–140/60–90	mmHg
Pulmonary arterial pressure	15–30/8–14	mmHg
Left ventricular geometry		
LV end-diastolic volume index	30–110	$ml\ m^{-2}$
LV end-systolic volume index	10–45	$ml\ m^{-2}$
LV mass index	60–124	$g\ m^{-2}$
LV wall thickness	7–12	mm
Left ventricular function		
Cardiac index (CI)	2.5–4.0	$l\ min^{-1}\ m^{-2}$
LV stroke volume index (SVI)	40–70	$ml\ m^{-2}$
LV ejection fraction (LVEF)	50–85	%
LV stroke work index (LVSWI)	40–80	$g.m\ m^{-2}$
Pulmonary and systemic vascular resistance		
SVR index (SVRI)	1970–2390	$dyne.s\ cm^{-5}\ m^2$
PVR index (PVRI)	225–315	$dyne.s\ cm^{-5}\ m^2$
Peak forward flow velocities (ECHO)		
Aortic valve	0.9–1.8	$m\ s^{-1}$
Mitral valve	0.6–1.4	$m\ s^{-1}$
Pulmonary valve	0.5–0.9	$m\ s^{-1}$
Tricuspid valve	0.4–0.8	$m\ s^{-1}$
Ascending aorta	0.7–1.4	$m\ s^{-1}$
Descending aorta	0.7–1.4	$m\ s^{-1}$
Abdominal aorta	0.5–1.7	$m\ s^{-1}$
Pulmonary artery	0.5–1.2	$m\ s^{-1}$

Coronary perfusion pressure (mmHg) = aortic diastolic pressure − mean right atrial pressure

Many of these parameters vary according to the patient's size and are expressed as an index of body surface area (BSA). For example, cardiac index = cardiac output/BSA:

$$\text{BSA (m}^2\text{)} = \sqrt{(\text{height (m)} \times \text{weight (kg)}/36)}.$$

THE CARDIAC CYCLE

Phase I: Isovolumic contraction
As the left ventricle begins to contract, coincident with the QRS complex, all four valves are closed. During this pre-ejection phase, LV and RV pressures do not exceed aortic and pulmonary artery pressures.

Phase II: Ventricular ejection
As the aortic valve opens the ejection phase begins. By the end of the T wave the left ventricle begins to relax and the aortic valve closes when LV pressure falls below aortic pressure.

Phase III: Isovolumic relaxation
All four valves are again closed as LV pressure continues to fall. The mitral valve does not open until left ventricular pressure falls below left atrial pressure.

Phase IV: Ventricular filling
During ventricular systole the atrioventricular ring is pulled down, augmenting atrial filling. Thus, when the mitral valve opens ventricular filling occurs rapidly – passive diastolic filling. Towards the end of diastole active filling occurs as a result of atrial contraction, which is coincident with the P wave.

REGULATION OF CARDIAC OUTPUT

Cardiac output is influenced by:

- Preload: Frank–Starling relationship
- Contractility: force and rate of contraction
- Afterload: resistance to ejection.

These factors all interact to maintain cardiac output and blood pressure and cannot be seen in isolation. For example, a fall in heart rate is associated with a rise in preload and left ventricular end-diastolic pressure, which in turn increases contractility and stroke volume owing to the Frank–Starling relationship. Under normal circumstances a fall in heart rate is not associated with more than a transient change in cardiac output. Similarly, a rise in systemic resistance and blood pressure will initially reduce stroke volume, but this serves to elevate preload due to incomplete left ventricular ejection, and again cardiac output normalizes. In disease these compensatory mechanisms may not function, or maladaptive responses may occur. For example, in

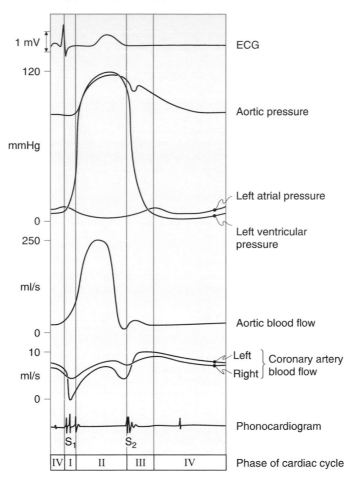

Fig. 1.4 Variations in the phonocardiogram, electrocardiogram, blood flow and pressure with the phases of the cardiac cycle.

cardiogenic shock compensatory vasoconstriction increases the work of an already failing heart.

CARDIOVASCULAR PHARMACOLOGY

TABLE 1.6 The principal classes of cardiovascular drugs and their pharmacological properties

Class of drug	Examples	$t_{1/2}$	Ex^n	Indication *	Mechanism of action	Side effects	Comments
I Sympathetic nervous system							
Selective α-blocker	Doxazosin Prazosin	22 h* 3 h	PH PH	Hypertension	Antagonize $α_1$ adrenoreceptors	Dizziness, hypotension and headaches	Doxazosin * $t_{\frac{1}{2}}$ now recognized as 22 h
Non-selective α-blocker	Phentolamine	1.5h*	B	Phaeochromocytoma, hypertensive crisis	Antagonize $α_1$ and $α_2$ adrenoreceptors	Dizziness, flushing, hypotension and headaches	*Haemodynamic response up to 12 h
Selective β-blockers	Atenolol Metoprolol Bisoprolol	6 h 3.5 h 11 h	R H HR	Angina pectoris, myocardial infarction, arrhythmias, hypertension, vasovagal syncope, chronic heart failure	Antagonize $β_1$ adrenoreceptor: negative inotropism and chronotropism	Lethargy, tiredness, exacerbate bronchial reactivity, impotence, cold peripheries	Esmolol is rapidly metabolized by erythrocyte esterases and can be used in circumstances where the effects of β-blockade are uncertain
	Esmolol	540 s	–	Short-term treatment of arrhythmias			
Non-selective β-blockers	Propranolol	4 h	P, B	Angina pectoris, myocardial infarction, arrhythmias, hypertension, vasovagal syncope	Antagonize $β_1$ and $β_2$ adrenoreceptors	Lethargy, tiredness, exacerbate bronchial reactivity, impotence, cold peripheries	
Combined α- and β-blockers	Labetalol Carvedilol	4 h 6 h	H PH	Aortic dissection, hypertension, eclampsia, chronic heart failure	Antagonize $α_1$, $β_1$ and $β_2$ adrenoreceptors	Dizziness, hypotension, bradycardia and headaches	

TABLE 1.6 (cont'd)

Category	Drug	Time	Route	Indications	Mechanism	Side effects	Notes
Selective α-agonist	Noradrenaline (epinephrine)	120 s	–	Septic shock, low peripheral vascular resistance, hypotension	Stimulates α_1 and α_2 adrenoreceptors	Headache, pallor, chest pain, sweating, hypertension and peripheral ischaemia	
Selective β-agonists	Dobutamine	120 s	–	Cardiogenic shock, acute cardiac failure, stress echocardiography	Stimulates β_1 adrenoreceptors	Tachycardia, ectopic beats, ventricular tachycardia, hypotension, headache, vomiting	Dopamine has direct dopaminergic agonist actions causing renal, mesenteric, cerebral and coronary vasodilatation. At high doses it also releases noradrenaline from storage sites
	Dopamine	120 s	–				
Non-selective β-agonists	Isoprenaline	300 s	–	Bradycardia, cardiogenic shock	Stimulates β_1 and β_2 adrenoreceptors	Tachycardia, ectopic beats, ventricular tachycardia, tremor, sweats, flushing	
Combined α- and β-agonists	Adrenaline	120 s	–	Circulatory collapse, cardiac arrest, anaphylaxis, septic shock	Stimulates α_1, α_2, β_1 and β_2 adrenoreceptors	Ventricular arrhythmias, hypertension, anxiety, restlessness, palpitations, sweats, tremor, headache	
2 Vasodilators							
Calcium antagonists	Nifedipine	2–6 h	P,B	Angina pectoris, non-Q wave myocardial infarction, arrhythmias (rate-limiting antagonists only), hypertension	Antagonize cellular calcium channels, causing vasodilatation	Negative inotropism, ankle swelling, flushing	Some demonstrate negative chronotropism (verapamil and diltiazem)
	Diltiazem	5 h	PH				
	Verapamil	5 h	PH				
	Amlodipine	40 h	PH				

TABLE 1.6 (cont'd)

Long-acting nitrates	Isosorbide mononitrate	4.5 h	H	Angina pectoris, heart failure	Release nitric oxide, causing predominantly venodilatation but also vasodilatation	Headaches, dizziness, hypotension	Dinitrate is subject to extensive first-pass metabolism
	Isosorbide dinitrate	1 h	H				
Potassium channel openers	Nicorandil	1 h	H	Angina pectoris	Stimulate cellular potassium channels causing vasodilatation. Also has a nitrate action causing venodilatation	Initial headaches (nitrate effect)	Theoretical benefits in ischaemic preconditioning
Long-acting peripheral vasodilator	Hydralazine	3 h	P, E	Hypertension, eclampsia, chronic heart failure	Arteriolar vasodilatation. Mechanism of action unknown	SLE-like syndrome particularly at higher doses, hypotension, skin rashes, impaired reaction times	Induces reflex sympathetic stimulation and sodium and water retention. Best given in combination with a β-blocker for hypertension and with a nitrate for heart failure
3 Thrombolytic, antiplatelet and anticoagulant agents							
Thrombolytics	Streptokinase Alteplase (tPA)	18 min 4 min	– H	Acute myocardial infarction, life-threatening pulmonary embolism, prosthetic valve thrombosis	Activates plasminogen to plasmin causing fibrinolysis	Haemorrhage, hypotension. Allergic reactions with streptokinase – urticaria and skin rashes	Tissue plasminogen activator is more thrombus specific but has greater risk of stroke
Antiplatelets Salicylate	Aspirin	4 h	P*, B	Secondary prevention, myocardial infarction	Platelet and prostaglandin inhibition	Gastric irritation, idiosyncratic allergic reactions	*Protein binding is variable

TABLE 1.6 (cont'd)

Thienopyridines	Clopidogrel Ticlopidine	8 h 10 h	P,B PH	Coronary stents, secondary prevention	Ticlopidine – ADP dependent. Inhibits platelet fibrinogen receptor	Clopidogrel – diarrhoea, rash, GI haemorrhage and rash occur frequently. Minor bleeding occurs occasionally. Bone marrow suppression. Can interact with theophylline	Blood count should be measured every 2 weeks during ticlopidine therapy
						Ticlopidine – diarrhoea	
Glycoprotein IIb/III receptor antagonists	Abciximab	600 s	–	An adjunct to heparin and aspirin in high-risk PTCA procedures, acute coronary thrombosis, unstable angina	Abciximab is a Fab fragment of a murine chimeric monoclonal antibody directed against the platelet glycoprotein IIb/IIIa receptor	Haemorrhagic complications, sheath site vascular haematomas and pseudoaneurysms, allergic reactions, thrombocytopenia	If severe bleeding needs correction, then consider platelet transfusion
Anticoagulants Parenteral: Thrombin inhibitors	Unfractionated heparin Low molecular weight heparin, e.g. Enoxaparin	0.5 h* 4.5 h	H R	Deep vein thrombosis, pulmonary and arterial embolism, unstable coronary syndromes and MI	Inhibits several clotting factors, including Factor X and thrombin. Low molecular weight heparins such as Enoxaparin have more selective anti-Xa activity	Haemorrhage, thrombocytopenia; long-term treatment associated with osteoporosis	$t_{\frac{1}{2}}$* range 0.5–2.5 h Enoxaparin does not require anticoagulant monitoring

TABLE 1.6 (cont'd)

Oral: Coumarins	Warfarin	36 h	P, E	Deep vein thrombosis, pulmonary embolism, prosthetic heart valves, atrial fibrillation, stroke, poor left ventricular function, endarterectomy	Inhibition of vitamin K-dependant carboxylation of Factors II, VII, IX, X and proteins C and S. Prevents binding of calcium ions necessary for the coagulation pathways	Main adverse effect of oral anticoagulants is haemorrhage. Check INR and omit doses when appropriate. Hypersensitivity reactions, skin rashes, alopecia, hepatic dysfunction, skin necrosis	Multiple drug interactions so therapeutic action may be potentiated. Reversal of anticoagulation by vitamin K and factor concentrates. Vitamin K treatment will make reheparinization difficult, taking possibly up to 72 h
	Phenindione	5–6 h	P, E				

4 Renin–angiotensin–aldosterone system

Angiotensin-converting enzyme inhibition	Captopril	1–2 h	R	Heart failure, post-myocardial infarction, hypertension, diabetic nephropathy	Antagonism of angiotensin-converting enzyme. Inhibits conversion of angiotensin I to angiotensin II	Cough, angio-oederna, skin rashes, taste disturbance, first-dose hypotension, renal impairment, hyperkalaemia	Confers symptomatic and prognostic benefits in patients with heart failure. Progression of diabetic nephropathy is inhibited by ACE inhibition
	Enalapril	11 h	B				
	Lisinopril	13 h	R				
	Ramipril	15 h	B				
	Fosinopril	12 h	H, R				
Angiotensin II receptor antagonists	Losartan	7 h	P, B	Hypertension, heart failure	Antagonism of the angiotensin type I receptor	Hypotension, renal impairment, hyperkalaemia	Does not cause cough. Prognostic benefits await confirmation
	Valsartan	9 h	P, B				
Aldosterone antagonists	Spironolactone	19 h	P, B	Heart failure, liver cirrhosis and ascites, nephrotic syndrome	Antagonism of aldosterone receptors causing a diuresis	Hyponatraemia, hypokalaemia, gynaecomastia, renal failure. Theoretical carcinogenicity	Usually reserved for cases of severe and resistant heart failure. Takes 2–3 days to have maximal effect. Spironolactone is also a potassium-sparing diuretic

TABLE 1.6 (cont'd)

5 Diuretics

Thiazide diuretics	Bendrofluazide Hydrochloro-thiazide	8.5 h 2.5 h	B* R	Hypertension, heart failure	Inhibits sodium and water resorption in the proximal tubules of the kidney	Electrolyte imbalance, gout, exacerbation of diabetes mellitus	*30% bendrofluazide excreted as unchanged drug in urine
Loop diuretics	Frusemide Bumetanide	2 h 1.5 h	P, B P, H, R	Cardiac, pulmonary, hepatic and renal oedema, hypertension	Inhibits chloride transport in the ascending limb of the loop of Henle	Electrolyte imbalance, hypotension, gout, muscle cramps, myalgia (bumetanide)	
Potassium-sparing diuretics	Amiloride Triamterene	8 h 2 h	R B	Cardiac, pulmonary, hepatic and renal oedema, hypertension	Increases sodium and chloride excretion, and decreases potassium excretion in distal tubules	Electrolyte imbalance (hyperkalaemia), hypotension, gout, muscle cramps GI disturbances	

6 Antiarrhythmic agents

Class Ia	Quinidine Disopyramide Procainamide	7 h 7 h 7 h	P, B H, R H, R	Paroxysmal supraventricular (AV nodal) tachycardia, WPW, prevention of atrial flutter/fibrillation, ventricular arrhythmias	Prolongs action potential and refractory period. Inhibits sodium channels	

TABLE 1.6 (cont'd)

Class Ib	Lignocaine Mexiletine	1.6 h 12 h	H B	Ventricular arrhythmias and fibrillation	Shortens action potential and refractory period. Inhibits sodium channels	Mexiletine causes frequent side effects: tremor, dysarthria, dizziness, paraesthesia, confusion, vomiting	
Class Ic	Propafenone Flecainide	3.6 h 14 h*	H B	Paroxysmal supraventricular tachycardia, ventricular arrhythmias	Reduces fast inward sodium currents decreasing electrical excitability and automaticity. Neutral effect on action potential and refractory period	Prolonged QT interval, arrhythmogenesis. Propafenone has a slight β-blocker action and is more likely to produce gastrointestinal upset	*In heart disease $t_{\frac{1}{2}}$ flecainide = 20 h
Class II	β-blockers			See above			
Class III	Amiodarone Sotalol Bretylium	50 d 17 h 14 h	PH R R	Ventricular arrhythmias, supraventricular tachycardias, (paroxysmal) atrial fibrillation	Prolongs action potential and refractory period. Inhibits slow ion channels	Prolonged QT. Amiodarone: multiple side effects, principally skin sensitivity, thyroid and liver dysfunction, pulmonary fibrosis, peripheral neuropathy Sotalol: β-blocker effects, torsades de pointes Bretylium: hypotension (transient initial hypertension)	Amiodarone also has class I, II and IV actions. It has a very long $t_{\frac{1}{2}}$ (~50 days) and has vasodilator properties. Bretylium initially causes, and then prevents, noradrenaline release. Sotalol interacts with many commonly prescribed drugs, e.g. erythromycin, cisapride, antihistamines

TABLE 1.6 (cont'd)

Class IV	Verapamil	5 h	PH	See above: calcium antagonists			
	Diltiazem	5 h					

7 Lipid-lowering agents

Statins	Simvastatin	<2 h	PH	Hypercholesterolaemia, primary and secondary prevention	HMGCoA reductase inhibitor – inhibits liver cholesterol synthesis	Derangement of liver function, rhabdomyolysis, gastrointestinal upset	LFTs should be performed before the initiation of treatment and periodically thereafter. *20% pravastatin renally excreted
	Pravastatin	2 h	H*				
	Atorvastatin	14 h	PH				
Fibrates	Bezafibrate	2 h	PR	Hypercholesterolaemia, mixed hyperlipidaemia	Reduces LDL-cholesterol and triglycerides, increases HDL-cholesterol	Derangement of liver function, rhabdomyolysis, gallstones, gastrointestinal upset	More suitable for mixed hyperlipidaemias and isolated low HDL cholesterol
	Clofibrate	16 h	PR				
	Ciprofibrate	60 h	PR				
Nicotinic acid group	Acipimox	1.5 h	R	Hypercholesterolaemia, mixed hyperlipidaemia	Inhibits cholesterol and triglyceride synthesis, increases HDL-cholesterol	Vasodilatation and flushing, gastrointestinal upset	Side effects limit their use, especially vasodilatation
	Nicotinic acid	45 min	HR				
Anion exchange resins	Cholestyramine	–	*	Hypercholesterolaemia	Bind bile acids and interrupt hepatoenteric circulation of cholesterol	Unpalatable, flatulence, gastrointestinal upset GI side effects predominate	May reduce fat-soluble vitamin absorption. Can increase triglycerides *not absorbed in GI tract, therefore excreted in faeces
	Colestipol						

TABLE 1.6 (cont'd)

8 Miscellaneous

Cardiac glycosides	Digoxin	36 h	P,E,	Control of ventricular rate in atrial tachycardias and fibrillation, heart failure	K^+/Na^+ ATPase inhibitor. Lengthens refractory period in AV node, shortens refractory period in ventricles and atria. Positive inotrope	Control ventricular rate but makes atrial and ventricular arrhythmias more likely. Toxicity (nausea, vomiting, anorexia, xanthopsia, ectopics and AV block) not only seen when above the therapeutic range	Lateral ST segment changes – 'reversed tick'. Improves symptoms and hospitalization rates in heart failure. No effect on mortality
Adenosine		15 s	–	Diagnosis and treatment of supraventricular tachycardias	Stimulates A_1 purine receptors. Transient AV block	Transient chest pain and flushing	Contraindicated in asthma. Action blocked by theophyllines and potentiated by dipyridamole
Phospho-diesterase inhibitors	Milrinone Enoximone	2 h 1.3 h*	P,R B	Severe cardiac failure	Selective inhibitors of cellular type III phosphodiesterases. Vasodilator and positive inotrope	Hypotension, headache, insomnia, vomiting, arrhythmias	For short-term use, particularly where filling pressures are high. Short-term therapy associated with improvement in cardiac failure. Long-term therapy causes an increased mortality. *Increased in chronic cardiac failure

$T_{\frac{1}{2}}$, plasma half-life of drug or principal active metabolite (d, days; h, hours; s, seconds).
Ex^n, plasma binding and main route of metabolism/excretion.
P, significant plasma protein binding (90%+).
H, significant excretion by the liver – as unchanged drug in faeces, or as active or inactive metabolite.
R, significant excretion by the kidney.
B, Hepatic metabolism, excreted renally.
*, licensed or unlicensed indications.

CHAPTER 2

CARDIOLOGY CONSULTATIONS AND REFERRALS

INTERDEPARTMENTAL REFERRALS

Referrals between departments are an essential form of communication in hospital medicine. Referrals give you, the trainee, an opportunity to expand your knowledge of medicine, both inside and outside cardiology. Properly carried out they ensure expert and prompt management of patients with problems that span the different specialties. Done badly they waste time, cause friction between doctors and departments, and do not help the patient. Making referrals calls for a degree of professional etiquette: after all, you are asking an expert in another field for help with your patient. It is important to be well prepared before making the call.

MAKING REFERRALS TO OTHER SPECIALTIES

Ask yourself the following questions before making your referral:

- Is the referral necessary? Can you institute basic investigations and treatment yourself?
- Are there hospital guidelines for the management of that condition?
- Can the referral be made after discharge, on an outpatient basis?
- When is the best time to refer? Ensure you have all the basic information and results ready, but don't wait until after working hours to refer a problem that was noticed earlier in the day.
- Are you the best person to make the referral? Does someone else know the case better? *Don't* delegate the task to a resident, who is the least able member of the team to answer complex questions about the case over the phone.
- Do you just need advice, or do you want the specialist to come and review the patient?
- To whom do you want to make the referral? If it is a general query a registrar-level member of the specialist team is appropriate. If it is a complex case well known to a specific doctor, contact that doctor.
- Other than in emergency, it is a matter of professional courtesy that you discuss the case with your consultant before referring the patient to another consultant.

Each specialty has its own idiosyncrasies, cardiology included! In general, make sure you know the patient's current history and relevant previous history and current treatments. In all cases you should also have basic results, such as U&Es and FBC. As well as this clinical information, specific specialties might expect you to have the following facts to hand:

Respiratory	CXR, blood gas, current O_2 therapy, PFTs, sputum culture
GI	LFTs, amylase, FOBs, fluid balance
Renal	U&Es, creatinine, calcium, phosphate, creatinine clearance, urinalysis/microscopy, urinary osmolality,

	previous U&E/creatinine, note of potentially nephrotoxic drugs, renal ultrasound
Diabetes	U&Es, creatinine, serial glucose measurements, acid–base status, urinalysis (ketones, protein, glucose), fluid balance
Haematology	Antiplatelet and antithrombotic therapy, markers of haemolysis (prosthetic valves), haematinics
Geriatric medicine	Mental state, mobility, independence, OT and physiotherapy assessment, family and home circumstances
General surgery	FBC, amylase, LFTs, fluid balance, AXR, erect CXR, rectal examination + FOBs, blood group
Orthopaedics	Relevant X-rays, social circumstances, previous operations, blood group
Vascular surgery	Possible source of embolism, assessment of pulses (Doppler pressures if possible), blood group
Cardiac surgery	Blood group, hepatitis B status, coagulation screen, angiography report, PFTs

DEALING WITH REFERRALS FROM OTHER SPECIALTIES

On your first day as 'cardiology registrar' you are all of a sudden assumed to be knowledgeable and competent to deal with a huge range of complex conditions. You may deal with a large number of referrals and need to be able to prioritize and work quickly. Most referrals are made after the morning ward round, so 10am to 2pm tends to be the busiest time. Less urgent cases can be deferred until later in the day. Also, some problems can legitimately be dealt with over the phone. In handling referrals you can learn a lot from other specialties and expand your knowledge of the cardiac complications of non-cardiac illness, surgery and pregnancy.

Doctors at all levels may call you for help. Although some referrals may seem trivial, unnecessary or garbled, do not lose your cool as this is unhelpful. Ask for a clear reason for the referral; if this is unclear, ask to speak to a more senior member of that team. Referrals are often (inappropriately) delegated to residents: don't give them a hard time, particularly if they are flustered and dealing with a sick patient. It's best to give help first and, if you have a criticism about the referral or their management, deal with it calmly later. It's easy to forget how stressful medical emergencies are to a newly qualified doctor! Similarly, if you feel out of your depth call for help from a senior member of your team. The following sections describe specific problems which are commonly referred to the cardiology team from other departments.

REFERRALS FROM THE CARDIAC SURGERY UNIT

Calls to the cardiac surgery unit account for a large proportion of the cardiology team's workload in centres with this facility. Although cardiothoracic anaesthetists usually coordinate patients' perioperative medical management, you will be called upon for advice about specific problems. In most centres the cardiology team also provides an emergency echo service. Postoperative problems generally fall into the following categories.

LOW CARDIAC OUTPUT/SHOCK

After cardiac surgery low cardiac output states may not be easy to recognize. Low output is associated with high postoperative mortality and early recognition and treatment are extremely important. Typical features of postoperative low-output state are cold extremities, mottling, tachycardia, reduced systolic pressure (<90 mmHg), acidosis, reduced urine output (<30 ml/h) and reduced mixed venous oxygen saturation (<50%; see Chapters 3 and 18, cardiac output measurement). However, hypotension may not be evident because blood pressure can be maintained by systemic vasoconstriction. In low-output states information gained by clinical and non-invasive assessment can be usefully supplemented by invasive haemodynamic monitoring (Chapter 3). This gives a direct measurement of filling pressures, cardiac output and pulmonary and systemic vascular tone.

TABLE 2.1 Causes of low-output state after cardiac surgery

Reduced preload
Hypovolaemia (intraop losses, postop haemorrhage)
Vasodilatation (rewarming, vasodilator drugs)

Pump failure	
Pre-existing LV dysfunction	perioperative MI
Myocardial ischaemia	$\downarrow$ contractility post cardiopulmonary bypass
Negatively inotropic drugs	failed correction of cardiac lesion (e.g. residual shunt after VSD repair)
Acid–base disturbance	electrolyte disturbance (e.g. $\downarrow K^+$, Ca^{2+})

Cardiac tamponade

Septic shock		
Wound infection	mediastinitis	endocarditis

Arrhythmias
Electrolyte disturbance (low K^+, Ca^{2+}, Mg^{2+}, high K^+).
Mechanical irritation (lines, drains, haematoma, effusions)
Myocardial ischaemia/infarction – hypotension
Proarrhythmic drugs (inotropes – post cardiopulmonary bypass (rewarming) noradrenaline, antiarrhythmics)

Pulmonary embolism

Investigation of low-output state after cardiac surgery

History and examination
Symptoms and signs of ischaemia, sepsis, hypovolaemia, cardiac failure

Check charts
Fluid balance, urine output, sudden drop in BP/heart rate (bleeding or septic episode), current treatment, -ve inotropic drugs

Check cardiac rhythm
Loss of atrial contribution to cardiac output (e.g. junctional rhythm, atrial fibrillation/flutter, inappropriate bradycardia/tachycardia)

Check for ischaemia/infarction
ECG, CK-MB

Assess cardiac function
Echo, CXR, mixed venous O_2 saturation

Assess metabolic status
U&Es, Ca^{2+}, Mg^{2+}, blood gases, lactate

Check for sepsis
↓SVR, low filling pressures, ↑WCC, sputum, blood, urine cultures, wound swabs, evidence of endocarditis?

Management of low-output states after cardiac surgery

Management is governed by the underlying cause of the low-output state.

- In cases of *reduced preload*, loading conditions should be optimized before driving the heart with inotropes. Hypovolaemia should be treated with plasma expander (and blood transfusion if Hb <10 g/dl) and vasopressors should be administered if systemic vascular resistance is low (e.g. in septic states).

- In cases of *normal or increased preload*, reversible causes of depressed cardiac function should be removed (e.g. negatively inotropic drugs). If significant myocardial ischaemia is present an intra-aortic balloon pump may be required to increase coronary perfusion and reoperation may be required if graft occlusion is suspected.

- *Postoperative tamponade* can be difficult to diagnose clinically, because features such as diminished heart sounds and pulsus paradoxus can be affected by mechanical ventilation. Non-constricting pericardial effusions are common, but tamponade should be suspected if diastolic collapse of the right-sided chambers is seen during echocardiography (Chapter 19). Pericardial aspiration is rarely useful because postoperative effusions tend to be loculated, with a solid, clot component. Surgical drainage is usually indicated in this situation.

ARRHYTHMIAS

Arrhythmias occur most commonly on the second to fifth postoperative days.

As with any situation, correct identification of the arrhythmia and its cause is necessary to enable appropriate management. Potential causes of postoperative arrhythmias are summarized in Table 2.1 (arrhythmias). **It is not sufficient to diagnose the arrhythmia based on monitor tracings alone**. A 12-lead ECG is required, supplemented by recordings from epicardial electrodes if present.

Supraventricular tachyarrhythmias

Atrial fibrillation affects up to 50% of patients who undergo valve surgery. DC cardioversion is not necessary unless it is associated with haemodynamic compromise, as most patients will cardiovert spontaneously within 48 hours. *Atrial flutter* is often associated with a rapid ventricular rate, is poorly tolerated and can be more resistant to rate-limiting drug therapy. Synchronized cardioversion at 50 J is usually successful. The possibility of digoxin toxicity should be considered if *ectopic atrial tachycardia* is diagnosed.

In patients with good LV function the following drug regimens are useful to limit the ventricular response to atrial flutter/fibrillation:

- **IV metoprolol**, 5 mg every 5 min, up to maximum of 15 mg
- **IV esmolol**, loading dose 500 µg kg^{-1} min^{-1} over 1 min, followed by infusion of 50–200 µg^{-1} kg^{-1} min^{-1}. Esmolol has a very short half life, so adverse effects usually resolve within 30 minutes of stopping the infusion
- **IV verapamil**, 5 mg every 10 min, up to maximum of 20 mg.

 Warning: IV verapamil should not be given to a patient who is β-blocked, nor should IV β-blocker be given to a patient already taking verapamil.

In patients with LV impairment the following treatments should be considered:

- **IV digoxin** is the safest agent for rate limitation.
- **IV amiodarone** is also rate limiting and may restore the patient to sinus rhythm, although it has a mild negatively inotropic effect.
- **DC cardioversion** should be performed if there is evidence of cardiac failure or haemodynamic compromise. Formal anticoagulation should be initiated if the arrhythmia does not resolve within 48 hours.

Postoperative *re-entrant SVT* (AV nodal re-entrant SVT) should be treated in the usual way with vagal manoeuvres, IV adenosine (3–12 mg) or IV verapamil (5–10 mg). If an epicardial electrode is left in place atrial overdrive pacing can be used to terminate the SVT. Atrial pacing is also useful for overdrive suppression in patients with recurrent postoperative supraventricular arrhythmias.

Ventricular tachyarrhythmias

These are common after cardiac surgery. If they occur, consider K^+, Ca^{2+} or Mg^{2+} abnormalities, digoxin toxicity, sepsis, volume overload, or the proarrhythmic effect of inotropes. There is no indication for the use of antiarrhythmic agents for isolated ventricular premature beats (VPBs).

Ventricular tachycardia (VT) does not require treatment if episodes are brief (less than 15 s) and do not compromise the patient. Longer episodes, or sustained VT, require treatment. Compromised patients should be treated as follows:

- **DC cardioversion**, 200 J; increase to 360 J if ineffective
- **IV lignocaine 100 mg** followed by repeat DC cardioversion at 360 J
- **Overdrive or underdrive right ventricular pacing** (see Chapter 3). Atrial or ventricular overdrive suppression can help prevent recurrences
- **Other antiarrhythmic agents** (β-blocker (see esmolol, above), bretylium tosylate 5–10 mg/kg over 15 min, flecainide 2 mg/kg (maximum 150 mg) over 20 min, procainamide 500–1000 mg over 20 min) amiodarone 5 mg kg^{-1} over 1–2 h.

The algorithms for treatment of VT in Chapter 7 should be followed for patients who are haemodynamically stable.

Ventricular fibrillation (VF) should be treated using the European Resuscitation Council guidelines (Chapter 4). Sudden VF or VT after coronary artery bypass surgery is associated with a high perioperative mortality, probably due to native vessel or graft occlusion and resultant ischaemia and pump failure. Emergency cardiopulmonary bypass or intra-aortic balloon pumping may help in this situation.

HYPERTENSION

Postoperative hypertension affects approximately 50% of patients after cardiac surgery. This is defined as systolic BP >150 mmHg or diastolic >90 mmHg. It is associated with an increased risk of postoperative haemorrhage, LV failure, bypass graft occlusion, stroke and aortic dissection. Causes include fluid overload, withdrawal of oral β-blockers, hypoxia, excessive sympathetic nervous system activity (e.g. pain, anxiety, heart failure), iatrogenic (especially noradrenaline) and baroreceptor responses (e.g. after correction of aortic coarctation). Hypertension is usually short-lived and the following treatments can be used:

- **IV labetolol** 1–2 mg min^{-1} or IV metoprolol 5–10 mg over 3–4 min
- **IV glyceryl trinitrate** 0.5–10 mg h^{-1}
- **IV sodium nitroprusside** 0.5–2.0 µg kg^{-1} min^{-1}
- **Nasogastric or sublingual nifedipine** 5–10 mg.

SEPSIS

Sepsis can be difficult to diagnose postoperatively, as fever can occur during normal recovery for 4 or 5 days. In addition, fever can accompany other conditions such as venous thromboembolism, drug reactions and postoperative Dressler syndrome. A source of sepsis should be sought in any patient with unexplained hypotension, high fever (>38.5°C), confusion, new cardiac murmur or rash. The following sources should be considered:

- **Wound infection** (check sternotomy and vein harvest sites) is usually caused by staphylococci, streptococci, or aerobic Gram-negative organisms. Occasionally fungal wound infections occur. Wounds should be swabbed and treatment commenced with a broad-spectrum agent, e.g. IV co-amoxiclav 1.2 g tid, IV erythromycin 1 g qid, or IV cefotaxime 1–2 g bd.
- **Mediastinitis** affects 1–2% of patients. It may be associated with pyrexia >39°C, evidence of systemic sepsis, leucocytosis and sometimes discharge from the sternotomy wound. CT or MRI scanning may help localize the infection. Staphylococci cause around 50% of cases; Gram-negative bacilli are also a common cause. Treatment is with IV antibiotics and sometimes mediastinal irrigation and surgical debridement.
- **Infective endocarditis** affects around 2% of valve surgery cases. Early prosthetic endocarditis is caused by staphylococcus in one-half of cases, with group D streptococci and *Streptococcus pneumoniae* also common. Diagnosis and treatment are discussed in Chapter 8. Early reoperation is indicated in the following circumstances:
  - significant cardiac failure or haemodynamic compromise caused by prosthetic dysfunction
  - evidence of perivalvular abscess formation
  - persistent evidence of, or recurrence of, infection despite adequate antibiotic therapy
  - recurrent embolization from prosthesis.
- **Postoperative pneumonia**
- **Infected central venous catheter.**

REFERRALS FROM NON-CARDIAC SURGERY UNITS

Surgical ward referrals are a source of continual frustration to the cardiology team. Most are for simple problems which are easily dealt with. Remember that most surgical colleagues have very little medical or cardiological experience and the threshold for referral is correspondingly low. Referrals are often made through junior residents, who may not fully understand the complexities of the case or the reason for referral. If the referral is unclear, contact a senior member of the surgical team and ask the resident to ensure that relevant results (ECGs, electrolyte and cardiac enzyme results, X-rays) are available. For seemingly trivial referrals it is better to try and educate the residents so that they know how to deal with the same problem next time.

PREOPERATIVE ASSESSMENT

The decision as to whether a patient is fit for surgery rests with the anaesthetist and surgeon, not with the cardiologist. A 'cardiology opinion' should be used to obtain the information needed for that decision to be made and to provide advice to minimize operative risk. The history, examination and ECG assessment should be used to identify prognostically important disorders, principally coronary artery disease, cardiac failure, electrical instability and valve disease. The AHA has published a useful and comprehensive document, 'Guidelines for perioperative cardiovascular evaluation for noncardiac surgery' *Circulation* 1996;93:1278–1317, from which Table 2.2 is derived.

TABLE 2.2 Clinical predictors of cardiac risk in non-cardiac surgery

Major predictors
Recent MI
Unstable or severe stable angina
Decompensated cardiac failure
Second- or third-degree AV block
Symptomatic arrhythmias due to underlying cardiac disease
Severe valvular heart disease

Intermediate predictors
Previous (remote) MI
Mild angina
Controlled cardiac failure
Diabetes mellitus

Minor predictors
Advanced age
Abnormal ECG in absence of cardiac symptoms
Absence of sinus rhythm
Uncontrolled hypertension
Poor functional capacity
Previous stroke

Ischaemic heart disease

Patients with known IHD can be divided into the following categories for preoperative assessment and management (Mangano DT, Goldman L. Preoperative assessment of the patient with known or suspected coronary disease. *N Engl J Med* 1995;333:1750):

● **Mild exertional angina** is associated with low perioperative mortality (<2%). Preoperative stress testing is not required. Postoperatively, ECGs should be performed on day 1 and before discharge to exclude MI.
● **If status is unclear**, e.g. when other pathology limits effort tolerance, stress testing (exercise ECG, stress myocardial perfusion scan, or stress echo) is indicated to identify whether early ischaemia occurs or significant territory is

at risk. Angiography may be indicated if ischaemia is easily induced, with a view to coronary revascularization prior to surgery. Otherwise, medical management should be intensified prior to, and reinstituted as soon as possible after, surgery.

● **Moderate or severe exertional angina** is associated with higher mortality and medical management should be optimized before surgery; if possible, surgery should be postponed. Patients who fail to respond should undergo angiography with a view to revascularization.

Cardiac failure

The risk of death during non-cardiac surgery increases with functional class of heart failure and is especially high in patients with overt pulmonary congestion and with a third heart sound, in whom perioperative mortality exceeds 15%. If possible, a period of inpatient medical management should be undertaken, avoiding excessive diuresis as hypovolaemia and hypokalaemia both increase operative risk.

Electrical instability

The perioperative risk associated with arrhythmias usually relates to the underlying heart disease rather than to the arrhythmia itself. For example, ventricular extrasystoles are of no consequence in patients without underlying heart disease, but reflect increased risk if associated with coronary disease. Thus, any investigations and treatment should be directed at the underlying disease; suppression of extrasystoles should not be seen as an end in itself.

Atrial fibrillation

Atrial fibrillation does not require preoperative cardioversion other than in situations where cardioversion would be carried out anyway. Risk factors for atrial arrhythmias are thoracic surgery in the elderly, mitral valve disease and a previous history of atrial arrhythmia. These patients may benefit from preoperative digitalization.

Atrioventricular block

AV block should be treated in exactly the same way as in the non-operative situation. In general, temporary pacing is only required if the patient has an indication for permanent pacing and non-cardiac surgery cannot be delayed. Patients with chronic bifascicular block do not require prophylactic pacing unless there is associated Mobitz type II AV block, transient complete AV block or syncope.

Permanent pacemakers

Pacemakers may require reprogramming in the perioperative period. In particular, ill patients undergoing major surgery may benefit from an increase in base rate. Diathermy can inhibit the function of demand pacemakers, and so if possible bipolar diathermy should be used. Otherwise, the indifferent electrode should be placed well away from the heart and pacemaker. If inhibition occurs, a magnet can be placed over most pacemakers to activate fixed-rate pacing; otherwise reprogramming to DOO or VOO mode may be required.

Valve disease

Valve disease is associated with perioperative heart failure, endocarditis, atrial arrhythmias and systemic embolism. Prognosis is largely predicted by functional capacity; patients with limiting or severe symptoms are at the highest risk. Patients with critical mitral or aortic stenosis cannot mount an adequate cardiac output in the face of systemic vasodilatation and may become critically unwell if arrhythmias develop. These patients should have valve surgery first if possible. If non-cardiac surgery is urgent then a pulmonary artery catheter should be used to guide fluid loading and estimate systemic vascular resistance. Patients with *prosthetic valves* should have warfarin stopped 3 days before surgery and restarted within 3 days of surgery. Ball and cage prostheses (e.g. Starr–Edwards) are at especially high risk of thrombosis. These patients should receive IV heparin until 6–8 hours before surgery and heparin restarted as soon afterwards as deemed safe by the surgeon until the INR is therapeutic.

Antibiotic prophylaxis before surgery is discussed in Chapters 8 and 12.

Patients with *hypertrophic obstructive cardiomyopathy* may be critically dependent on high ventricular filling pressures because of reduced ventricular compliance, and so tolerate hypovolaemia poorly. Also, cardiac output may fall in the face of systemic vasodilatation because of outflow tract obstruction. Atrial fibrillation may precipitate hypotension because of loss of atrial contribution to ventricular filling; if so, immediate cardioversion is indicated. Invasive haemodynamic monitoring is indicated in symptomatic patients undergoing major surgery.

PERIOPERATIVE CARDIOVASCULAR COMPLICATIONS

Myocardial ischaemia/infarction

Perioperative MI is often asymptomatic because of anaesthesia and postoperative analgesia. It may be precipitated by a perioperative increase in cardiac work, or by postoperative hypercoagulability. The ECG often does not reveal classic ST elevation and Q waves and non-Q wave MI is common. Cardiac enzyme levels can be difficult to interpret because of injury to skeletal muscle during surgery, although MB-CK, troponin T and troponin I are relatively cardiospecific and may be helpful. Threshold levels depend on the assay method used, so local laboratory reference ranges should be consulted. Thrombolysis is contraindicated, but otherwise conventional medical therapy with aspirin and β-blockade is helpful. In patients with ST elevation MI affecting a large (usually anterior) territory, cardiac catheterization should be considered with a view to target lesion angioplasty. Also, in patients with unstable angina or non-Q wave MI and chest discomfort refractory to conventional treatment (Chapter 5), angiography is indicated. The follow-up of patients after perioperative MI does not differ from that of other patients with MI.

Cardiac failure

Postoperative cardiac failure is most common in patients with poor cardiac reserve. It is diagnosed from clinical examination and the chest X-ray. It may be difficult to distinguish from postoperative atelectasis, chest infection and adult respiratory distress syndrome (ARDS). In septic patients or patients with 'third-space' losses (e.g. in acute pancreatitis) fluid balance can be difficult to assess and a central venous catheter or pulmonary artery catheter may help establish a diagnosis.

Most cases are due to overhydration of patients with impaired cardiac function. Fluid restriction (to 1500 ml/24 h) and IV diuretics usually correct this. Sometimes previous oral diuretic or digoxin therapy may not have been restarted, especially if the patient is 'nil by mouth'. These agents should be given intravenously in the perioperative period. Other causes of postoperative cardiac failure are listed below.

Arrhythmias

Sinus tachycardia

This is the most common postoperative rhythm disturbance. It is sometimes confused with atrial flutter (and 2:1 AV block) and with AV node re-entrant

---

Checklist for postoperative cardiac failure

Fluid balance chart
Indices of renal function
Haemoglobin
Evidence of perioperative MI
New atrial fibrillation
Failure to restart diuretics
Hypertension
Sepsis

Checklist for postoperative arrhythmias

Fluid balance chart (overhydration → atrial arrhythmias; hypovolaemia → sinus tachycardia)
Evidence of perioperative MI
Serum K^+, Mg^{2+}, Ca^{2+}
Oxygenation/acid–base balance
Evidence of sepsis/pneumonia
Failure to restart digoxin/antiarrhythmic medication

tachycardia. Treatment is directed at the underlying cause (pain, anxiety, hypoxaemia, cardiac failure, hypovolaemia, sepsis, pulmonary embolism, anaemia etc.).

Atrial fibrillation

This is often precipitated by overhydration, especially in patients with mitral valve disease or left ventricular dysfunction. Treatment of the underlying cause often results in spontaneous conversion to sinus rhythm; **digoxin** and/or a **β-blocker** may be needed to control the ventricular rate. Early cardioversion is only indicated if there is haemodynamic compromise. **IV heparin** can be given until underlying causes have been adequately treated and if atrial fibrillation persists, cardioversion is used. *Atrial flutter* is often associated with a rapid ventricular response and may require early cardioversion. Treatment is as for atrial fibrillation.

Treatments for resistant atrial fibrillation, *ventricular arrhythmias* and postoperative *hypertension* were discussed earlier.

CARDIOLOGY AND PREGNANCY

During pregnancy cardiac output and blood volume both increase by an average of 50%. Diastolic blood pressure normally falls, especially in the second trimester, along with peripheral resistance. During labour, cardiac output and blood pressure increase dramatically. These physiological changes can unmask previously undiagnosed heart disease and can compromise patients with manifest heart disease.

PRE-PREGNANCY COUNSELLING

It is better to discuss pregnancy issues with women of childbearing age who have cardiac disease before conception than to counsel and manage problems afterwards. The key to counselling is an accurate evaluation of the nature and severity of the patient's disease, which allows a risk assessment to be made.

Key issues in pregnancy counselling and heart disease

Contraception
Maternal risk from pregnancy
Maternal long-term prognosis
Fetal risk from pregnancy
Fetal risk of inherited disease
Anticoagulation
Antibiotic prophylaxis (valvular and congenital heart disease)

Valvular heart disease
- **Mitral stenosis** is associated with decompensation during pregnancy

because of limitation of cardiac output, increased valve gradient and left atrial pressure and the development of atrial fibrillation. With severe mitral stenosis (valve area <1.0 cm^2), the risks of pregnancy need to be carefully balanced against the risks of valve replacement, followed by pregnancy with a prosthetic valve (see below). With moderate mitral stenosis (valve area <1.5 cm^2) pregnancy is usually well tolerated. Diuretics may be needed to reduce plasma volume and β-blockers or digoxin to control heart rate. Strenuous exertion should be avoided as it increases left atrial pressure significantly. During and immediately after delivery invasive haemodynamic monitoring is helpful because left atrial pressure rises with increased cardiac output; venous return and left atrial pressure increase when the inferior vena cava is decompressed; and postpartum haemorrhage is poorly tolerated.

● **Mitral regurgitation** does not usually cause problems during pregnancy, as peripheral resistance falls physiologically, thereby reducing afterload. Digoxin and diuretics can be used in symptomatic patients; hydralazine is a relatively safe and effective afterload reducer and can also be used.

● **Aortic regurgitation** is similarly well tolerated.

● **Aortic stenosis** is usually associated with a bicuspid valve in women of childbearing age. Unless valve stenosis is severe, pregnancy is normally well tolerated. Pulmonary oedema, presyncope and syncope during pregnancy herald a high risk of maternal death and may necessitate termination of the pregnancy or valve replacement.

● **Prosthetic valves** are associated with an increased incidence of thromboembolism, teratogenicity of warfarin (3–5% of cases) and rapid deterioration in bioprosthetic valve function. Patients without limiting symptoms generally tolerate pregnancy well. Bioprostheses avoid the risks of anticoagulation, but may need to be replaced after only a few years. Some centres advocate a meticulous heparin regimen during the first trimester and last month of gestation and consideration of elective caesarian section at 38 weeks. In the UK most centres advocate counselling, the continuation of warfarin throughout pregnancy, antenatal ultrasound screening and conversion to heparin in the third trimester prior to elective caesarian section.

Ischaemic heart disease

Ischaemic heart disease is uncommon in women of childbearing age. The risk of MI is increased in heavy smokers who have used oral contraception.

● **Myocardial infarction** can occur in the absence of obstructive disease and may be due to coronary artery spasm, dissection or thrombosis. Spasm can occur with ergometrine and oxytocin and with some prostaglandin preparations. If a large territory is threatened, limited reports indicate that thrombolysis or PTCA can be used successfully and relatively safely.

● **Suspected angina** should be investigated non-invasively, to avoid radiation exposure. Asymptomatic resting ST segment depression is recognized in pregnancy: echocardiography should be used to identify any associated wall motion defect. Otherwise a submaximal exercise test can be used for risk stratification. Fetal monitoring is advisable during exercise testing to identify fetal bradycardia. **Aspirin 75 mg** daily is safe; higher doses are associated with maternal bleeding. β-**Blockers** can be used for symptom control, but may cause intrauterine growth retardation.

● **Refractory angina** is uncommon but may necessitate coronary angiography and/or angioplasty or bypass surgery. Termination of pregnancy may be needed if the maternal risk is considered high.

Congenital heart disease

Patients with *non-cyanotic* congenital heart disease tend to have a good prognosis in pregnancy. *Cyanotic* patients may decompensate as the pregnancy progresses and fetal development can be retarded because of intrauterine hypoxia.

Adverse prognostic factors in pregnancy in patients with congenital heart disease
Systemic hypoxaemia
High haematocrit
Pulmonary hypertension
Poor functional capacity

Risk should be assessed on an individual basis, taking into account potential high-risk indicators and the specific condition in question.

TABLE 2.3 Pregnancy and common congenital heart defects

Condition	Pregnancy/labour	Action
Atrial septal defect	Usually well tolerated as pulmonary hypertension not usually present at childbearing age	
Ventricular septal defect	Usually well tolerated. Risk of shunt reversal if hypotensive peripartum. Up to 20% risk of congenital HD in offspring	May need fluid replacement and vasopressors postpartum
Tetralogy of Fallot	Risk of shunt reversal high if VSD not surgically corrected. Up to 20% fetal risk of congenital HD	Consider corrective surgery before planning family. Avoid hypotension during delivery: local nerve block, inhalation analgesics
Eisenmenger syndrome	Maternal mortality approx 40%. Many deaths occur in few days postpartum	Consider termination of pregnancy. Otherwise, anticoagulate during third trimester, invasive haemodynamic monitoring peripartum, avoid hypotension, consider use of vasopressors postpartum

Antibiotic prophylaxis should be used at the time of vaginal delivery in patients with prosthetic valves and with most forms of congenital heart disease. It is not necessary in patients with native valve disease, secundum ASD or corrected patent ductus arteriosus. Caesarian section is usually only needed for obstetric reasons, although maternal haemodynamic deterioration may necessitate it. Antibiotic prophylaxis is not needed in that event.

Cardiomyopathies

- **Idiopathic dilated cardiomyopathy** is uncommon in young women. The prognosis is predicted by functional capacity. Maternal long-term prognosis may be limited. Digoxin, diuretics and hydralazine are the mainstay of treatment in the event of arrhythmic or haemodynamic deterioration during pregnancy. Anticoagulation is advised because of the high incidence of thromboembolic events in pregnancy.
- **Hypertrophic cardiomyopathy (HCM)** is associated with an up to 5% risk of maternal ventricular arrhythmia during pregnancy and up to 25% risk of worsening cardiac failure. The fetal risk of inherited HCM is 50% in familial cases. β-Blockers and/or verapamil may be needed if there is symptomatic outflow obstruction. Diuretics can also be used. Vaginal delivery is allowed, but vasodilatation during delivery can increase outflow tract obstruction. Spinal and epidural anaesthesia, prostaglandins and volume depletion should be avoided.
- **Peripartum cardiomyopathy** affects 1 in 10 000 pregnancies, causing left and right heart dilatation, heart failure and sometimes atrial fibrillation. Its onset is usually from 3 months before to 6 months after delivery. It is commoner in multiple pregnancies and tends to recur in subsequent pregnancies; 50% of patients recover completely and the remainder run a chronic course, sometimes requiring transplantation. For treatment, see **Dilated cardiomyopathy**, above.

Hypertension

Chronic hypertension (BP ≥ 140/90 mmHg) is associated with an increased incidence of pre-eclampsia and eclampsia, fetal growth retardation, premature birth and placental abruption. Drug treatment is indicated if the diastolic BP exceeds 100 mmHg. The treatment of pre-eclampsia and eclampsia is usually the domain of the obstetrician and intensivist and is beyond the scope of this manual.

Arrhythmias

- **Extrasystoles**, both ventricular and supraventricular, are common and do not need treatment.
- **AV node re-entry tachycardia** is exacerbated in susceptible patients because of this and can be terminated with IV adenosine. Recurrent episodes may necessitate treatment with oral digoxin or β-blockers.
- **Accessory pathway tachycardias**: recurrent troublesome episodes can be

treated with a β-blocker or calcium channel antagonist.

● **Atrial flutter and fibrillation** are rare in pregnancy and usually accompany rheumatic heart disease. Treatment is with digoxin and/or β-blockers.

● **VT** is also rare and may reflect impending eclampsia or previously undetected structural heart disease. Drug treatment is only indicated if there are severe symptoms or life-threatening episodes.

● **Congenital AV block** should be treated by permanent pacing before pregnancy if possible. If the patient is already pregnant pacing may not be needed, so unnecessary exposure to radiation should be avoided; a pacemaker can be implanted later in pregnancy if limiting symptoms develop.

TABLE 2.4 Common cardiac drugs and pregnancy

Drug	Suitability in pregnancy
Digoxin	Safer than most; can cause growth retardation
Diuretics	Use only if volume excess; reduces placental blood flow; hyponatraemia
ACE inhibitors	**Contraindicated.** High risk of fetal defects, spontaneous abortion
Hydralazine	Safe. Useful in heart failure during pregnancy
Nitrates	Safe. Short-acting nitrates may cause reflex fetal bradycardia
Adenosine	Safe
β-Blockers	Relatively safe. Can cause growth retardation, fetal bradycardia, hypoglycaemia at birth
Calcium channel blockers	Intravenous or short-acting versions can cause maternal hypotension. Fetal abnormalities rare. High levels excreted in breast milk
Amiodarone	**Avoid if possible.** Causes growth retardation, neonatal hypothyroidism, premature birth

CHAPTER 3

EMERGENCY CARDIOLOGICAL PROCEDURES

CENTRAL VENOUS ACCESS

INDICATIONS

- CVP monitoring
- Central access for drug or fluid administration
- Pulmonary artery catheterization
- Transvenous pacing wire insertion.

CHOICE OF ACCESS ROUTE

There are three main approaches to central venous access: via the internal jugular, subclavian and femoral veins. The choice depends on several factors:

- The experience of the operator and their preferred route.
- The femoral approach is preferable if there is:
  - coagulopathy (platelets $<50 \times 10^{12} \, l^{-1}$, or prothrombin time $>2 \times$ control) post thrombolysis. There have been deaths after neck line insertion in such patients, where tracheal obstruction made intubation impossible. Bleeding is more easily controlled with pressure at the groin than at the other insertion sites.
  - a hyperinflated chest or respiratory compromise (the high subclavian
  - approach can also be used, to avoid pneumothorax).

METHOD

- Explain the procedure to the patient; obtain written consent if possible.
- Position patient head down for internal jugular and subclavian approaches to ensure target vein is filled and to avoid air embolism.
- If fluoroscopic screening required (e.g. pacing wire or PA catheter insertion), wear a lead apron and thyroid collar.
- Scrub; use a sterile gown and gloves.
- Cleanse insertion site and position sterile drapes.
- Infiltrate local anaesthetic as appropriate for access route (below). **Do not** inject it into the vein (or worse, the artery) and give it a few minutes to take effect.
- Locate the target vein by aspirating with small needle.
- Insert access sheath using the Seldinger technique (see below).

Tip: Use all of your drapes to make as big a work surface as possible. It is difficult to keep a long catheter or pacing wire sterile otherwise.

Internal jugular approach (Fig. 3.1)
- Extend patient's neck slightly and turn head to left (for right-sided puncture).

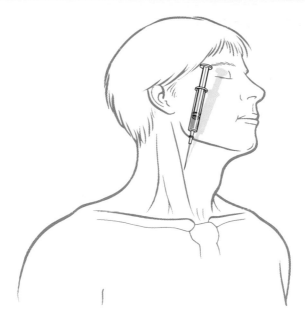

Fig. 3.1 Internal jugular vein puncture.

- Locate midpoint of sternomastoid muscle, between right mastoid process and suprasternal notch.
- Slide finger off thyroid cartilage to feel carotid artery pulsation.
- Infiltrate c 5 ml 1% lignocaine into subcutaneous tissues, lateral to artery.
- Insert access needle at this site, at 45° to skin; aim for ipsilateral nipple.

Subclavian approach (Fig. 3.2)
- Turn patient's head to left (for right-sided puncture).
- Locate midpoint of clavicle (use sternoclavicular and acromioclavicular joints as landmarks).
- Infiltrate c 5–10 ml 1% lignocaine into subcutaneous tissues, 1–2 cm below this point; infiltrate towards sternal notch. Aspirate each time the needle is advanced, as the subclavian vein may be encountered at this point.
- Insert access needle at same site; aim almost horizontally across chest towards sternal notch.
- Vary angle slightly if vein is missed at first pass. Too superior an angle risks arterial puncture; too inferior or posterior an angle risks pneumothorax.

Femoral approach
This is located midway between the anterior superior iliac spine and the pubic

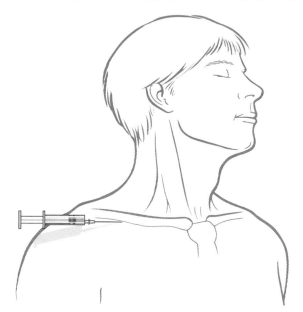

Fig. 3.2 Subclavian vein puncture.

symphysis. Remember your femoral canal anatomy: from medial to lateral – vein, artery, nerve.

● Palpate femoral artery just below the inguinal ligament.
● Infiltrate *c* 5–10 ml 1% lignocaine into the subcutaneous tissues, about 2–4 cm below the inguinal ligament and medial to the femoral pulse. Angle needle 45° to skin, point in direction of umbilicus and infiltrate carefully. The femoral vein may be encountered during infiltration.
● Insert access needle (16–18 gauge Cook's needle) at same site and aim in same direction to puncture femoral vein.

Sheath insertion – the Seldinger technique
When the site of the vein has been identified the introducer needle is inserted using the same technique. Following the flashback of blood the syringe is disconnected and a soft-tipped guidewire advanced down the lumen of the needle and into the vein. The needle is withdrawn over the stationary wire. **At no time should control of the guide wire be lost**. A small (1 cm) skin incision is made with a scalpel and the tract dilated with a dilator. The sheath is then introduced over the guidewire and into the vein.

TROUBLESHOOTING

Inability to cannulate the vein

This is unusual when the CVP is high and the veins well filled, but can be a problem in hypovolaemic patients. For subclavian and jugular approaches, increase head-down tilt to maximize venous filling. The subclavian approach has the highest failure rate: sometimes it helps to use a more lateral approach than normal. If unsuccessful, use another route. **Never attempt cannulation of the contralateral vein if ipsilateral pneumothorax is suspected**: use the femoral approach instead.

Resistance to guidewire insertion

The guidewire should slide in without resistance. If there is resistance the wire is probably extravascular: withdraw it and ensure blood can still be freely aspirated. If there is continued resistance angle the needle in a slightly different direction, or rotate it through 90–180° to change the direction of the bevel. The guidewire may not advance because it is misshapen (replace with a new wire), or because the vein is tortuous. Fluoroscopy often helps in these circumstances as the wire can be steered under X-ray guidance. Contrast agent injection helps delineate abnormal anatomy (e.g. SVC obstruction), but ensure the needle is properly in the vein before you inject.

Arterial puncture

Accidental arterial puncture is fairly common, especially with the femoral approach. It can lead to haematoma, pseudoaneurysm formation and local pressure effects (e.g. femoral nerve compression), especially if clotting is abnormal. If the artery is punctured and there is concern about the risk of bleeding (e.g. after thrombolysis), a vascular sheath should be inserted into the artery (using the Seldinger technique) until clotting has normalized, to limit bleeding and haematoma formation. This may prove useful for arterial pressure monitoring. In shocked patients accidental cannulation of the artery may go unrecognized until the pressure waveform is examined.

COMPLICATIONS

Serious complications are uncommon but include pneumothorax, haemorrhage, infection, neuropraxia and arrhythmias.

> Warning: Tension pneumothorax can complicate subclavian or internal jugular line insertion. Dyspnoea, chest pain and haemodynamic compromise (or worse, cardiac arrest) may occur. Treat by immediately inserting a small cannula into the second or third intercostal space, in the midclavicular line. Chest drain insertion is essential.

Tachyarrhythmias (especially non-sustained VT) suggest mechanical irritation of the tricuspid valve. This often occurs during pacing wire or pulmonary artery catheter insertion, but if it occurs during CVP line insertion the line is too far in and should be pulled back 4–5 cm (to the junction of the right atrium and SVC).

SWAN–GANZ CATHETERIZATION

Swan–Ganz or PA flotation catheters are useful in the assessment of critically ill patients with haemodynamic compromise, allowing estimation of cardiac output, pulmonary and systemic vascular resistance, venous oxygen saturation, right and left atrial pressure and PA pressure. There are two main types of PA catheter, both of which have an inflatable balloon at the tip to allow flotation:

- **Basic**: a single lumen, which opens at the catheter tip and allows pressure measurements only. It is possible to measure PA pressure and pulmonary capillary wedge pressure (PCWP). Inflation of the balloon in a branch pulmonary artery occludes antegrade PA flow. In the absence of pulmonary vascular disease, the pressure at the catheter tip equilibrates with left atrial pressure.
- **Thermodilution**: two lumina on the tip (PA) and shaft (CVP) of the catheter. The proximal lumen is used to measure CVP (required to calculate systemic vascular resistance) and for the injection of cold fluid, which is detected by a thermocouple at the distal end of the catheter. The *thermodilution curve* is used to estimate cardiac output.

INDICATIONS

A PA catheter may be helpful in the following circumstances:

- Cardiogenic shock
- Pulmonary oedema
- Shock of unknown origin
- Right ventricular infarction
- Suspected acquired VSD (helps estimate size of left-to-right shunt)
- Management of sepsis, hypovolaemia, or major surgery in patients with impaired LV function
- After cardiac surgery
- Life-threatening pulmonary embolism.

METHOD

PA catheterization should only be performed where full resuscitation facilities are available. Fluoroscopy is used to position the catheter. ('Blind' PA catheterization is sometimes carried out by experienced operators, using the pressure trace as a guide to position. This should only ever be attempted using a jugular or subclavian approach and should only be done if fluoroscopy is difficult to arrange.) Peripheral IV access should be obtained first and ECG monitoring is essential. Central venous access should be obtained as described earlier.

- Flush all catheter lumina.
- Test flotation balloon before introducing into vein.
- Zero pressure transducer (at height of right atrium).
- Pass catheter down venous sheath; guide into right atrium.
- Inflate balloon to float catheter into RV and then PA.
- Advance catheter, with balloon inflated, until PA pressure trace damps or until catheter tip lodges into branch PA (Fig. 3.3).
- Record pressure readings and (if intracardiac shunt suspected) oxygen saturations, from right atrium, RV and PA.
- Arrhythmias are common when the catheter crosses the tricuspid valve. Ventricular ectopic beats or non-sustained VT are most common, but in the setting of acute MI ventricular fibrillation may occur.

The final position of the catheter should be stable (catheter not moving much in PA), with a reproducible 'wedge' tracing with the balloon inflated and a clear PA tracing with the balloon deflated.

- Never pull the catheter back through the pulmonary or tricuspid valve with the balloon inflated – you may damage a valve leaflet.
- Always watch the pressure tracing when inflating the balloon. Do not inflate if there is resistance, or beyond the point where wedging occurs.
- Patients with severe mitral regurgitation have a marked systolic wave on the wedge tracing, which may resemble a PA trace.
- Continually monitor pressure through catheter when it is in the PA, as spontaneous wedging and pulmonary infarction can occur.

TROUBLESHOOTING

Unable to position catheter in the pulmonary artery

From the jugular or subclavian approach the PA catheter naturally curves round into the RV and its outflow tract and it is usually fairly easy to float it into the PA. If it will not 'turn' in the body of RV, advance it while applying torque. Occasionally the catheter may not turn down into the SVC, but advances towards the right arm. If so, withdraw the sheath slightly and angle it caudally to point the catheter towards SVC and the right atrium. Rarely, SVC obstruction necessitates a femoral approach.

From the femoral approach, the PA catheter tends to arch into the RV apex and does not readily turn up into the outflow tract. Try the following:

- Torque the catheter anticlockwise as it crosses the tricuspid valve.

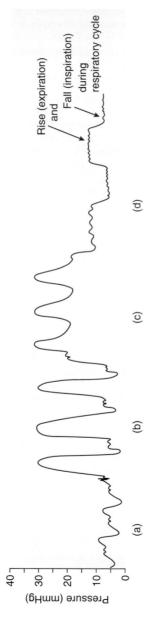

Fig. 3.3 Pressure tracings obtained during right heart catheterization: (a) right atrium, (b) right ventricle, (c) pulmonary artery and (d) pulmonary artery wedge. Pulmonary artery wedge pressure is measured during expiration, since inspiration causes a fall in pressure due to the reduction in intrathoracic pressure.

● Make an anticlockwise loop in the right atrium so that the catheter naturally curves upwards after crossing the tricuspid valve. Be careful not to make a knot in the catheter.

● Use a long, *soft-tipped*, curved-ended guidewire once catheter is just through the tricuspid valve, to 'find' the PA.

Knotting the catheter

Expletives may relieve operator stress but don't help the patient! If a knot is produced, do not pull the catheter tight. Knots can be undone by a combination of advancing the catheter (which loosens the knot), torsion, deflating the balloon and manipulation with a long guidewire. If the knot becomes irretrievable it should *not* be pulled out through the neck veins; a Dotter retrieval snare should be used to capture the knot, the catheter cut at the insertion site and the ensnared catheter removed via the femoral vein.

Failure to obtain satisfactory wedge trace

Balloon rupture or catheter displacement

Lack of resistance to balloon inflation suggests rupture. This can be confirmed with fluoroscopy. Catheter displacement is usually remedied by advancing the catheter slightly. If there is significant pulmonary vascular disease or mitral valve disease, it may not be possible to obtain a satisfactorily damped wedge tracing.

Overwedging

Here the pressure trace rises inexorably when the balloon is inflated. If this occurs, the distal end of the catheter is impacted in a small PA branch and further inflation may cause pulmonary artery rupture. Retract the catheter a few centimetres and advance again to find another wedge position.

Damped pressure trace

Damped traces result from catheter kinking, intraluminal thrombosis or distal impaction. A badly kinked catheter will not record pressures accurately, even when straightened out, and will need to be replaced.

COMPLICATIONS

This includes those listed earlier, but also includes:

● Ventricular arrhythmias
● PA rupture and pulmonary haemorrhage
● Pulmonary infarction (from persistent branch occlusion)
● Trauma to tricuspid/pulmonary valves (retraction of catheter with balloon inflated).

INTERPRETATION OF DATA

The CVP and wedge pressures indicate the filling state of the right and left atria, respectively.

- **Hypovolaemia and peripheral venodilatation** are associated with reduced left and right atrial pressures (left atrial pressure typically <8 mmHg).
   - Fluid replacement augments preload in this situation.
- **LV failure** is associated with increased right and left atrial pressures; if there is pulmonary oedema, the wedge pressure usually exceed 20 mmHg.
   - Nitrates reduce the wedge pressure through preload and afterload reduction.
   - Loop diuretics both venodilate and reduce intravascular volume.
- **Cardiogenic shock** is usually associated with a normal or high wedge pressure (but see RV infarction, below).
   - Inotropes increase cardiac output and blood pressure at the expense of cardiac work.
   - intra-aortic balloon pump augments diastolic BP, coronary perfusion and cardiac output.
- **RV infarction** is a cause of cardiogenic shock and is associated with high CVP, but because of reduced right-sided output the wedge pressure may be low.
   - Fluid (crystalloid) should be given to raise left atrial pressures to 14–18 mmHg, to optimize left-sided preload. A very high CVP (>20 mmHg) may be needed to achieve this.

Estimating cardiac output

Thermodilution
Cardiac ouput can be measured using a thermodilution catheter. A fixed volume of chilled saline is rapidly injected through the CVP lumen and the rate of temperature change at the catheter tip is used to calculate cardiac output. An average of three to five injections is used. Moderate or severe tricuspid regurgitation renders this type of measurement meaningless.

Fick principle (see Chapter 18 for method)
Here, cardiac output is estimated by measuring oxygen extraction from arterial blood. Mixed venous oxygen saturation is measured from a pulmonary artery blood sample (assuming there is no intracardiac shunt). A saturation of ~75% is normal. Lower saturations are are associated with low-output states and result from increased tissue oxygen extraction. Measurement of mixed venous saturation is a useful way of assessing response to treatment in these patients. In high-output states, such as septic shock, mixed venous oxygen saturation may be increased owing to arteriovenous shunting and low oxygen extraction relative to cardiac output. Remember, however, that high mixed venous saturations in the

presence of a low cardiac output state may indicate a left-to-right shunt, e.g. acquired VSD.

Both pulmonary vascular resistance (PVR) and systemic vascular resistance (SVR) can be calculated if cardiac output and intracardiac pressures are known (see Chapter 1). Knowledge of SVR helps diagnose possible causes of shock and helps in the choice of drug therapy:

- **Shock with ↑ SVR and normal or high wedge pressure**. This is due to low cardiac output, or cardiogenic shock. A vasodilating inotrope, e.g. dobutamine, may help to increase cardiac output and reduce afterload.
- **Shock with ↑ SVR and low wedge pressure**. If CVP is also low the patient is likely to be hypovolaemic and requires fluid resuscitation. If CVP is normal or high the patient may have had an RV infarct. Fluid resuscitation is also indicated in this situation.
- **Shock with ↓ SVR**. This usually indicates sepsis, although vasodilator medication can also produce this pattern. Fluid replacement ± vasoconstrictor (e.g. noradrenaline) is indicated.

TABLE 3.1 Interpretation of right heart catheterization data. A-V SaO$_2$ = the difference in arterial and mixed venous oxygen saturations

	Hypovolaemia	Sepsis	LV failure	RV failure	Tamponade	Acquired VSD
CVP	↓	↓	↑	↑	↑	↑
PCWP	↓	↓	↑	↓	↑	↑
CO	↓	↑	↓	↓	↓	↓
SVR	↑	↓	↑	↑	↑	↑
A-V SaO$_2$	↑	↓	↑	↑	↑	↓

TEMPORARY CARDIAC PACING

INDICATIONS

Temporary pacing should be considered in the following situations.

Acute MI

AV block is common with inferior MI because the right coronary artery supplies both the inferior surface of the heart and the AV nodal artery. The block usually occurs high in the conducting system, near the compact AV node. Mobitz type I (Wenckebach) second-degree AV block may be partly due to excess vagal tone and often responds to IV **atropine** 0.5–1 mg. Mobitz type II second-degree AV block is very rare with inferior MI, since this type of block is *infranodal*. Third-degree AV block is usually associated with a relatively rapid (>40 bpm) narrow complex rhythm. It is reasonable, in this setting, to withhold temporary pacing if the patient is stable and thrombolysis is being administered, to expedite therapy and to avoid the risks of instrumentation.

Anterior MI complicated by AV or intraventricular block carries a poor prognosis because the infarct is usually large and involves the bundle branches and/or fascicles. The level of block is infranodal and can result in Mobitz type II second-degree AV block, or third-degree AV block with a slow escape rhythm. The risk of asystole is high. Pacing is indicated in:

- Inferior MI with:
    third-degree or Mobitz type II second-degree AV block and haemodynamic compromise
    prolonged third-degree AV block
    sinus/junctional bradycardia with inadequate response to atropine and associated with haemodynamic compromise
    asystole.
- Anterior MI with:
    second- or third-degree AV block
    bifascicular block
      RBBB + left or right axis deviation
    trifascicular block
      RBBB + left axis deviation + first-degree AV block
      LBBB + first degree AV block
    alternating LBBB and RBBB
    sinus/junctional bradycardia with inadequate response to atropine and associated with haemodynamic compromise
    asystole.

Prior to general anaesthesia

The indications for pacing prior to general anaesthesia encompass the general indications for permanent pacing (see Chapter 17) when, if possible, a permanent system should be implanted in preference to a temporary one. There is considerable disagreement about the need for temporary pacing in patients with bifascicular block, but those with trifascicular block should have a temporary wire placed prophylactically.

Other indications

- Symptomatic sinus or AV node disease, where further evaluation is required before decision made re implantation of a permanent pacemaker (e.g. to exclude MI or to allow effects of medication to wear off)
- Heart failure or haemodynamic compromise associated with inappropriate bradycardia
- Profound bradycardia associated with drug overdose, e.g. digoxin, β-blockers
- Asystole or ventricular standstill

- Cardiac surgery which may affect AV node or His bundle, e.g. aortic valve replacement, AV canal defects, tricuspid surgery with Ebstein's anomaly (epicardial electrodes normally placed intraoperatively)
- Aortic valve or root endocarditis with evidence of AV block
- Overdrive suppression of bradycardia-mediated ventricular tachycardia
- Overdrive termination of recurrent or persistent tachyarrhythmias.

TEMPORARY PACING METHODS

Transcutaneous ventricular pacing

This is reserved for the emergency treatment of a severe bradycardia or asystole. Two large pads are attached to the chest, one on the anterior chest wall at the V_3 position and one posteriorly beneath the left scapula. The procedure is very distressing for patients, who often require sedation and analgesia. Transcutaneous pacing is a temporizing measure prior to transvenous pacing.

Transvenous pacing

- Atrial pacing is useful for treating sinus or junctional bradycardias in the absence of AV block. AV synchrony is maintained, which improves cardiac output in patients with low cardiac output, in whom the atrial contribution to ventricular filling is important.
- Ventricular pacing is useful in AV block and as prophylaxis where the risk of AV block is anticipated, e.g. trifascicular block in anterior MI. Ventricular pacing is also indicated for bradycardias associated with atrial fibrillation/flutter, in which atrial pacing is not possible.
- Dual-chamber pacing is indicated for patients with AV block and significant haemodynamic compromise.

A single-lead temporary VDD system can be used which senses atrial activity and paces the ventricles. This avoids the need to insert atrial and ventricular pacing wires (see Chapter 17, pacing modes).

Epicardial pacing

At the time of cardiac surgery both atrial and ventricular epicardial wires can be inserted. These fine small-calibre wires are only useful for a short period as the pacing threshold often rises postoperatively.

METHOD

Central access and sheath insertion should be performed as previously described. The femoral approach is advisable for patients who have had thrombolysis for acute MI. To avoid extravasation of pacing leads, all manipulation should be done under fluoroscopic guidance. If permanent pacing is anticipated do not site the temporary lead at the same access site as you normally implant your permanent pacemakers.

Atrial lead insertion

The atrial 'J' wire is shaped to hook into the right atrial appendage. The lead is fed into the right atrium and pulled back with the tip pointing anteriorly (use RAO view to confirm; Fig. 17.13c). The lead tip should catch in the appendage; further withdrawal causes it to straighten out. Atrial appendage motion makes the tip of the wire swing, or to trace out an 'anticlockwise square'. Atrial leads are quite prone to displacement and stability should be checked during coughing and deep inspiration. J-leads cannot be inserted via the femoral vein; a straight ventricular lead can be aimed at the atrial appendage in this situation, although lead displacement is common.

Ventricular lead insertion

Ventricular temporary leads are either straight or slightly angulated near the tip. Once in the right atrium, the lead is torqued so that the tip points towards the cardiac apex. Ventricular arrhythmias, usually transient, may occur when the lead is advanced through the tricuspid valve. The lead may curve upwards into the RV outflow tract, in which case it should be withdrawn and torqued so that it points towards the RV apex (Fig. 17.12). The lead is advanced to the RV apex and enough 'belly' is left so that it does not displace during deep inspiration.

Checking lead function

- Connect lead to pacing box (polarity is not important).
- Set temporary pacemaker to *demand pacing* at 2 V, with demand rate 20 bpm faster than the patient's intrinsic heart rate. Capture is confirmed by an increase in heart rate and (with ventricular pacing) complexes with LBBB morphology. Capture is more difficult to confirm with atrial leads, as paced P waves may not be clearly seen.
- Reduce output gradually until pacing does not occur. The minimum output needed to achieve capture is the pacing *threshold*. The threshold should be <1.0 V for ventricular leads and <1.5 V for atrial leads (at standard pulse width of 1.0 ms). If these targets are not achieved, a small adjustment in lead position may be sufficient to improve the threshold.
- Check sensing: set demand rate below patient's intrinsic heart rate. If the temporary pacemaker senses properly, pacing should not occur. *Undersensing* and *oversensing* are discussed further in Chapter 17.
- Set the demand rate according to clinical need. A low demand rate (e.g. 40 bpm) should be used if pacing is for prophylaxis against bradycardia (e.g. anterior MI with trifascicular block). A high demand rate may be needed for patients with inappropriate bradycardia (e.g. cardiogenic shock with bradycardia).
- Set the output of the pacing unit to 2.5–3.0 V (or three times the pacing threshold, if >1.0 V).
- Check threshold daily.

PACING FOR TACHYARRHYTHMIAS

Recurrent or persistent VT may respond to or be suppressed by temporary pacing. Full resuscitation facilities, including defibrillation, must be immediately available.

- **Overdrive pacing**, to terminate VT, is done by setting the ventricular pacing rate slightly faster than the arrhythmia rate. Pacing is continued only for a few seconds, to ensure capture is achieved. Pacing can either be stopped abruptly, or the paced rate can be gradually reduced below that of the VT. If this fails to terminate VT faster overdrive rates can be used, but at the risk of accelerating VT or causing VF.
- **Underdrive pacing** (fixed-rate ventricular pacing, at a rate slower than the VT rate) may interrupt VT by interrupting the circus intraventricular depolarization which often perpetuates VT.
- **Overdrive suppression** is used to prevent VT, especially when secondary to bradycardia. Overdrive atrial or ventricular pacing, at a rate higher than the patient's sinus rate, suppress the ectopic beats that initiate VT episodes.

TROUBLESHOOTING

Unable to position pacing lead

Torque should be used to steer the pacing lead to the correct site. Slow, controlled torsion should be used; small movements only are needed. Excessive twisting may soften, fatigue or even fracture the wire. Some sheaths have a haemostatic valve which can be tightened to prevent lead displacement. Ensure that the valve is loose during lead manipulation. The pacing wire may become entangled in the tricuspid apparatus; if it does not advance freely, it should be withdrawn to the tricuspid valve before readvancing. Lead displacement is much more likely in patients with right-sided cardiac dilatation and tricuspid regurgitation; in these cases a stiffer lead may be needed to secure position in the RV apex. These leads are more likely to perforate the ventricle and should only be used if absolutely necessary.

High threshold, or failure to capture/sense

Before adjusting lead position check the lead's connections, the pacing box function (including batteries) and settings. If these are correct, the problem is usually lead position. Occasionally the RV apex is infarcted and fibrosed and satisfactory apical thresholds cannot be achieved. The RV outflow tract, or a more medial position on the floor of RV, can be tried, although lead displacement is quite common from these sites. Pacing thresholds are higher than normal in patients taking amiodarone or class Ic antiarrhythmic drugs (e.g. flecainide).

Rising threshold

The pacing threshold usually rises after lead insertion. Repositioning is not usually needed unless the threshold rises over 2.0 V, but the output should be reset to three times the threshold to ensure an adequate margin of safety. A rapid or large rise in threshold is most often caused by lead displacement, or perforation through the RV wall. Repositioning can be done if the lead is protected by a sterile sheath; otherwise, lead replacement is needed.

Perforation
The pacing threshold rises rapidly and diaphragmatic (ventricular leads) or phrenic nerve (atrial leads) pacing may occur. The patient may feel 'rabbit kicks' or 'hiccups'. Surprisingly, perforation is only rarely associated with tamponade, even after withdrawal of the lead. Tamponade is more likely to occur in patients with RV infarction. If perforation is suspected, the lead should only be withdrawn where there are facilities for echocardiography, pericardial aspiration and, if necessary, surgical drainage. Perforation may be confirmed by recording the intracardiac electrocardiogram from the temporary wire: a narrow 'surface' QRS complex is seen.

Pyrexia
This usually indicates local infection at the insertion site and is especially common with femoral access. *Staphylococcus aureus* and *Staph. epidermidis* are the most common culprit organisms. As a matter of routine, temporary leads should be resited from femoral access sites after 48 hours and from other sites after 4–5 days, to prevent infection. If infection is suspected swab the access site, take blood cultures and insert a new lead from another access site. Antistaphylococcal antibiotics (e.g. oral flucloxacillin 500 mg qid for 1 week) should be given, pending culture and sensitivity results.

Other complications
Sustained ventricular arrhythmias are most common during instrumentation in patients with acute MI. Bradycardias may also occur, and include complete heart block and ventricular standstill. These assist in focusing on the job in hand! An isoprenaline infusion may be needed to maintain a perfusing rhythm until the temporary lead is positioned (see Chapter 17).

PERICARDIAL ASPIRATION

INDICATIONS
- Cardiac tamponade
- Symptomatic pericardial effusion
- Diagnostic pericardiocentesis.

METHOD

Percutaneous
Aspiration should be performed under echo guidance if possible, although

this may not be possible in an extreme emergency, e.g. EMD cardiac arrest. Echo is helpful because it identifies the best approach to drainage: effusions are often localized to the inferior surface or apex, which can then be targeted. The procedure below should be followed:

- Explain the procedure to the patient, including risks; obtain informed consent.
- Obtain IV access.
- Position patient so that the effusion is accessible (confirm with echo).
- Scrub, wear gown and gloves. Clean and drape access site.
- Infiltrate skin and subcutaneous tissues with local anaesthetic (e.g. 5–10 ml 1% lignocaine). You may find the pericardial space during infiltration; withdraw needle immediately.
- Using access needle, a soft J guidewire and dilator, insert a pericardial pigtail drain into the pericardial space using the Seldinger technique (subxiphoid and apical approaches described below).
- Collect pericardial fluid for cytology, protein content and microbial assessment (including *Mycobacterium tuberculosis*).
- If blood is aspirated, use echo or fluoroscopy to confirm that catheter is in the pericardial space rather than the RV cavity.
- Aspirate fluid until no more can be removed, or until the patient begins to experience discomfort.
- Unless rapid reaccumulation is anticipated, remove the pericardial drain straight away to minimize the risk of introducing infection.

Subxiphoid approach
Position the patient either semirecumbent or supine. After local anaesthesia, a pericardial needle is inserted 1–2 cm beneath the xiphisternum and advanced towards the left shoulder at ~45° to the midline, until pericardial fluid is aspirated. The drain is inserted as described above.

Apical approach
Position patient semirecumbent, inclined to ~45°. Confirm precise access site and angle of approach using echo probe (a sterile sleeve can be used over the transducer head and lead). After several practice approaches using the probe, the access needle is inserted along the same path.

Surgical
Malignant and postsurgical pericardial effusions should be drained surgically, especially if loculated. Chronic inflammatory effusions may necessitate surgical fashioning of a pericardial window to allow drainage into the pleural cavity. Without surgical drainage and pericardiectomy, inflammatory pericardial effusions may lead to constrictive pericarditis.

Percutaneous balloon pericardiotomy
Chronic drainage of a (usually malignant) pericardial effusion can also be

performed using percutaneous balloon pericardiotomy. Percardial aspiration is done using the xiphisternal approach, leaving at least 200 ml of fluid in place. A long (30–40 mm) balloon is inserted along the aspiration tract and, when positioned across the parietal pericardium, in the trefoil of the diaphragm, inflated to a diameter of 2–3 cm. The pericardial effusion drains into the abdominal cavity, avoiding the need for surgical intervention.

TROUBLESHOOTING

Unable to insert drain
Sometimes the pericardial drain will not advance over the guidewire, either because the tract has not been sufficiently dilated, or because the guidewire has displaced. Recheck guidewire position using fluoroscopy or echo. If the wire is displaced it should be withdrawn and reintroduced.

Drain inserted in wrong place
It can be difficult to tell whether a pericardial drain is correctly positioned if there is a coexisting pleural effusion (common with pathologies that cause pericardial effusion). If haemodynamic improvement does not occur with aspiration, check the position of the pericardial drain with echo or fluoroscopy.

Perforation of the free wall of the heart can be a serious complication, but it is difficult to distinguish this from successful aspiration of a haemorrhagic effusion! The following may help:

● Check the haematocrit of the aspirated fluid.
● It is often claimed that haemorrhagic pericardial fluid will not clot after aspiration. This is not invariably true, but it can be a helpful distinguishing feature.
● Attach the aspiration needle to an ECG terminal. ST segment elevation is seen if the myocardium is entered.
● Using fluoroscopy, inject X-ray contrast into drain/needle (ensure that blood/fluid can be freely aspirated, to avoid intramyocardial injection).

COMPLICATIONS

In addition to the complications seen with central line insertions, pericardial aspiration can be complicated by myocardial perforation, cardiac tamponade, coronary artery dissection, arrhythmias, trauma to the abdomen (especially the liver) and death.

 Warning: Never rethread the access needle over the guidewire as this can shear off its tip.

INTRA-AORTIC BALLOON PUMP INSERTION

An intra-aortic balloon pump (IABP) consists of a large (30–50 ml) helium-filled balloon which is positioned in the thoracic aorta and attached to a pneumatic pump. The balloon is inflated in diastole and has two main haemodynamic effects:

- Augmentation of diastolic blood pressure (and thus coronary perfusion)
- Afterload reduction.

The IABP is used to support the circulation in patients with haemodynamic compromise or profound myocardial ischaemia.

INDICATIONS

Intra-aortic balloon pump insertion is used either as a bridge to definitive intervention (e.g. CABG or cardiac transplantation), or as a short-term treatment to support coronary perfusion.

- Cardiogenic shock, especially after acute MI or cardiac surgery
- Unstable angina with haemodynamic compromise or recurrent ventricular arrhythmias – bridge to revascularization
- Acquired VSDs or mitral regurgitation complicating acute MI
- High-risk PTCA and CABG
- Bridge to cardiac transplantation.

CONTRAINDICATIONS

- Aortic dissection/aneurysm
- Aortic regurgitation
- Patent ductus arteriosus
- Severe femoral or aortoiliac peripheral vascular disease.

METHOD

Insertion

The femoral artery is cannulated as described in Chapter 18. The balloon requires a large diameter sheath (9–12 Fr) for insertion, although with some modern balloons sheathless insertion can be used. Before insertion the balloon should be purged with helium and its integrity tested. The balloon is inserted over a J-shaped guidewire into the descending thoracic aorta and positioned with its distal radio-opaque marker just below the junction of the aorta with the left subclavian artery. The balloon is secured in position by suturing its shaft to the leg.

Operation

Diastolic counterpulsation is usually triggered by the ECG signal, although

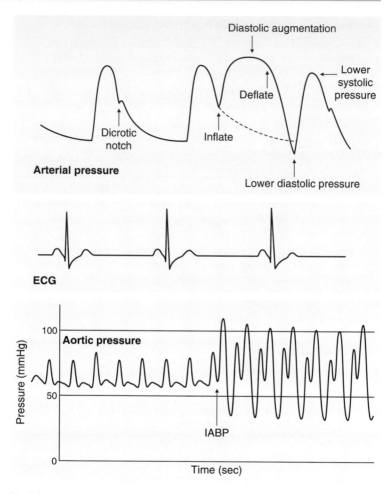

Fig. 3.4 Intra-aortic balloon counterpulsation. Augmentation of aortic pressure during diastole is gated to the electrocardiogram. Overall mean aortic pressure falls but coronary blood flow is enhanced owing to the augmented diastolic aortic pressure.

the aortic pressure waveform can also be used (Fig. 3.4). Counterpulsation is usually done every cardiac cycle (1:1 augmentation). The timing (relative to the ECG) can also be adjusted to optimize diastolic pressure. If the patient improves counterpulsation can be weaned by reducing the synchronization ratio to 1:2 or 1:3. If the patient tolerates this it is usually appropriate to remove the balloon. While the balloon is in place the patient should be heparinized to prevent arterial thromboembolism.

Removal

The balloon and sheath are removed as described in Chapter 18. As the puncture is usually large it is sensible to use a mechanical clamp for at least 30 minutes to achieve haemostasis.

COMPLICATIONS

- Limb ischaemia (5–19%). Usually responds to removal of IABP, but may require surgical repair or embolectomy
- Aortic dissection (<5%)
- Aortoiliac perforation
- Infection
- Haemorrhage and haematoma formation.

MANAGEMENT OF IN-PATIENT CARDIAC PROBLEMS

ACUTE CARDIAC EMERGENCIES

CARDIAC ARREST

The UK Resuscitation Council operates specific courses to train medical and paramedical staff in advanced life support skills. Most countries operate similar courses, based on national resuscitation guidelines. These skills are fundamental to the practice of medicine and all trainees, regardless of specialty, should undertake an advanced life support training course.

Figures 4.1 and 4.2 describe the treatment algorithms for basic and advanced life support. In certain circumstances a modified approach needs to be taken which will potentially result in an improved outcome.

CARDIAC ARREST – SPECIAL CIRCUMSTANCES

Anaphylaxis

This is an exaggerated IgE-mediated hypersensitivity reaction which results in cardiovascular collapse due to a profound fall in systemic vascular resistance, capillary integrity and blood pressure.

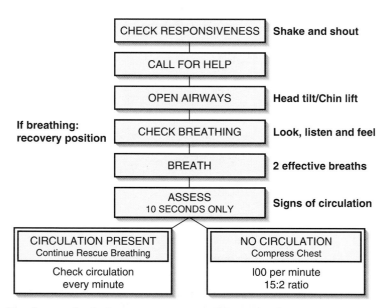

ADULT BASIC LIFE SUPPORT

Send or go for help as soon as possible according to guidelines

Fig. 4.1 European Resuscitation Council algorithm for adult basic life support.

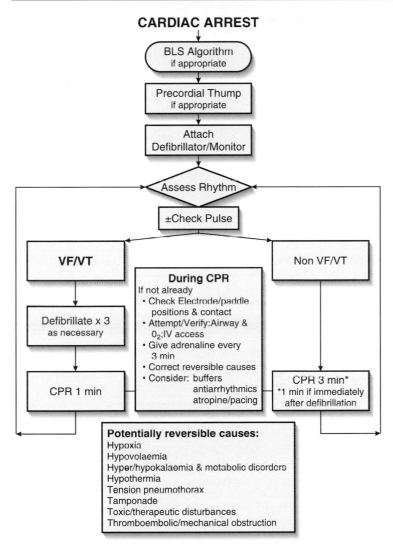

CARDIAC ARREST

BLS Algorithm
if appropriate

Precordial Thump
if appropriate

Attach
Defibrillator/Monitor

Assess Rhythm

±Check Pulse

VF/VT

Non VF/VT

Defibrillate x 3
as necessary

During CPR
If not already
• Check Electrode/paddle
  positions & contact
• Attempt/Verify:Airway &
  O₂;IV access
• Give adrenaline every
  3 min
• Correct reversible causes
• Consider: buffers
           antiarrhythmics
           atropine/pacing

CPR 1 min

CPR 3 min*
*1 min if immediately
after defibrillation

Potentially reversible causes:
Hypoxia
Hypovolaemia
Hyper/hypokalaemia & metabolic disorders
Hypothermia
Tension pneumothorax
Tamponade
Toxic/therapeutic disturbances
Thromboembolic/mechanical obstruction

The ALS Algorithm for the management of Cardiac Arrest in Adults

Note that each successive step is based on the assumption that the one
before has been unsuccessful

Fig. 4.2 European Resuscitation Council algorithm for adult advanced life support.

Shock may be accompanied by flushing, urticaria, GI upset and respiratory compromise (laryngeal angio-oedema and bronchospasm). Anaphylaxis can be precipitated by exposure to a variety of antigens, sometimes in food (e.g. peanuts, seafood), bee stings, drugs etc.

Specific management
Maintain airway and give high-flow oxygen. Drug treatments are:

- **IM adrenaline** 500 µg (0.5 ml of 1:1000 solution) or, if cardiac arrest is imminent, 300–500 µg slowly IV. This may need to be repeated at 5 min intervals.
- **IV antihistamine**, e.g. chlorpheniramine 10–20 mg.
- **IV hydrocortisone** 100–500 mg by slow injection.

IV colloid 500–1000 ml, should be given rapidly to augment blood pressure.

Electrocution
This can occur because of a lightning strike or, more commonly, from a mains electricity supply. Electricity tends to pass along excitable tissues (e.g. muscle and nerves) and may cause respiratory muscle paralysis or cardiac arrest. In general, direct current tends to cause asystole and alternating current (especially at 50 Hz) ventricular fibrillation. Standard resuscitation protocols apply, but beware of 'arcing' electricity when approaching the casualty.

Hypothermia
The hypothermic patient (core temperature <35°C) may appear dead and often has a slow, irregular low-volume pulse. Hypothermia is most common in the elderly and the very young; in young adults drugs and alcohol are common associations.

Specific management
Rewarming is essential. Replace cold, wet clothes with warm blankets or clothes. If the victim is conscious and able, immerse in a bath (40°C) until comfortably warmed. If the patient is unconscious, or if core temperature <28°C, consider:

- ventilation with warm humidified oxygen
- warm (40°C) IV fluids
- gastric, peritoneal or pleural lavage with warm (40°C) fluids
- heated blankets or cradle
- blood rewarming with cardiopulmonary bypass or haemodialysis.

Hypovolaemia is common during hypothermia and warm IV fluids should be given (with caution in patients with impaired LV function). Arrhythmias are common and, as core temperature falls, the patient may develop sinus bradycardia, atrial fibrillation, VF or asystole. Moving or intubating the patient may cause VF. If core temperature is less than 30°C VF may be resistant to cardioversion. Rewarming during CPR may be necessary to raise core temperature sufficiently to permit successful cardioversion.

Drug overdose/toxicity

Drug overdose/toxicity can cause both arrhythmias and direct myocardial depression. Information about the management of specific drug toxicities can be obtained from drug data sheets or (in the UK) the National Poisons Information Bureau.

Specific management

Oral activated charcoal may reduce drug absorption. Gastric lavage has fallen out of favour for most overdoses because it can hasten the passage of tablets into the small intestine and enhance absorption. Some non-protein bound drugs can be removed using haemofiltration.

Bradycardias should be treated as normal with IV atropine, isoprenaline or temporary pacing (see Chapter 7). β-Blocker toxicity should be treated in addition with IV glucagon 5 mg. Digoxin toxicity can be treated with Fab fragment antibody specific for digoxin (Digibind). Profound bradycardia and asystole secondary to digoxin toxicity may be resistant to pacing. Tachycardias may also occur, commonly atrial fibrillation, sinus or atrial tachycardias, or ventricular tachycardia.

Digibind treatment	
Acute overdose	
Unknown amount ingested	800 mg
Known amount ingested	amount ingested (µg)/15
Toxicity from chronic dosing	
Serum digoxin concentration (ng ml^{-1}) × weight (kg) × 0.4	

Toxicity or overdose with drugs that cause QT interval prolongation (which predisposes to atypical or polymorphic VT, e.g. torsades de pointes VT) are often difficult to treat. See Chapter 7 for management.

Tachycardias caused by tricyclic antidepressant drugs often respond to β-blockade (e.g. **IV esmolol, propranolol**), although myocardial depression may occur. **IV physostigmine salicylate** (1–3 mg) is occasionally used for life-threatening overdoses. Patients with severe toxicity should undergo ECG monitoring for 4–5 days. Shock and metabolic acidosis are treated using standard measures. Convulsions may also occur and can be treated with **IV diazepam** (10 mg), paraldehyde or anaesthesia. Dialysis does not help in tricyclic overdosage. Antiarrhythmics may worsen arrhythmias.

Pregnancy

The welfare of both mother and fetus needs to be considered.

Specific management

Call the obstetric and pediatric teams immediately. Early intubation and displacement of the uterus (using a Cardiff wedge under the patient's right side) to aid venous return are essential. If cardiac arrest persists for more than 5 minutes in the third trimester of pregnancy emergency caesarean section should be performed to rescue the fetus and to improve maternal venous return by decompressing the IVC.

The most likely cause of cardiac arrest in pregnancy is hypovolaemia secondary to occult blood loss (placental abruption, aortic dissection) or pulmonary embolism (thrombotic or amniotic). Vigorous IV fluid ± blood infusion may be needed. Management is otherwise according to standard protocols.

PERI-ARREST ARRHYTHMIAS (See also Chapter 7)

Many patients suffer cardiac arrest because of a serious illness which is complicated by malignant arrhythmias. Also, most patients initially resuscitated from cardiac arrest experience bradycardias or tachycardias which require treatment to prevent further circulatory collapse. 'Peri-arrest arrhythmias' encompass rhythm disorders which occur at these times and can be divided into three main categories:

- Bradycardia (relative to clinical state)
- Broad-complex tachycardias
- Narrow-complex tachycardias.

The management algorithms given in Figures 4.3, 4.4 and 4.5 are based on the guidelines published by the European Resuscitation Council (*Resuscitation* 1996;31:281). These algorithms all include the statement 'Seek expert help'. If you *are* the duty cardiologist, then you *are* the expert help!

BRADYCARDIA

Although bradycardia is often defined as a heart rhythm disorder with rate <60 bpm, in this setting it refers to a heart rate which is slow relative to the clinical situation – 'relative bradycardia' – e.g., a patient with cardiogenic shock and heart rate 70 bpm is relatively bradycardic. The principles underlying the management of these patients are as follows:

- If there is no perceived risk of asystole but the haemodynamic state of the patient is poor, give atropine and pace only if this is ineffective.
- If there is no perceived risk of asystole and the patient is not compromised, then only observation is needed.

Risk of asystole is highest in patients with previous asystole. Patients with evidence of high-grade AV nodal or infranodal block are also considered at high risk. Mobitz type I (Wenckebach) AV block does not carry the same risk of asystole.

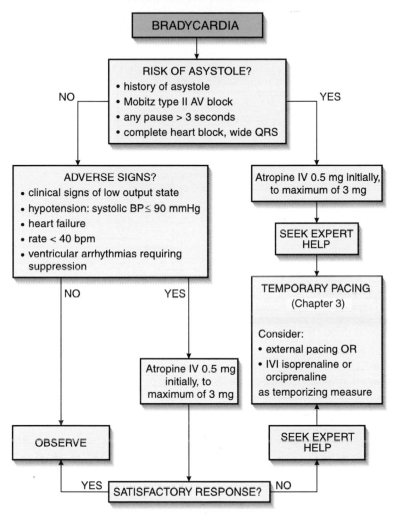

Fig. 4.3 Management of peri-arrest bradycardia.

BROAD-COMPLEX TACHYCARDIAS

Tachycardias are divided into 'broad'- and 'narrow'-complex varieties rather than SVTs and VT because this is how the tachycardia presents itself in the acute setting. Differentiation of SVTs and VT is discussed in Chapter 7. The

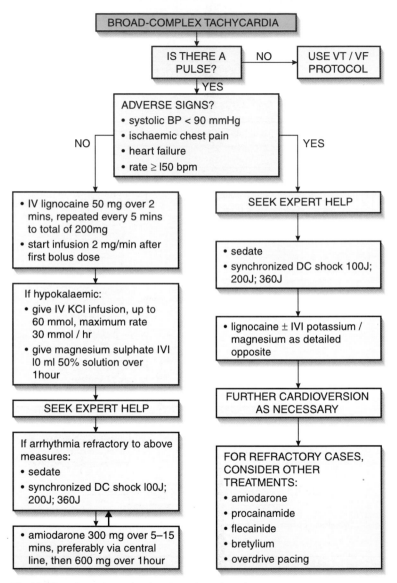

Fig. 4.4 Management of peri-arrest broad-complex tachycardia.

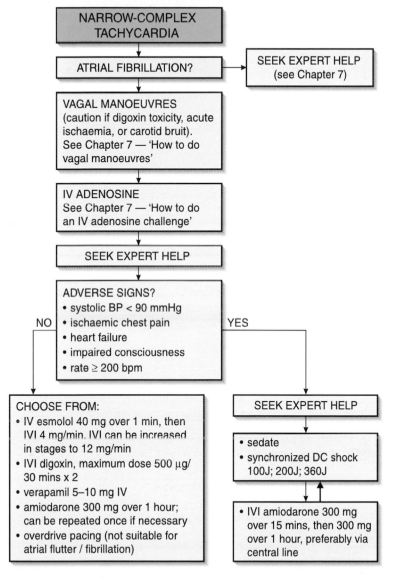

Fig. 4.5 Management of peri-arrest narrow-complex tachycardia.

principles underlying the management of patients with broad-complex tachycardia are as follows:

● If there is no pulse, treat using the VT/VF algorithm for cardiac arrest (see previous section).
● If there is a pulse but the patient is compromised, cardiovert as soon as possible.
● If there is a pulse and the patient is not compromised, antiarrhythmic drug therapy should be used, with cardioversion only if this fails.

Broad-complex arrhythmias and their management are discussed further in Chapters 7 and 12.

NARROW-COMPLEX TACHYCARDIAS

These are almost always supraventricular in origin and do not carry as hazardous a prognosis. In susceptible patients they can trigger malignant arrhythmias, e.g. during myocardial ischaemia. The principles underlying the management of patients with narrow complex tachycardia are as follows:

● For regular SVTs, vagal manoeuvres or adenosine can be tried first.
● In the presence of adverse signs, if these are not successful, the first-line treatment is cardioversion.
● In the absence of adverse signs a choice of antiarrhythmic agents can be tried, including short-acting β-blocker, digoxin, verapamil and amiodarone.

Narrow-complex tachycardias and their management are discussed further in Chapters 7 and 12.

CARDIAC TAMPONADE

Tamponade occurs when a pericardial effusion compromises ventricular filling by increasing end-diastolic pressure and reducing compliance in all cardiac chambers. This reduces cardiac output and further elevates ventricular filling pressures. Acute tamponade is life-threatening and often requires emergency pericardial aspiration (see Chapter 3).

CAUSES OF PERICARDIAL EFFUSION

● Cardiac rupture (post-MI (Chapter 5), iatrogenic (cardiac catheterization, pacing wire, myocardial biopsy), chest trauma)
● Type A aortic dissection (Chapter 4)
● Cardiac surgery (acute inflammation, infection, anastamotic leak, post-pericardiotomy syndrome)
● Malignancy
● Hypothyroidism
● Pericarditis – infection (viral (e.g. Coxsackie B), bacterial, TB, fungal), MI,

inflammatory (e.g. rheumatoid arthritis, Dressler syndrome, post-pericardiotomy syndrome), uraemia, trauma, idiopathic
- Anticoagulant therapy.

DIAGNOSIS

Tamponade is a clinical diagnosis, made by checking for specific clinical signs in association with a pericardial effusion. Many patients with a pericardial effusion do not have tamponade, especially when the effusion is chronic, and it is important not to expose these patients to the risks of pericardial drainage.

Tamponade can cause clinical signs of low cardiac output (e.g. shock, low-volume pulse, poor peripheral perfusion), oliguria and a raised JVP with a pronounced x-descent. The JVP may rise on inspiration (Kussmaul's sign; see Chapter 1). The main discriminating physical sign is pulsus paradoxus, which should always be sought if tamponade is suspected, although atrial fibrillation can render its identification difficult. The differential diagnosis of shock associated with elevated JVP includes pulmonary embolism, RV infarction, end-stage cardiac failure, constrictive pericarditis, restrictive cardiomyopathy and tension pneumothorax.

INVESTIGATIONS

ECG   if the effusion is large, ↓ QRS voltage and sometimes electrical alternans (due to movement of heart in pericardial space)
CXR   globular cardiac silhouette ± pulmonary oedema
Echo   shows location of effusion, whether loculated, fibrinous
        May show RV collapse in diastole, RA collapse
        Helps identify best access route for drainage (see Chapters 3, pericardial aspiration and 19, echocardiography).

The size of the effusion is not necessarily a good guide as to the presence or absence of tamponade because a small effusion can cause tamponade if it develops rapidly, or if it selectively compresses the right ventricle.

Tamponade is occasionally caused by the erosion of a central line through the right atrial wall. This should be considered in patients who suddenly collapse with a central line in situ. Aspiration from the catheter may temporarily reduce the size of the effusion.

MANAGEMENT

Tamponade usually necessitates urgent pericardial aspiration (see Chapter 3). However, if cardiac rupture or aortic dissection are implicated as the cause, pericardial aspiration may precipitate further, fatal, intrapericardial bleeding. Emergency surgery is the treatment of choice in these cases. After successful aspiration a pericardial drain can be left in place to prevent the reaccumulation of fluid. Subsequent management depends on the aetiology of the effusion, but may ultimately require surgical correction or pericardiodesis.

ACUTE MITRAL AND SEPTAL RUPTURE

Both of these conditions are most often encountered in the first week after acute MI and usually cause sudden and major haemodynamic compromise. Other causes are less common:

● Acute mitral valve failure can also occur because of myxomatous degeneration of a floppy mitral valve, trauma, infective endocarditis (Chapter 8) or prosthetic valve failure (Chapter 4).
● Acquired VSDs may occur after direct cardiac trauma, e.g. after stabbing or RV biopsy. Presentation may be delayed because oedema initially limits the amount of shunting through the VSD.

CLINICAL PRESENTATION

Symptoms
● Sudden severe breathlessness
● Autonomic activation: sweating, nausea, vomiting
● Chest pain.

Signs
● Haemodynamic compromise: shock, tachycardia, acute pulmonary oedema
● Systolic murmur, often loud and harsh. The murmurs of acute mitral regurgitation and acute septal rupture can be difficult to differentiate, but:
  VSD murmur often radiates to right side of chest
  anterior leaflet mitral murmur often radiates to the back
● Parasternal heave (due to RV overload or systolic left atrial expansion)
● Palpable thrill
● Elevated JVP.

The following points may help distinguish acute VSD from acute mitral regurgitation, although it is usually very difficult to differentiate the two:

● Acute mitral regurgitation more often causes severe dyspnoea and pulmonary oedema.
● JVP is usually elevated with acute VSD, but may not be elevated with mitral regurgitation.
● Inferior MI favours mitral regurgitation, anterior MI favours acute VSD. However, either pathology can occur with either infarct territory.

INVESTIGATIONS

- Arterial blood analysis
  metabolic (lactic) acidosis due to systemic hypoperfusion
  hypoxia associated with pulmonary oedema
- Serum biochemistry
  acute renal failure
- ECG
  often shows recent Q-wave MI with persistent ST segment elevation
- CXR
  pulmonary oedema (mitral regurgitation) or plethora (acute VSD)
- Echo
  prolapsing or flail mitral valve leaflet, sometimes with a chunk of
  papillary muscle attached
  mitral regurgitation jet (see Chapter 19).
  VSDs are easy to miss and failure to identify a defect does not exclude the
  diagnosis. Colour flow mapping and Doppler assessment of the
  intraventricular septum are essential (see Chapter 19)
  RV function is a strong predictor of outcome in acute VSD
- Swan–Ganz catheterization
  with VSD, step up in O_2 saturation at RV/PA level. This confirms the
  diagnosis and allows quantification of the shunt (see Chapter 18)
  with acute mitral regurgitation, large systolic pressure waves in PCWP trace
- Left heart catheterization
  allows better characterization of location and severity of pathology
  document coronary anatomy prior to surgery.

MANAGEMENT

The mortality from acute VSD and acute mitral regurgitation is high,
especially after acute MI (50–90%). Early medical management centres on
treating any associated cardiac failure and haemodynamic compromise.

- **Cardiogenic shock** is treated using standard therapy (see Chapter 5).
- **Pulmonary oedema** is treated with IV diuretics and peripheral vasodilators
  (to reduce afterload), if blood pressure allows. In acute VSD this reduces the
  shunt volume and in acute mitral regurgitation the regurgitant volume is
  reduced. One of the following can be used:
  IVI GTN 10–200 µg min^{-1}
  IVI sodium nitroprusside 10–15 µg min^{-1}, titrated to maximum of
  200 µg min^{-1}
  IVI hydralazine 150–300 µg min^{-1}.
- **An intra-aortic balloon pump** may help stabilize the patient before surgery
  by reducing afterload and augmenting diastolic blood pressure.
- **Arrhythmias**, such as atrial fibrillation, are usually not well tolerated and
  should be treated aggressively with digoxin and/or amiodarone.

Urgent corrective surgery is usually indicated, unless comorbidity precludes it. Some patients can survive with small VSDs without early surgery, but there is a significant risk of death owing to extension of the VSD. Operative mortality is very high (up to 50%), but long-term prognosis is good in those who survive.

Patients with acute mitral regurgitation who stabilize well with medication can be treated with semielective valve replacement a few weeks later. This allows the infarct zone to demarcate and heal and reduces the operative risk.

SINUS OF VALSALVA RUPTURE

This rare condition occurs either because of a congenital aneurysm of the sinus of Valsalva, or because of infective endocarditis affecting the aortic root. Sinus of Valsalva rupture usually creates a fistula into the right atrium, but can also form a fistula with the right ventricle or left atrium.

CLINICAL PRESENTATION

Aneurysms and abscesses usually affect the non-coronary cusp of the aortic valve; when rupture occurs the patient develops sudden chest pain and dyspnoea. There may be clinical signs of volume overload and a loud, continuous murmur is often heard, associated with a precordial thrill. There may also be clinical signs of infective endocarditis (see Chapter 8). Sinus of Valsalva rupture may occur after aortic valve replacement if a secondary abscess forms.

INVESTIGATIONS

- ECG
  AV block may occur as a result of septal or AV nodal involvement
- CXR
  pulmonary oedema, often with normal cardiac size
- Echo
  transthoracic echo may not demonstrate a ruptured sinus of Valsalva: transoesophageal echo is the modality of choice
  a high-velocity jet is usually seen passing over the posterior surface of the tricuspid valve leaflets into the right atrium
- Swan–Ganz catheterization
  step up in O_2 saturation at RA, or sometimes RV, level
  allows quantification of the shunt (Chapter 18).
- Left heart catheterization and aortography
  contraindicated if infective endocarditis is suspected
  confirms diagnosis and location of fistula
- Magnetic resonance imaging
  helps confirm diagnosis and demonstrates site of the fistula
- Investigate for infective endocarditis (see Chapter 8).

MANAGEMENT

As with acute VSD, the initial medical management centres on minimizing shunt volume and managing associated haemodynamic compromise and cardiac failure (see Chapter 4). Peripheral vasodilators should be used to reduce afterload and to reduce shunting by decreasing systemic vascular resistance and aortic pressure. Surgical ligation and repair with or without valve replacement is the definitive treatment.

ACUTE AORTIC DISSECTION

Aortic dissection usually occurs because of an intimal tear which is propagated along the media of the aorta and its main branches. Occasionally the tear may re-enter the aortic lumen, resulting in the so-called *double barrelled aorta*. Unfortunately, the aorta can also rupture outwards, resulting in catastrophic haemorrhage and death. Occasionally aortic dissection occurs as a consequence of an intramural haemorrhage from the vasa vasora, which then perforates through the intima and into the lumen. Indeed, one in eight aortic dissections do not have an identifiable intimal tear and represent an intramural haematoma. Diagnostic difficulties can arise when trying to distinguish intramural haematoma from aortic dissections; this is a practical problem because subsequent management depends on the underlying pathology.

CLASSIFICATION

There are two main classifications for aortic dissection:

- The **Stanford classification** is the most clinically useful and divides aortic dissections into type A (involving the ascending thoracic aorta) and type B (involving the descending, but not the ascending, thoracic aorta).
- The **DeBakey classification** subdivides type A dissection into type I, which involves both the ascending and the descending thoracic aorta and type II, which is confined to the ascending thoracic aorta only. DeBakey type III dissection is equivalent to Stanford type B dissection.

AETIOLOGY

Aortic dissection often follows the formation of cystic medial necrosis, which leads to a weakening of the collagen and elastin components of the aortic media. The following factors predispose to, or are associated with, aortic dissection:

- Hypertension (80% of cases)
- Aortic atherosclerosis
- Advanced age (common in 60–80-year-olds)
- Collagen disorders: Marfan syndrome, Ehlers–Danlos syndrome, SLE

- Pregnancy (usually third trimester and possibly due to hyperoestrogenaemic state)
- Trauma
- Aortic coarctation
- Bicuspid aortic valve
- Turner or Noonan syndromes
- Infective or inflammatory aortitis: syphilitic aortitis or giant cell arteritis
- Iatrogenic: previous cardiac surgery (aortic vent sites), intra-aortic balloon pump, cardiac catheterization, penicillamine therapy.

CLINICAL PRESENTATION

Symptoms

The classic presentation is with very sudden onset of severe, tearing interscapular pain which appears to migrate along the path of the dissection. The distribution of pain may mirror the site of dissection, although this cannot be relied upon.

- Type A dissections tend to present with anterior chest pain, which may radiate to the face.
- Type B dissections are more often associated with back pain.

The presentation can be very variable and aortic dissection can present painlessly with dizziness (hypovolaemia), sudden collapse or acute limb ischaemia. If severe aortic regurgitation occurs (with type A dissection), acute cardiac failure may follow. Other symptoms relate to areas of vascular compromise, e.g. paraplegia (anterior spinal artery), stroke (carotid artery dissection), abdominal pain (mesenteric/renal ischaemia), anuria or haematuria. Rarely, hoarseness may result from aortic dilatation and left recurrent laryngeal nerve compression.

Signs

The patient may be extremely distressed and there may be severe haemodynamic compromise. Check airway, breathing and circulation. Look for signs of poor peripheral perfusion and low cardiac output.

- Pulse   usually tachycardic; may be low volume
                    peripheral pulses may be absent because of subclavian or iliac artery dissection
                    check for arterial bruits
- Blood pressure   may be high (predisposing factor); hypotension signifies tamponade or aortic rupture
                    unequal upper limb BP (>20 mmHg) may indicate subclavian artery dissection, or simply peripheral vascular disease
                    check for pulsus paradoxus (tamponade)

- Precordium   aortic regurgitant murmur
  precordial pulsation (aortic root dilatation)
- Chest   pleural effusion (aortic leak or reactive, due to aortic
  inflammation)
  pulmonary oedema
- Abdomen   palpable mass (abdominal aorta)
  tenderness
  absent bowel sounds (mesenteric ischaemia)
- CNS   hypertensive retinopathy
  focal/lateralizing signs
  Horner syndrome/hoarseness.

Aortic regurgitation is an ominous sign, suggesting aortic root dilatation, a
flail valve or distortion of the aortic root by haematoma. Rarely (1–2%),
dissection compromises one of the coronary ostia (usually the right) and
causes acute MI. Thrombolytic therapy is likely to kill the patient;
approximately one-third of cases of aortic dissection go unrecognized and are
often misdiagnosed as acute MI.

INVESTIGATIONS

- ECG
  - sinus tachycardia
  - LVH criteria often seen, due to hypertension
  - (rarely) acute MI due to coronary ostial dissection
- CXR (10% of patients have a normal CXR)
  - widened aortic silhouette seen in 90% of type A dissections, but is
    easily confused with unfolded aorta
  - disruption of aortic knuckle calcification is often cited as a sign of
    dissection, but this is a misleading and unreliable sign
  - left-sided pleural effusion may represent aortic leak or may be
    'sympathetic' – inflammatory
- Echo
  Transthoracic echo is helpful but lacks specificity and sensitivity. Only the
  proximal part of the aorta is seen. Useful signs are:
  - dissection flap in aortic root/aortic root dilatation
  - Doppler evidence of aortic regurgitation
  - pericardial effusion
  - wall motion abnormality (may signify coronary artery compromise)
  Transoesophageal echo (TOE) provides more information but should not
  be done if another definitive imaging modality (e.g. MRI) is planned – it
  wastes time and benzodiazepine sedation may cause haemodynamic
  collapse. TOE is very useful if CT or MRI are not accessible. It has very
  high sensitivity and specificity, although visualization of the aortic arch is
  sometimes difficult because of the interposition of the trachea
- MRI and ultrafast spiral CT scanning

These are very useful diagnostic modalities, with high sensitivity and specificity. CT scanning is done with and without contrast enhancement. The 'plain' scan identifies areas of high attenuation in the aortic wall – intramural haematoma. The contrast scan outlines the dissection flap. MRI scanning does not require contrast injection and can detect aortic regurgitation. Both modalities can show:

- classic 'tennis ball' sign in transverse views, with intimal flap crossing the aorta in an arc. The false lumen is usually the larger of the two
- head and neck vessel involvement can be identified
- distal extent of dissection/renal involvement can be identified
- lumina and the entry site commonly arise in the arch of the aorta at the branch points of the head and neck vessels

- Cardiac catheterization and aortography
  Aortography identifies the site of the intimal tear and the extent of the dissection. It also allows the assessment of branch vessels, the severity of aortic regurgitation and the patency of the coronary arteries. Intramural haematomas may, however, be missed and the sensitivity for detecting aortic dissection is inferior to that of CT or MRI. The procedure carries significant risk, including instrumentation of the false lumen, contrast agent load and the associated time delay.

MANAGEMENT

Untreated, acute aortic dissection is often fatal: 25% die within 24 hours, 50% within a week and 90% within a year. Mortality is significantly greater with type A than type B dissection. Urgent surgery should be undertaken if possible, because the attrition rate is up to 5% per hour. Delays should be avoided by expediting essential investigations and contacting the surgical team as soon as the diagnosis is known.

All patients with aortic dissection require aggressive medical treatment to minimize the extent of propagation of the medial tear. Patients should be managed in a high dependency area, with facilities for invasive haemodynamic monitoring considered. Blood pressure and urine output should be carefully monitored. The mainstay of medical therapy is analgesia and antihypertensive drug therapy. To stabilize the dissection while maintaining organ perfusion, aim for a target systolic blood pressure of 100–120 mmHg. Antiemetics may help because retching may cause acute aortic wall stress.

Antihypertensive therapy

Shear stress, the rate of pressure rise in the aorta and heart rate are important factors in determining the extent of propagation of the dissection. Negatively inotropic, negatively chronotropic agents minimize these effects and are preferable to vasodilators, which may increase the shear force and pulse pressure and cause reflex tachycardia.

- **IVI labetalol** 1–2 mg min^{-1}, total dose 50–200 mg, is useful as it is a negative inotrope, negative chronotrope and has additional vasodilator actions through α-blockade.
- If β-blockade is contraindicated, consider rate-limiting calcium antagonists such as oral **diltiazem** or **verapamil**.

Refractory hypertension may indicate renovascular disease or renal artery dissection, with associated renin–angiotensin system activation. ACE inhibitors or angiotensin-receptor antagonists may help control blood pressure, but risk precipitating acute renal failure. Renal failure can also complicate aortic dissection because of renal ischaemia due to renal artery dissection, a sudden reduction in chronically elevated blood pressure, or shock due to hypovolaemia or tamponade.

Haemopericardium and cardiac tamponade is a common mode of death in patients with type A dissection. Pericardiocentesis should **not** be performed in patients with haemopericardium who are relatively stable (see earlier); this should be reserved as a treatment of last resort.

Surgical repair

Surgical repair is indicated for type A dissection because of the risk of retrograde dissection into the pericardium and fatal tamponade. Aortic root replacement, reimplantation of the coronary arteries and valve resuspension or replacement may be necessary. In most cases the main aim of surgery is to secure the proximal entry point of the dissection; this usually prevents the dissection from propagating. It is sometimes possible to resect a diseased segment and to interpose a prosthetic vascular graft. Surgical repair is indicated for :

- type A dissection
- type B dissections complicated by rupture, saccular aneurysm formation, limb ischaemia, vital organ ischaemia or persistent pain
- dissection associated with Marfan syndrome.

ACUTE PROSTHETIC VALVE FAILURE

Acute prosthetic valve failure is rare but often catastrophic. It can occur because of mechanical failure, valve dehiscence or thrombosis. Prompt diagnosis, assessment and treatment is essential.

MECHANICAL FAILURE

The Bjork–Shiley 60°CC (concavoconvex) is the valve most associated with acute failure. This single tilting disc prosthesis is associated with mechanical failure because of mechanical fatigue of the strut which supports the valve disc. The annual risk of failure is low at 7 per 10 000 patients, but is more likely in the following cases:

- Valves manufactured between January 1981 and July 1982
- Size 31–33 mm valves
- Valves implanted in the mitral position.

Other valve designs may also fail acutely, although this is rare. Given the low event rate, prophylactic valve replacement or strut screening is not indicated unless the patient falls into one of the above three categories. With the Bjork–Shiley design mechanical failure results from embolization of the disc into the aorta and patients present with catastrophic circulatory collapse, acute LVF and absent prosthetic heart sounds. CXR, fluoroscopy or echocardiography may reveal the absence of the valve disc. Immediate valve re-replacement is mandatory.

VALVE DEHISCENCE

Prosthetic valve dehiscence presents with acute valve regurgitation and is usually seen in the period immediately following surgery. More rarely, it is associated with prosthetic endocarditis (see Chapter 8). Valve dehiscence is also seen in patients with Marfan syndrome because of the friability of the tissues that support the prosthesis. Valve dehiscence requires emergency valve replacement. Medical treatment and intra-aortic balloon pumping (see Chapters 3 and 6) may stabilize the patient prior to definitive surgery.

VALVE THROMBOSIS

Valve thrombosis usually affects mechanical valves when anticoagulant control is inadequate. Tricuspid prostheses are especially prone to thrombosis and present with right heart failure: ↑↑ JVP, hepatomegaly and peripheral oedema. Mitral and aortic valve thrombosis usually present with pulmonary oedema and signs of low cardiac output. Prosthetic valve sounds are quiet or absent. Fluoroscopy or echocardiography may show marked restriction of valve movement, or intermittent valve opening.

Emergency valve replacement during the acute episode is associated with a mortality rate of ~30%. Thrombolysis is an acceptable alternative and is the treatment of choice for tricuspid valve thrombosis. Thrombolysis is associated with a significant risk of embolism (5–20%) and recurrence of thrombosis (10%). It is less ideal for mitral and aortic valve thromboses, but should be considered for patients in whom surgery is contraindicated or carries a particularly high risk.

CHAPTER 5

ACUTE CORONARY
SYNDROMES

UNSTABLE ANGINA/NON-Q WAVE MYOCARDIAL INFARCTION

Patients with suspected unstable angina require rapid assessment to identify those at risk of MI which, in its early stages, is indistinguishable from non-Q wave MI.

AETIOLOGY/PATHOPHYSIOLOGY

The *clinical* diagnosis of unstable angina is defined as typical ischaemic chest pain occurring at rest, abrupt onset of effort-limiting angina, or rapid deterioration of previously stable chronic angina. Of patients with clinical unstable angina 85% have significant obstructive coronary artery disease. In these patients plaque rupture leads to platelet aggregation, thrombus formation and vasoconstriction. These form the therapeutic targets for drug therapy. *Crescendo angina* (rapidly worsening exertional angina) is sometimes distinguished from unstable angina because it may be caused by plaque expansion rather than rupture. A minority of patients have angiographically normal coronary arteries or non-obstructive coronary lesions, or have unstable angina secondary to increased cardiac work (e.g. anaemia, thyrotoxicosis, fever, accelerated hypertension).

CLINICAL FINDINGS

Symptoms
Symptoms vary widely between patients and their severity does not always reflect the severity of underlying coronary disease.

- 'Classic' central ischaemic chest pain
- Pain or heaviness in the arm(s) (most commonly left)
- Discomfort in neck or jaw
- Back pain
- Autonomic upset (nausea, vomiting, sweating)
- Breathlessness – due to ischaemic LV dysfunction or dynamic mitral regurgitation.

Some patients present solely with breathlessness: this is sometimes referred to as 'angina equivalent'.

Signs
Examination is usually unremarkable but can give helpful information about exacerbating factors and complications.

- Signs of autonomic upset: pallor, sweating
- Signs of exacerbating factors: fever, hypertension, cyanosis, clinical anaemia
- Signs of complications: irregular pulse, hypotension, evidence of LVF.

Clinical risk stratification

High-risk clinical features
  Hypotension
  (New) cardiac failure
  Ventricular arrhythmias

INVESTIGATIONS

In the initial assessment of patients with suspected unstable angina a 12-lead ECG and cardiac enzyme estimation are mandatory.

ECG

The ECG allows early identification of patients with ST-elevation MI, for whom treatment should not be delayed. The ECG should be repeated frequently in patients with persisting symptoms to identify worsening ischaemia or evolving infarction.

Risk stratification from the ECG

Low-risk ECGs:	normal ECG (present initially in 25% of cases)
	T-wave flattening, or inversion <1 mm
Medium-risk ECGs:	ST segment depression 1 mm or less
	T-wave inversion >1 mm
High-risk ECGs:	transient ST segment elevation
	ST segment depression >1 mm
	deep symmetrical T-wave inversion

Cardiac enzymes

The measurement of cardiac enzymes allows differentiation between unstable angina and non-Q wave MI. Sensitivity is maximized if the enzymes are measured every 6 hours during the first day of admission. Most centres use creatine kinase (CK) and its cardiac isoform (CK-MB), which has greater specificity. In patients who present more than 36 hours after the onset of symptoms, serum lactate dehydrogenase (LDH) is useful for retrospective identification of MI. More recently the cardiac isoforms of troponin T (TnT) and troponin I (TnI) have been found to be released in unstable angina and can aid risk stratification.

Other non-invasive tests

- CXR: assess for signs of LVF
- Echo: wall motion defects support cardiac diagnosis
  LV impairment indicates adverse prognosis
  Aortic stenosis, LV outflow tract obstruction and LVH may be aggravating factors

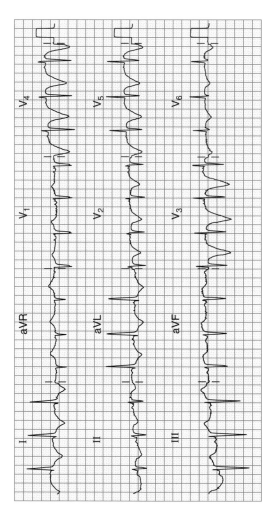

Fig. 5.1 Unstable angina with high-risk ECG features: the deep symmetrical T-wave inversion in the anterior leads suggests proximal LAD or left main stem disease.

- Full blood count: anaemia
- Biochemistry: U&Es, TFTs (lipids).

Risk stratification from maximum troponin T – FRISC study		
	Serum TnT	5-month risk of death or MI
Low risk	<0.06 µg l^{-1}	4.3%
Medium risk	0.06–0.18 µg l^{-1}	10.5%
High risk	>0.18 µg l^{-1}	16.1%

DIFFERENTIAL DIAGNOSIS

The differential diagnosis is that of acute chest discomfort. A careful history helps distinguish ischaemic chest discomfort from that of non-cardiac origin. This is covered in Chapter 1.

- Cardiovascular
  - MI
  - variant angina
  - syndrome X
  - aortic dissection/aneurysm
  - pericarditis
- Respiratory
  - pulmonary embolism
  - lobar pneumonia
  - pneumothorax
  - acute asthma
  - pneumomediastinum
- Gastrointestinal
  - oesophagitis
  - oesophageal spasm
  - hiatus hernia
  - peptic ulcer disease
  - biliary colic
  - pancreatitis
- Other
  - chest wall pain/musculoskeletal
  - costochondritis
  - cervical spondylosis
  - psychogenic pain
  - Bornholm's disease

COMPLICATIONS

The major complications of unstable angina relate to its tendency to progress to acute MI. With antithrombotic and antiplatelet therapy up to 5% of patients with unstable angina develop fatal or non-fatal acute MI within a week; another 3% have refractory angina despite optimal medical therapy. A further 5% die within 6 months of admission. Haemodynamic instability (cardiogenic shock or LVF) can occur in the absence of infarction, if the ischaemic territory is large. This often reflects plaque rupture in the left main stem or left anterior descending coronary artery, or multivessel disease. Papillary muscle ischaemia sometimes causes dynamic mitral regurgitation, which may contribute to instability. Malignant ventricular arrhythmias also occur without infarction. Sinus or junctional bradycardia and AV block can result from sinus or AV node ischaemia; this most often reflects plaque rupture in the proximal right coronary artery.

EARLY MEDICAL MANAGEMENT

Low-risk patients can be managed in a non-intensive medical unit. Medium-risk patients should be managed in a unit with ECG monitoring. High-risk patients should ideally be managed in a cardiac or intensive care unit.

Basic management
- Bedrest, ECG monitoring
- Inhaled O_2 oximetry
- Opiate analgesia if pain not controlled with nitrate and β-blocker
- Anxiolytic if required.

Antiplatelet therapy
Aspirin reduces the risk of death and non-fatal MI very substantially (relative risk 0.3 aspirin vs placebo, in some studies). Oral aspirin 300 mg then 75 mg d should be given. The only absolute contraindications are *true* aspirin allergy or a clear risk of major haemorrhage (e.g. recent GI bleeding). **Clopidogrel** 75 mg d (an ADP receptor antagonist) is effective at reducing mortality in patients with atherosclerotic vascular disease (CAPRIE study) and is a useful substitute for aspirin-intolerant patients.

Antithrombotic therapy
IV heparin, aiming for an aPTT ratio of 1.5–2.5, reduces the incidence of MI and refractory angina. Combined treatment with heparin and aspirin is superior to either agent alone. Treatment should continue at least 24 hours after symptoms have resolved. Discontinuation of heparin may be associated with recurrence of angina ('rebound angina') as a result of increased thrombin activity.

Low molecular weight heparins have greater anti-Factor-Xa activity. They

Warning: Urgent cardiac catheterization should be considered in patients with high-risk clinical features, or with ECG features of severe or worsening ischaemia.

are administered by SC injection without the need for aPTT monitoring and are at least as safe and effective as unfractionated heparin. **SC enoxaparin** 1 mg kg^{-1} bd reduces the risk of refractory angina and MI in patients with unstable angina. The extra cost of this drug has to be weighed against savings in anticoagulant monitoring and the convenience of administration. Direct thrombin inhibitors (e.g. hirudin and hirulog) are currently the subject of large-scale trials.

β-Blockers

β-Blockers reduce heart rate, blood pressure and myocardial oxygen demand and have antiarrhythmic properties. Oral β-blockers (e.g. **metoprolol** 25–100 mg bd) are usually adequate, but in high-risk patients or patients with sinus tachycardia >90 bpm or hypertension, IV agents can be given as follows:

- IV **metoprolol** 5 mg over 2 min, repeated every 5 min up to 15 mg, or until HR <60 bpm or systolic BP <100 mmHg.
- IVI **esmolol** (an ultrashort-acting β-blocker) is useful if there is a relative contraindication to β-blockade (e.g. H$_x$ of bronchospasm) but heart rate or BP is elevated. The initial dose is 0.1 mg kg^{-1} min^{-1}, increased by 0.05 mg kg^{-1} min^{-1} every 10 min until either pain is relieved, HR <60 bpm, systolic BP <100 mmHg, or a dose of 0.2 mg kg^{-1} min^{-1} is reached.
- Once stabilized, treatment may be converted to a once-daily preparation, e.g. oral **atenolol** 50–100 mg d^{-1}.

Vasodilators

Vasodilators do not reduce MI or death rates but are effective at relieving symptoms.

- **Nitrates**, such as **GTN**, are commonly used (buccal GTN 1–5 mg or IVI GTN 5 μg min^{-1}, titrated according to response), but tolerance may develop after 24 hours. Patients may be converted to oral preparations (e.g. sustained-release **isosorbide mononitrate** 30–180 mg d^{-1}) when stable.
- **Calcium channel antagonists**, e.g. oral **amlodipine** 5–10 mg d^{-1} or **diltiazem** 120–480 mg d^{-1}, are also effective. Short-acting agents should be avoided because of concerns over the increased incidence of adverse coronary events.
- **Potassium channel openers**, e.g. oral **nicorandil** 10–20 mg bd, may be used instead of or in addition to oral nitrate preparations after initial stabilization.

The importance of repeated clinical and ECG assessments during initiation of these therapies cannot be overemphasized. Failure to respond to medical therapy is a high-risk indicator and these patients should proceed to angiography.

INVASIVE VERSUS CONSERVATIVE TREATMENT STRATEGIES

The role of cardiac catheterization in unstable angina is poorly defined. The degree to which angiography and intervention are used is partly determined by facilities and operators in individual centres. Two approaches are commonly practised, early conservative management and early invasive management.

Early conservative management

This involves stabilization with aspirin, heparin, β-blockers and/or calcium channel antagonists and a 'watch and wait' strategy. Cardiac catheterization is only used if ischaemic symptoms and high-risk ECG features persist after 48 hours. High-risk clinical indicators also prompt early assessment with angiography. Patients whose symptoms settle and who are considered low risk for MI, are assessed with a low workload stress test (e.g. modified Bruce protocol treadmill ECG). This allows further risk stratification, leading to medical management of low-risk patients or elective cardiac catheterization of high-risk patients.

Early invasive management

This involves cardiac catheterization of all patients with unstable angina in the first few days of admission, followed by revascularization if the coronary anatomy is suitable. Clinical trials do not give a clear answer: in the TIMI IIIB study an invasive strategy did not reduce deaths or MI within the first 42 days, but late ischaemia, the need for medication and rehospitalization were all reduced. In the VANQWISH study an early invasive approach in non-Q wave MI was associated with worse outcome. However, the more recent FRISC II study showed that early intervention can reduce serious events in unstable angina.

ACUTE MYOCARDIAL INFARCTION

AETIOLOGY/PATHOPHYSIOLOGY

Acute MI is usually caused by the formation of occlusive thrombus in an atheromatous coronary artery. A sequence of plaque rupture, platelet aggregation, fibrin deposition and vasoconstriction underpins the pathogenesis of vessel occlusion. MI is often caused by thrombotic occlusion at the site of a mild or moderate stenosis, so the patient may not have prodromal angina. The volume of myocardium at risk depends on the size and territory of the infarct-related vessel, collateral blood supply from other vessels, coronary perfusion pressure, arterial O_2 saturation and time from onset of coronary occlusion. Necrosis spreads from the endocardium to the epicardium and usually reaches its limit after around 12 hours. Without treatment mortality approaches 40% in the first month and half of deaths occur because of sudden VF within 2 hours of the onset of symptoms. Treatment of early MI at home is inappropriate except in areas remote from resuscitation facilities, or in patients who otherwise would not be resuscitated.

In patients who survive this early phase, in-hospital mortality is around 10%. When out-of-hospital cardiac arrest occurs, bystander CPR and early defibrillation dramatically improve survival rates.

DIAGNOSIS

Early diagnosis is based mainly on the history and ECG. Cardiac enzymes serve to confirm the diagnosis later on.

Symptoms

Symptoms of myocardial ischaemia are described in Chapters 1 and 5. Patients with MI are more likely to have severe chest pain and autonomic symptoms. The differential diagnosis of chest pain was described earlier. Elderly and diabetic patients may present with 'silent' or painless infarction.

Signs

Physical signs may be absent early on but autonomic disturbance is common (pallor, sweating, bradycardia or tachycardia). Mechanical dysfunction may result in shock, cardiac failure and mitral regurgitation: check for hypotension ± tachycardia, dyskinetic apical impulse, elevated JVP (may signify right ventricular infarction – see below), S_3 and basal crepitations. Patients who present more than 12 hours after the onset of symptoms may have a pericardial rub, or a murmur suggesting mitral incompetence or septal rupture. Because time is of the essence, the initial assessment should be targeted at identifying patients who are likely to benefit from thrombolysis or primary angioplasty.

ECG

The sequential ECG changes of transmural MI should be well known to the cardiology registrar, but these features are often absent in the early stages of infarction. **The ECG should be repeated every 15–30 minutes in patients with suspected AMI who have ongoing symptoms**. In the absence of diagnostic features certain ECG changes may support a diagnosis of MI, such as axis deviation (indicating fascicular ischaemia) or new bundle branch block. Successful thrombolysis often accelerates the development of Q waves and T-wave inversion. If reperfusion occurs very early (within an hour of onset of symptoms) the ECG may normalize, signifying an aborted MI. Non-Q wave MI and unstable angina are indistinguishable in the early stages; their clinical and ECG features and management were discussed earlier.

Identification of the infarct site is important because it provides information about prognosis and likely complications. Recording from additional leads may give extra information.

- If **RV infarction** is suspected (typically inferior MI, hypotension, clear lungs and elevated JVP), record right chest leads that correspond with left-sided lead positions – V_2R, V_3R, V_4R etc., and look for ST elevation.

● If **posterior infarction** is suspected (see Fig. 5.5), record posterior leads (correspond to V_7, V_8, V_9 positions, which are an extension of V_1–V_6 layout).

ECG evolution in 'classic' transmural MI

1. Hyperacute phase (0–30 min). Peaked T waves and upsloping ST elevation (Fig. 5.2).
2. Acute phase. ST elevation is usually accompanied by ST depression in the 'opposite' lead group, e.g. inferior leads in anterior MI. This is usually an electrical phenomenon and does not necessarily indicate ischaemia in that territory (Fig. 5.3).
3. Postacute phase. Q waves develop. Pathological Q waves are >25% of R-wave height and are >1 mm wide and >2 mm deep. Subtle abnormalities, such as loss of R-wave height, may also occur (Fig. 5.4).
4. T-wave inversion. This is a non-specific feature which may accompany transmural MI or may occur in isolation in non-Q wave MI.

Look at previous ECGs. ECG changes may persist from previous MI. Some units keep an archive of predischarge ECGs, as case notes may be slow in arriving. It also helps to give patients a copy of their predischarge ECG to keep in their wallet or handbag, in case of subsequent admission.

TABLE 5.1 Main infarct sites, with associated prognosis and complications

Infarct site	ECG features	Prognosis	Associated complications
Inferior	Typical changes in II, III, aVF. May extend to lateral (I, aVL, V5–6) or posterior	Good (but some inferior MIs involve RV, or cause acute mitral regurgitation)	AV block (usually temporary), inferior aneurysm (uncommon, but associated with severe mitral regurgitation)
Posterior	ST depression and evolution of R waves in V_1, V_2 ('mirror image' of classic MI changes)	Often accompanies inferior MI; intermediate	As inferior MI; cardiogenic shock due to RV dysfunction (RV infarction syndrome)
Anterior	Typical features in V_1–V_2; may extend to V_3–V_4 (anteroseptal) or V_5–V_6 (anterolateral), ± I, aVL	Usually more extensive LV impairment, with increased morbidity and long-term mortality	LV failure, anterior aneurysm, cardiogenic shock due to LV dysfunction

Cardiac enzymes

These are released from myocytes during and after MI. Blood levels depend on the infarct volume, molecular weight of the marker and reperfusion of the

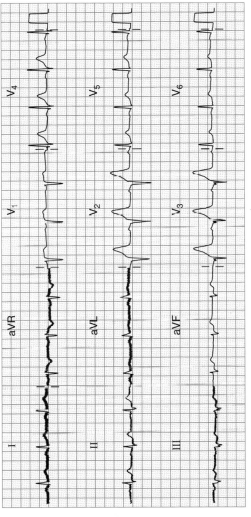

Fig. 5.2 Hyperacute changes of MI. Note peaked anterior T waves.

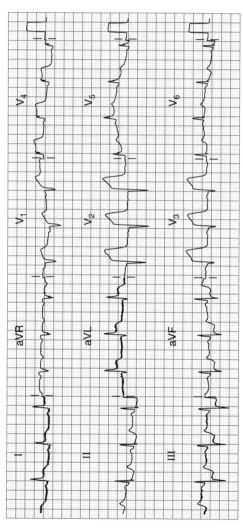

Fig. 5.3 Acute anteroseptal MI <8 hours: note ST segment elevation.

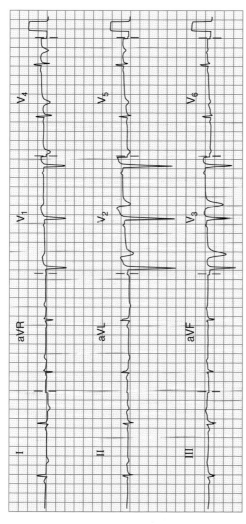

Fig. 5.4 Established anteroseptal MI >48 hours with anterior Q waves and T-wave inversion.

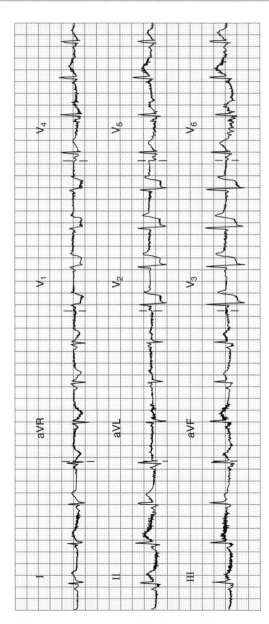

Fig. 5.5 Acute inferoposterior MI. Note anterior ST depression and tall R waves.

infarct zone ('washout' effect). To fulfil the WHO definition of MI, enzyme levels should rise above twice the upper limit of the reference range. Laboratory ranges vary according to the method used, so **local reference ranges should be referred to**. Cardiac enzymes are of no value in excluding MI in the initial phase, but may provide supportive information in patients who present several hours (or days) after the onset of symptoms. Also, the area under the curve described by sequential enzyme estimations gives a useful estimate of infarct size. Enzyme levels should be measured **as a minimum** on admission, 8–12 hours after onset of symptoms and at 24 and 48 hours.

- **Myoglobin** is a small molecule, and so is released into the circulation between 1 and 4 hours after the onset of AMI. Skeletal muscle injury due to trauma, IM injection, CPR or DC shock leads to falsely elevated myoglobin levels.
- **Total creatine kinase (CK)** activity rises to diagnostic levels within 6–8 hours of onset of MI and returns to normal within 2–3 days. It is sensitive, but suffers the same specificity limitations as myoglobin.
- **Creatine kinase MB (CK-MB)** is the main cardiac isoenzyme and can be measured using a mass or activity assay. This assay is more cardiospecific. Where significant skeletal muscle injury has occurred, a CK-MB:total CK activity ratio greater than 6% signifies probable myocardial infarction.
- **Aspartate aminotransferase (AST)** is not often used. It is detectable within 18–24 hours and peaks 2–3 days after AMI. Like LDH, it lacks cardiospecificity.
- **Lactate dehydrogenase (LDH)** is a late marker, detectable after 24–48 hours and peaking after 3–4 days. It lacks specificity as it is found in skeletal muscle and is released during haemolysis, in megaloblastic anaemia, liver disease, pulmonary embolism and renal disease. **Hydroxybutyrate dehydrogenase** refers to the LDH-1 isoenzyme found in the heart and in erythrocytes.
- **Cardiac troponin T** is detectable in blood within 8 hours of onset of symptoms, peaks at 24–36 hours and can remain elevated for up to 10 days. It is cardiospecific and is also released in some patients with unstable angina who do not fulfil the WHO criteria for MI. Using these criteria, troponin T lacks specificity for diagnosing MI. In reality, elevated troponin T in unstable angina may reflect watershed injury or microinfarction. What is important is that it is a strong risk predictor for subseqent MI or death in these patients. Elevated admission troponin T is also an adverse prognostic marker in MI itself, independent of duration of symptoms.
- **Cardiac troponin I** is a similar marker with approximately equivalent sensitivity, specificity and clinical applications.

Chest X-ray

The chest X-ray may show cardiomegaly, pulmonary oedema or LV aneurysm. In cases of undiagnosed chest pain it may show other pathology,

e.g. broadened mediastinum, lobar collapse or pleural effusion. If the
diagnosis of acute ST elevation or LBBB MI is made and you do not suspect
aortic dissection, the chest X-ray may be deferred until thrombolysis is
underway.

Echo

Echo is not essential early after MI but is helpful if the ECG is difficult to
interpret (e.g. LBBB). A regional wall motion defect suggests regional
ischaemia or infarction. Echo is useful *after* MI to assess LV function and is
mandatory in EMD arrest after AMI, to identify patients with tamponade, in
whom emergency pericardial aspiration is indicated. Patients with a new
murmur or sudden haemodynamic compromise require an echo to identify
acute mitral regurgitation or septal rupture (see Chapter 4).

EARLY MEDICAL MANAGEMENT

This section outlines the management of patients with definite MI. For
patients with suspected MI or unstable angina, the protocols outlined in the
previous section should be referred to.

Basic management

- Cardiac monitoring prior to and during transfer to CCU/ICU
- Inhaled O_2; oximetry
- Aspirin 300 mg. In the ISIS-2 study, **aspirin treatment had almost as much
  effect on 30-day mortality in AMI as streptokinase** and the effects were
  additive. Aspirin can be given IV to patients who are unconscious or who
  cannot swallow.
- IV access, bloods for U&Es, glucose, FBC, cardiac enzymes
- Analgesia if continuing pain (morphine 10 mg or diamorphine 5 mg IV)
- Antiemetic (avoid cyclizine in cardiogenic shock – can cause
  vasoconstriction)
- Anxiolytic if required (e.g. diazepam 5–10 mg orally).

Thrombolysis

Whereas aspirin inhibits platelet adhesion and aggregation at the site of
plaque rupture, thrombolytic agents promote the breakdown of fibrin through
conversion of the endogenous proteolytic enzyme plasminogen into the active
enzyme plasmin. The ISIS-2 and GISSI-1 trials both demonstrated that

**Warning: Administration of aspirin and thrombolysis should not be
delayed by waiting for CXR or transfer equipment. Ideally these
treatments should be started in the emergency room.**

streptokinase reduces the risk of death after AMI (overall approximately 20 lives saved per 1000 treated, in the first month).

Thrombolysis: indications	
• Typical ischaemic chest pain, onset within previous 12 h	AND
• ECG shows either :	
1 mm ST elevation in two or more adjacent limb leads	OR
2 mm ST elevation in two or more adjacent chest leads	OR
new left bundle branch block	

Thrombolysis should also be considered in patients with ongoing symptoms who fulfil ECG criteria and who present 12–24 hours after symptom onset. Although right bundle branch block is not a hard indication for thrombolysis, it is sometimes possible to identify infarct changes through this pattern.

Thrombolysis: contraindications	
Absolute	
Recent GI haemorrhage	Abdominal, neurological or eye surgery in past 1 month
Trauma with risk of major haemorrhage	Recent symptoms suggesting active peptic ulcer
Stroke within past 6 months	
Lumbar puncture, visceral biopsy or dental extraction in past 1 month	Haemorrhagic diathesis
	Aortic dissection
Acute pancreatitis	Oesophageal varices
Coma	Severe liver disease

Relative
Active menstruation (risk very low after first 2 days of menstruation)
Pregnancy
Hypertension (systolic >200 mmHg or diastolic >100 mmHg)
Concurrent anticoagulant therapy
Known intracardiac thrombus (thrombolysis may dislodge clot from LV or LA)
Known abdominal aortic aneurysm

Caution
Requirement for instrumentation (e.g. bradycardia requiring pacing – use femoral access site in case of bleeding – pressure can be applied in this instance)

Streptokinase or **anistreplase** are contraindicated if either has been given >4 days previously (neutralizing antibodies may reduce efficacy) or in cases of allergy. If hypotension develops the infusion should be stopped until BP normalizes, and then restarted. Recurrent or profound hypotension necessitates the use of an alternative thrombolytic, e.g. tPA, consider first the possibility of occult haemorrhage. A tPA-based thrombolytic should be used in preference to streptokinase if the patient presents with systolic BP <100 mmHg.

Thrombolytic regimens

● **IV streptokinase** (1.5 million units over 1 h) is the first-line agent in most centres. 1999 UK cost: £85.

● **'Accelerated' recombinant tissue plasminogen activator (rtPA)** (15 mg bolus, then 0.75 mg kg^{-1} (up to 50 mg) over 30 min, then 0.5 mg kg^{-1} over 60 min) confers a small mortality advantage over streptokinase at the expense of an increased incidence of major haemorrhage (GUSTO-I; overall, 10 additional lives (over streptokinase) per 1000 patients treated; groups shown below benefit most). This regimen used concomitant **IV heparin 5000 U**, followed by **IVI 1000 U h^{-1}**, adjusted to achieve APTT 60–85 s. Patients <75 years with anterior MI benefit most, especially if rtPA administered within 4 hours of AMI onset. 1999 UK cost: £395.

● **Anistreplase** (30 units over 5 min) is a modified streptokinase– plasminogen complex which is activated at the site of clot. It is administered as a bolus injection but is expensive. 1999 UK cost: £495.

● **Reteplase** (10 units over 2 min, repeated after 30 min) is a modified form of rtPA which is given by double bolus injection, so is convenient for out-of-hospital or emergency room administration. Mortality reduction is similar to that for rtPA. 1999 UK cost: £400.

● **Urokinase** is rarely used and has not been validated in large trials.

Failed thrombolysis reflects failure of the infarct-related vessel to reperfuse. Clinical markers are failure of symptoms to resolve and failure of elevated ST segments to resolve to 50% of initial level within 30–60 minutes of completion of infusion. There is currently little trial evidence to determine the best strategy in these patients. 'Rescue' angioplasty, or repeat thrombolysis with tPA (with significant added risk of bleeding) in patients treated with streptokinase, may be appropriate if within 6 hours of symptom onset.

Subcutaneous heparin

Other than those receiving heparins for non-Q wave MI or after tPA therapy, patients with MI should be given SC **unfractionated heparin** 15 000–25 000 U d^{-1} (in 2–3 doses) for at least 48 h, or until ambulant. Low molecular weight heparins are less well validated in the post-MI setting.

β-Blockers

β-Blockers have several beneficial effects in acute MI. By antagonizing the hyperadrenergic state that often accompanies MI, blood pressure and heart rate are reduced. This reduces myocardial O$_2$ demand, limits infarct size and relieves ischaemic pain. The incidence of free wall rupture is also reduced. When immediate IV β-blockade is followed by oral therapy, trials show a relative reduction of 15% in death, non-fatal reinfarction and non-fatal cardiac arrest. These benefits substantially outweigh the relatively uncommon adverse effects of hypotension, bradycardia and provocation of cardiac failure.

Patients with sinus tachycardia (>90 bpm) or hypertension (systolic BP >150 mmHg or diastolic >90 mmHg) are particularly suited to early IV β-blocker therapy.

β-Blocker regimens

- IV **metoprolol** 5 mg over 2 min, repeated every 5 min up to 15 mg, or until HR <60 bpm or systolic BP <100 mmHg
- IVI **esmolol** is useful where there is a relative contraindication to β-blockade (e.g. H_x of bronchospasm), but heart rate or BP elevated (see earlier for dosing regimen)
- Oral **metoprolol** 50 mg, given 15 min after last IV dose; repeat every 6 hours for 24 h then convert to 50 mg bd and titrate to heart rate response
- Once-daily β-blockers, e.g. oral **atenolol** 50 mg d^{-1}, can be given once appropriate dose determined using metoprolol
- **Avoid β-blockers with intrinsic sympathomimetic activity (ISA) in MI**, e.g. oxprenolol.

ACE inhibitors

There is considerable evidence that ACE inhibitors reduce mortality after acute MI.

- In *non-selective trials* (i.e. all MI patients with systolic BP >100 mmHg selected, see Table 5.2), the mortality gain was 5 patients per 1000 treated, over 4–6 weeks of therapy. One-third of this benefit was in the first 48 hours.
- In *selective trials*, targeting patients with LV failure, LVEF <40%, anterior MI or poor echo wall motion scores, the benefit was around 50 lives per 1000 treated.

Who should receive an ACE inhibitor?

Although net benefit is achieved with non-selective use of ACE inhibitors it is sensible to target patients with heart failure and/or AMI with anterior ST elevation or LBBB. Patients without these should have LV function assessed before discharge. Patients with LVEF <40%, or large wall motion defects, or at least 'moderate' global impairment on echo, should receive an ACE inhibitor.

ACE inhibitors can be given within 24 hours of onset of AMI unless there is hypotension (systolic BP <100 mmHg). The recent HOPE study has indicated that ACE inhibition may benefit most patients after AMI, regardless of LV function.

Which ACE inhibitor regimen?

Enalapril is effective at reducing acute coronary events in patients with asymptomatic LV dysfunction (SOLVD trial), but has not been proven effective in the MI setting (CONSENSUS-II trial showed no benefit against placebo).

TABLE 5.2 ACE inhibitor trials and regimens which show mortality reduction after AMI. Any of these regimens can be used

ACE inhibitor	Trial	High-risk pts selected*	Days after MI	Starting regimen	Target dose
Captopril	SAVE	yes (LVEF <40%)	3–16	6.25 mg, 12.5 mg	25 mg tid
	ISIS-4	no	<1	6.25 mg, 12.5 mg	50 mg bd
Lisinopril	GISSI-3	no	<1	5 mg od	10 mg od
Ramipril	AIRE	yes (clinical LVF)	3–10	2.5 mg bd	5 mg bd
Trandolapril	TRACE	yes (echo)	<7	1 mg od, 2 mg od	4 mg od

*Anterior MI, clinical signs of LVF, LVEF <40%, or reduced wall motion score.

Diabetic patients with MI

Diabetic patients with MI have higher mortality (relative risk 1.5–2.2) and morbidity than non-diabetics. An insulin/glucose infusion during MI, followed by long-term insulin therapy, was associated with an *absolute* mortality reduction of 11% in the DIGAMI study over 3 years. The study did not show whether the mechanism was early limitation of infarct size, late prevention of reinfarction/sudden death, or both. Consensus has not been reached about long-term insulin use in these patients. Long-term insulin should be considered in well motivated patients previously on oral hypoglycaemic agents, or with an abnormal fasting glucose/oral glucose tolerance test after the acute event.

Suggested insulin protocol (adapted from DIGAMI protocol)

ELIGIBILITY	acute MI with admission blood glucose >11 mmol/l
EARLY INFUSION	80 IU soluble insulin in 500 ml 5% glucose, with 20 mmol KCl, *or* equivalent
(24–48 hours)	Start at 5 U insulin/h (30 ml/h using above dilution). If glucose 7–10 mmol/l, check each 2 h; otherwise after 1 h. Use sliding scale below:

BLOOD GLUCOSE mmol/l	ACTION (1 u/h = 6 ml/h using above dilution)
>15	8 IU insulin bolus, increase infusion rate by 1 u/h
11–14.9	Increase infusion rate by 1 u/h
7–10.9	No change
4–6.9	Decrease infusion rate by 1 u/h
<4	Stop infusion for 15 min. Test blood glucose every 15 min until >7 mmol/l. Restart IVI at rate 1 u/h less than previous rate
Symptomatic hypoglycaemia	20 ml of 50% glucose IV
LONG-TERM INSULIN	Medium–long-acting insulin in evening tid soluble insulin using pen device

Prophylactic treatments for which there is *no* clear evidence of benefit

● **IV magnesium** does not significantly affect outcome when given as a prophylactic therapy in MI (ISIS-4 study). It may help in specific patients with ventricular arrhythmias associated with electrolyte disturbance (see Chapter 7).

● **IV nitrates** are similarly unhelpful as prophylactic therapy. Their role is limited to patients with LVF and for symptom control in post-infarct angina.

● **Calcium channel antagonists** have not been proved beneficial after MI. Early trials which implied benefit from verapamil and diltiazem were very limited in their inclusion criteria and took place before aspirin and ACE inhibitors were widely used. Short-acting dihydropyridines (e.g. nifedipine capsules) can be harmful in acute coronary syndromes because of the potential for reflex tachycardia.

EARLY COMPLICATIONS (<1 WEEK POST MI)

Acute cardiac failure

Cardiac failure after MI can be caused by LV systolic dysfunction (low output, low ejection fraction, sometimes hypotension), diastolic dysfunction (impaired LV filling, high LA pressure, pulmonary oedema) or both. An absence of pulmonary oedema does not necessarily imply good LV function, as the patient may have concomitant RV infarction or may be hypovolaemic. In first 48 hours after MI, assess the patient frequently for signs of low cardiac output and LV failure.

The management of acute cardiac failure is discussed in Chapter 6. Cardiac failure is also of long-term prognostic importance, as LV ejection fraction predicts long-term mortality after MI. Patients with EF <30% suffer 15–40% mortality at 1 year, compared to less than 5% mortality for those with EF >60%.

Cardiogenic shock

Cardiogenic shock is the most serious haemodynamic complication of MI and is usually caused by extensive LV injury. It is defined as a state of hypotension (systolic BP <90 mmHg) due to low cardiac output and resulting in impaired organ perfusion. Its management is discussed fully below and in Chapter 3.

Arrhythmias

Arrhythmia management in MI differs from that in other situations because many acute arrhythmias are a manifestation of ischaemia or reperfusion, resolve rapidly and do not necessarily require intervention. Management of the more common arrhythmias is described below.

Supraventricular arrhythmias

● **Sinus tachycardia** can reflect increased sympathetic drive or cardiac failure. In the absence of failure, β-**blockers** reduce rate and myocardial O$_2$ demand.

Ward round assessment of haemodynamic status after MI

● Heart rate	e.g. sinus tachycardia may be sign of ensuing LVF
● Rhythm	new AF is a cause and consequence of cardiac failure
● Pulse volume	↓ pulse volume indicates ↓ output; check for pulsus paradoxus (tamponade)
● Blood pressure	can mislead because normal BP can accompany very low output because of peripheral vasoconstriction ('compensated shock'). Also, BP <90 mmHg can accompany good output if vasodilated
● Respiratory rate	↑ in low perfusion states (systemic acidosis) and pulmonary oedema
● O₂ saturation	Use finger/earlobe oximeter. Desaturation breathing room air can indicate pulmonary congestion (but some patients chronically desaturated, e.g. COAD)
● Feel peripheries	cold peripheries, peripheral cyanosis and poor capillary refill accompany peripheral vasoconstriction
● JVP	elevated JVP with sharp y-descent may indicate RV infarction (see below).
● Chest	check for gallop rhythm (S₃), new murmurs of acute mitral regurgitation/VSD, basal crepitations
● CXR	pulmonary oedema, pleural effusions, heart size
● ECG	check for AV block, reinfarction/infarct extension
● Renal function	fluid balance (may need to catheterize if suspicious of low urine output), daily U&Es, creatinine

● **Sinus bradycardia** is common in inferior MI. Treatment is only needed if patient is haemodynamically compromised: use **IV atropine 0.5 mg**, or atrial pacing if persistent.

● **Junctional bradycardia** is treated in the same way as sinus bradycardia.

● **Atrial ectopic beats** do not require treatment but may signify atrial wall stretch in patients who are developing LVF. Atrial ectopics often herald atrial fibrillation.

● **Atrial fibrillation/flutter** may reflect atrial distension due to ventricular impairment. These rhythms aggravate cardiac failure and if ventricular rate is rapid, ischaemia may worsen and haemodynamic compromise may occur. Cardiovert if there is significant haemodynamic compromise. Treatment is similar to that in other settings (see Chapter 7). If rapid rate control is needed use **IV β-blockers** as long as hypotension/pulmonary congestion are not present. **IV esmolol** is especially helpful (for regimen see *Unstable angina*). Otherwise, consider **IVI digoxin 500 μg over 30 min**, or **IVI amiodarone 5 mg kg⁻¹ over 60 min** via central line.

Ventricular arrhythmias

● **Ventricular ectopic beats** do not require treatment, but may reflect increased sympathetic drive, ventricular wall stress or electrolyte disturbance. Check for signs of cardiac failure and hypokalaemia.

- **Accelerated idioventricular rhythm** is a broad-complex automatic ventricular rhythm, rate 60–110 bpm. It is common in the first 48 hours after MI and rarely causes compromise. It is usually seen during successful reperfusion. If compromised, use **IV atropine 0.5 mg** to accelerate sinus rate above ventricular rate; otherwise, do not treat.

- **VT** is also common in the first 48 hours of AMI. *Non-sustained* episodes <30 s duration which do not cause serious haemodynamic compromise do not require specific treatment. *Sustained* VT, or VT associated with significant compromise, requires treatment:

    – if VT well tolerated, give **IV lignocaine 100 mg** (50 mg if <50 kg) over 2 min, then infuse at 4 mg min^{-1} for 30 min, 2 mg min^{-1} for 2 h, 1 mg min^{-1} for up to 24 h. **IVI amiodarone 5 mg kg^{-1}** (via central line) over 30–60 min is a sensible alternative if evidence of LV failure.

    – if VT associated with hypotension (systolic BP <90 mmHg), try precordial thump, then cardiovert under sedation (e.g. **IV diazepam 5–10 mg**) or general anaesthesia. Use 100 J synchronized shock, increase to 200 J, then 360 J if ineffective. (Chapter 7 covers DC cardioversion for ventricular arrhythmias.)

Recurrent or incessant VT may signify continuing ischaemia and is an indication for early cardiac catheterization after MI. Late VT, >48 hours after MI, can occur because of persisting ischaemia, or the development of an arrhythmia focus adjacent to the infarct zone. The risk of late, fatal arrhythmia is high in these patients. Early cardiac catheterization is needed to identify potential 'culprit' vessels which require revascularization; thereafter, antiarrhythmic drugs and devices should be considered.

AV block and intraventricular block

- **First-degree AV block** requires no treatment.

- **Second-degree AV block** rarely requires treatment. If associated with marked bradycardia (<50 bpm) or hypotension, **IV atropine 0.5 mg** should be tried in case excessive vagal tone is a mechanism. Anterior MI with Mobitz type II block is an indication for temporary pacing because it often progresses to CHB with an unstable escape rhythm. Otherwise, temporary pacing is needed only if compromised.

- **Third-degree (complete) AV block** has a variable prognosis, depending on whether it occurs with inferior or anterior MI.

    – In *inferior MI*, block usually occurs at or above the AV junction and is often associated with a narrow-complex escape rhythm. Asystole is rare. It usually resolves within 3–4 days. It is sensible to give thrombolysis and not to pace in narrow-complex CHB, if escape rate >40 bpm and patient is normotensive, as reperfusion is likely to restore AV node function. Temporary pacing is indicated if hypotension or cardiac failure occur, or if CHB persists after thrombolysis/angioplasty. Permanent pacing is only required if CHB persists for >10 days.

    – In *anterior MI*, block often occurs in the His bundle or bundle branches, resulting in a broad-complex slow escape rhythm with a high risk of asystole. It signifies extensive infarction with a high risk of in-hospital death. Temporary pacing is mandatory and permanent pacing is almost always required (the exception is when CHB resolves without residual bundle branch block, an uncommon event).

● **Bifascicular block** (RBBB with left or right axis deviation) occurs more often in anterior than inferior MI. It is an indication for temporary pacing because there is a significant risk of progressing to CHB, with the risk of asystole. Permanent pacing is not needed unless episodes of Mobitz type II AV block or CHB occur.

● **Trifascicular block** (Long P–R interval and either RBBB with axis deviation or LBBB) also usually occurs in anterior MI and is an indication for temporary pacing.

● **Alternating LBBB and RBBB** signifies serious intraventricular block and always merits temporary pacing.

See also Chapter 7 for management of acute arrhythmias.

Mitral regurgitation

Mitral regurgitation can occur after MI because of papillary muscle ischaemia or rupture, or LV dilatation. Acute mitral regurgitation should be suspected in any patient with MI who abruptly develops pulmonary oedema or cardiogenic shock. The most obvious clinical sign is the development of a new systolic murmur. An echo should be performed to differentiate it from acute VSD. Treatments are summarized below; see Chapter 4 for details.

Treatment of acute mitral regurgitation complicating MI		
Papillary muscle ischaemia	anti-ischaemic R_x	– β-blockers
		– nitrates
		– revascularization
Papillary muscle rupture	stabilize with offloading agents	– Na^+ nitroprusside
		– IV nitrate
		– diuretic if pulmonary oedema
	mechanical support	– intra-aortic balloon pump to offload
EITHER:	mitral valve repair/replacement	
OR:	long-term drug R_x if surgery not possible	– hydralazine
		– ACE inhibitor
		– diuretic
Left ventricular dilatation	afterload reduction	– ACE inhibitor OR
		– hydralazine + nitrate

Digoxin may be helpful in acute mitral regurgitation because it limits the ventricular rate if atrial fibrillation ensues.

Rupture of the interventricular septum

Acute VSD should also be considered in patients who rapidly decompensate after acute MI. It affects about 2% of patients with AMI and usually presents on the second or third day with hypotension and a harsh, pansystolic murmur, with a thrill, radiating to the right sternal border. Echo is used to confirm the diagnosis, but VSD can be difficult to detect. Right heart catheterization may be needed to confirm a left-to-right shunt at ventricular level. Management is discussed in Chapter 4.

Cardiac tamponade

Myocardial rupture, causing tamponade, usually occurs on the first to fourth days after *transmural* MI. It is more common in elderly and in hypertensive patients. Steroid and non-steroidal anti-inflammatory drugs have been implicated as factors. Early thrombolysis reduces the risk of rupture. It presents with sudden catastrophic hypotension, often leading to electromechanical dissociation. Immediate echocardiography is needed to confirm the diagnosis (pericardial aspiration can be used if echo not available). Diagnosis and management are discussed fully in Chapter 4.

Post-infarct angina

Persistent ischaemic chest discomfort after MI usually denotes continuing ischaemia in the territory of the infarct-related vessel, although ischaemia can occur elsewhere because of 'steal' from collaterals arising from non-infarct-related vessels. Medical management of postinfarct angina is essentially the same as for other types of unstable angina (see earlier), although a lower threshold is often applied for early angiography and revascularization. *Stable exertional angina* affects approximately 25% of patients after MI; a low-intensity (e.g. modified Bruce) predischarge ETT should be considered to exclude critical ischaemia in these patients (see Chapter 16 – treadmill exercise testing).

Pericarditis

Pericarditis most often develops within 72 hours of *transmural* MI. It is characterized by a sharp, pleuritic chest pain which may radiate to the shoulder and may be accompanied by a pericardial friction rub. Echo should be performed to determine whether a pericardial effusion is present. If so, anticoagulant therapy should be discontinued to avoid pericardial

 Warning: Pericardial aspiration can be used to stabilize critically compromised patients, but should otherwise be avoided as decompression of the pericardial space could lead to further, fatal bleeding. Contact the cardiac surgery team immediately with a view to surgical repair.

haemorrhage unless there is a pressing indication to use it (e.g. unstable postinfarct angina). Other than aspirin, NSAIDs should be avoided as they may interfere with infarct healing and increase the risk of rupture. Opioid analgesics, e.g. oral **dihydrocodeine 60 mg**, may help to relieve symptoms; otherwise, oral **aspirin 600 mg qid** is effective.

Mural thrombus

Without SC heparin therapy mural thrombus affects about 20% of patients after MI. Patients with anterior MI involving the LV apex are at highest risk. High-dose SC **unfractionated heparin** (e.g. 12 500 units bd) reduces its incidence by about 50% and patients who have received thrombolysis also have a lower incidence. Around 10% of patients with mural thrombi have symptomatic embolic events. This provides a good argument for routine echocardiography of all patients before discharge. Patients with LV aneurysm and mural thrombus should receive lifelong warfarin R_x. Warfarin may also prevent embolic events in patients who have a large wall motion abnormality without visible thrombus.

Patients with mural thrombus should receive:

- **IV unfractionated heparin** (aiming for APTT 1.5–2.0) then
- **warfarin** (aiming for INR 3.0–4.5) for a minimum of 6 months.

LATE COMPLICATIONS (>1 WEEK POST MI)

Post-MI (Dressler) syndrome

This usually occurs 1–3 weeks after MI and is characterized by fever, pleuritis and pericarditis. It affects 2–3% of patients after MI and is distinct from early post-MI pericarditis. The cause is not clear, but may be an autoimmune reaction to myocardial antigens released after infarction. A similar syndrome can follow cardiac surgery involving pericardiotomy.

- Symptoms malaise, fever and (often severe) pleuritic chest pain
- Examination pleural or pericardial rub and pleural effusion. Cardiac tamponade can occur: check JVP and for pulsus paradoxus
- Echo check for pericardial effusion/tamponade
- CXR may show cardiomegaly, pleural effusions, lung infiltrates
- Bloods ↑ ESR, leucocytosis, normochromic normocytic anaemia antiphospholipid/antimyocardial antibody titres may be elevated, but are often so after uncomplicated MI.

Management is with NSAIDs (e.g. **aspirin 600 mg qid**); anticoagulants should be withheld if possible. Severe episodes merit admission, bedrest and monitoring for signs of increasing pericardial effusion. Pericardial aspiration may be required. Corticosteroids are needed in resistant cases.

Pericardiectomy is occasionally used in severe, intractable cases. Constrictive pericarditis is a recognized complication.

LV aneurysm

LV aneurysm is a complication of transmural MI in which part of the infarcted segment dilates and moves paradoxically in systole. Aneurysm formation begins early after MI and can be minimized by the use of ACE inhibition in patients with LV impairment. More than three-quarters of aneurysms form in the anteroapical position following anterior MI. It is more common after failed reperfusion.

Associations with LV aneurysm formation
- Reduced efficiency of LV systolic function → cardiac failure
- Refractory angina
- Mural thrombus and systemic embolization
- Symptomatic ventricular arrhythmias (15% of cases)

LV aneurysm should be suspected if:

- Late post-MI ventricular arrhythmias
- Embolic events after MI
- Persistent ST elevation on ECG
- Bulge on left heart border on CXR.

Echo usually confirms the diagnosis. Radionuclide ventriculography or LV angiography can also be used. LV angiography delineates residual viable myocardium and aids decision making for surgeon, but carries the risk of dislodging thrombus. Long-term anticoagulation is indicated especially if mural thrombus is seen or if thromboembolic events have occurred. Aneurysm resection is indicated if symptoms are refractory to medical R_x, the aneurysm is well circumscribed and there is sufficient viable myocardium to reconstruct LV.

Chronic cardiac failure
See Chapter 6.

Physical and psychological rehabilitation
See Chapter 15.

Secondary prevention
See Chapter 12 (risk factor management, post-MI follow-up, hypertension and hyperlipidaemia).

Driving after MI
In the UK the driving authorities recommend that patients should not drive

for 1 month after MI. Also, patients should not drive if symptoms are provoked by driving, or if episodes of syncope or presyncope occur. Specific stringent recommendations exist for heavy-goods and public service vehicle drivers, which means that the majority have their licence revoked. Only patients who are free of symptoms and can manage at least 9 minutes of a Bruce protocol treadmill test without ischaemic ECG changes (off antianginal medication) can regain their licence. Regulations vary widely between countries.

CARDIOGENIC SHOCK AND RIGHT VENTRICULAR INFARCTION

See also acute myocardial infarction (earlier) and Chapter 4 (acute mitral regurgitation/ruptured interventricular septum).

CARDIOGENIC SHOCK

Cardiogenic shock is one of the most serious conditions dealt with by cardiologists: mortality is in excess of 80% *with treatment*. It is usually caused by pump failure due to massive MI; cardiogenic shock from other causes is dealt with in separate sections. The recognition of cardiogenic shock, accurate assessment of the patient's haemodynamic status and identification of the cause are the key to its management.

Definition
Cardiogenic shock is a state of hypotension, with reduced end-organ perfusion due to low cardiac output. It is unhelpful to base its diagnosis purely on a threshold blood pressure, as many stable patients without cardiogenic shock are hypotensive but do not have reduced tissue perfusion. A checklist for bedside assessment of the patient's haemodynamic state was given earlier.

Aetiology/pathophysiology
In the acute MI setting over 80% of cases of cardiogenic shock are caused by extensive LV infarction. Other causes are shown in Figure 5.6.

Most patients with cardiogenic shock have three-vessel or left main stem disease, associated with infarction of at least 40% of the LV myocardium. Cardiogenic shock is more common in elderly patients and those with a history of heart failure.

As diastolic blood pressure falls coronary perfusion reduces, further worsening LV function. Systemic vasoconstriction increases afterload and lactic acidosis can occur which further impairs cardiac performance.

Clinical assessment of cardiogenic shock
There *is* a role for checking the history in suspected cardiogenic shock! Shock

Clinical diagnosis of cardiogenic shock

● **Blood pressure**	hypotension, systolic BP usually <90 mmHg
● **Pulse**	sinus tachycardia (may be absent if β-blocked, sinus node disease, ↑ vagal tone)
● **Peripheral circulation**	cool skin, low-volume pulse, poor capillary refill, peripheral cyanosis
● ↓ **End-organ perfusion**	oliguria or anuria
	confusion or impaired conscious level
	abdominal pain (mesenteric ischaemia – underdiagnosed)
● ↓ **Mixed venous O$_2$ saturation**	<70% (due to ↑ O$_2$ extraction in tissues)
● **Lactic acidosis**	if tissue perfusion very poor, may occur (↓ venous and arterial bicarbonate, ↑ arterial pH, ↑ venous lactate)
● **Echo**	large ventricular wall motion abnormality, or other cause for shock evident (e.g. tamponade, VSD, mitral regurgitation)

Haemodynamic features of cardiogenic shock

● Low cardiac index	(usually <1.8 l min^{-1} m^{-2})
● Persistent hypotension	(systolic BP <90 mmHg for >30 min)
● Elevated LV filling pressure	(PCWP >20 mmHg)

Shock also occurs in MI when PCWP is low (e.g. overdiuresis, dehydration, GI bleed after thrombolysis), due to reduced LV filling ± LV systolic impairment.

Key points from the history

- **Recent MI**? If so, which territory (inferior/posterior associated with RV infarct).
- **Previous heart failure?**
- **Valve disease or prosthesis, or cardiomyopathy?**
- **Thrombolysis** given? Any symptoms of internal/GI bleeding? Anaphylaxis?
- **Timing.** Days 2–3 post MI, suspect myocardial rupture.
- **Sudden onset** when previously stable: suspect rupture, VSD, acute mitral rupture.
- **Fluid balance.** Is patient dehydrated/overdiuresed?
- **Drugs.** Any negative inotropes, e.g. β-blocker, verapamil, diltiazem? Excessive opiate analgesia?

in cardiac patients can be multifactorial; focus on identifying underlying causes, especially reversible ones.

Examination

This should be brief, looking for signs of reduced tissue perfusion and of potential causes of shock:

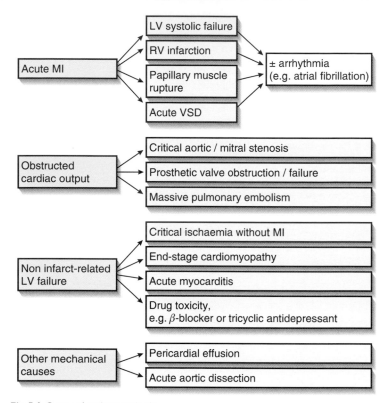

Fig. 5.6 Causes of cardiogenic shock.

- **General examination**
    ↓ conscious level, confusion
    central or peripheral cyanosis
    tachypnoea
    dehydration
    cool peripheries, reduced capillary refill
- **Pulses**
    tachycardia, low-volume pulse, pulsus alternans
    pulsus paradoxus (tamponade)
    unequal/absent pulses (aortic dissection OR peripheral atherosclerosis)
- **Blood pressure**
    equal or unequal between arms
- **JVP**

high in RV infarction, massive pulmonary embolism

often normal in LV infarction

- **Precordium**

    apex dyskinetic in anterior MI/LV aneurysm

    apex hyperdynamic in VSD and mitral regurgitation

    thrills/murmurs of mitral regurgitation/VSD

    S_3 when LA pressure high

- **Chest**

    combination of pulmonary oedema + shock heralds very poor prognosis

    chest infection can cause or exacerbate shock.

Investigations

Echo is the most important test, as it usually reveals the cause of cardiogenic shock. If LV function does not look badly impaired, consider other causes.

Transthoracic echo in suspected cardiogenic shock	
● **LV function**	– usually extensive wall motion abnormality in infarct territory
● **RV function**	– hypokinetic free wall in RV infarct
	dilated, poor function in massive pulmonary embolism
● **Pericardial effusion**	– signs of RV compression/tamponade
● **VSD**	– colour and continuous wave Doppler of septum in all views; can be easy to miss
	– pulmonary:systemic flow >1.5
● **Valves**	– flail, prolapsing mitral valve
	– coexisting valve stenosis/regurgitation
● **Aortic root**	– dilated in type A (proximal) dissection
	– TOE, fast CT or MRI scan if suspicious

- **CXR**

    coexisting pulmonary oedema/chest infection

    position of Swan–Ganz catheter; identify iatrogenic pneumothorax

    aortic root and mediastinal diameter

- **Laboratory tests**

    arterial blood analysis (acid–base balance, blood gases). If thrombolytic has been given, defer to avoid arterial bleeding or use pressure bandage

    U&Es, creatinine, LFTs (renal failure and 'shock' liver may develop)

    FBC

- **ECG**

    confirm ischaemia or infarct zone/infarct extension

    arrhythmias, especially atrial fibrillation, exacerbate shock.

Management

Rapid correction of haemodynamic compromise is essential to avoid organ damage from hypoperfusion: acute tubular necrosis, myocardial infarct extension, 'shock' liver.

Oxygenation
- High-flow (100%) O_2 via mask, unless type II respiratory failure/COAD
- Consider continuous positive airway pressure (CPAP) mask, or mechanical ventilation if inadequate with O_2 mask
- Finger oximetry may not reflect central oxygenation (↓ peripheral perfusion). If in doubt, take arterial blood sample.

Monitoring
- ECG/blood pressure
- Urinary catheter
- Swan–Ganz catheter (for details of insertion and interpretation of data, see Chapter 3) allows:
    - CVP measurement
    - PCWP measurement
    - central administration of drugs
    - mixed venous O_2 saturation measurement (calculate cardiac output)
    - confirmation of VSD (step-up in O_2 saturation between RA and PA) and shunt volume estimation
    - thermodilution catheters especially useful if suspected mixed picture (e.g. sepsis and LV impairment).

Optimize filling pressures
Optimum LV filling pressure (assessed as PCWP) is the highest that can be achieved without causing pulmonary oedema – usually 16–20 mmHg. Low PCWP, which accompanies RV infarction and reduced blood volume, is corrected by giving aliquots of 100–200 ml plasma expander (e.g. Haemaccel) and remeasuring PCWP. Although large volumes may be needed to optimize LV filling, PCWP may rise quickly once a critical volume has been infused. High PCWP in the presence of shock necessitates inotropic or mechanical support.

Improve cardiac output
If the condition persists despite optimal LV filling, inotropic support is usually needed. Dobutamine (2.5–15 $\mu g\ kg^{-1}\ min^{-1}$) has a combined inotropic/vasodilator effect which reduces afterload. It is less prone to cause tachycardia than dopamine. Low-dose dopamine (2.5–5 $\mu g\ kg^{-1}\ min^{-1}$) improves renal blood flow, improves cardiac output and can be used in conjunction with dobutamine. Higher doses may cause renal and peripheral vasoconstriction.

Treat reversible myocardial ischaemia
- **Thrombolysis** with rTPA is indicated in cardiogenic shock caused by acute MI, within 12 hours of symptom onset. Benefit may be conferred between 12 and 24 hours if there is continued chest discomfort.

- **Emergency cardiac catheterization**, with a view to urgent PTCA, may help in certain circumstances:
    - primary treatment of MI complicated by cardiogenic shock (in centres with rapid access to cardiac catheterization facilities)
    - after failed thrombolysis. Cardiogenic shock is one of the few situations in which 'rescue' angioplasty may be beneficial after failed thrombolysis
    - acute ischaemia with an ECG pattern unsuitable for thrombolysis (e.g. ST segment depression).
- **Intra-aortic balloon pump (IABP)** counterpulsation is helpful prior to and during PTCA. It augments coronary perfusion pressure and may reverse shock and limit infarct size in patients with critical ischaemia.

Treat other reversible causes
- **Surgical repair** of VSD and flail mitral leaflet carries a high operative mortality but is the only treatment option if cardiogenic shock ensues. IABP may help stabilize the patient before surgery.
- **Arrhythmias** should be corrected to optimize cardiac output. Atrial fibrillation can cause severe compromise and DC cardioversion should be considered. **IV amiodarone 5 mg kg^{-1}** over 30 minutes limits heart rate and may restore sinus rhythm; it is also the treatment of choice for ventricular arrhythmias.
- **Pericardial aspiration** (see Chapter 3) is used to treat cardiac tamponade, unless caused by aortic dissection or myocardial rupture. In these situations aspiration may trigger catastrophic bleeding and is used only if the patient is rapidly decompensating. Otherwise, surgery is the treatment of choice.

RIGHT VENTRICULAR INFARCTION

Definition
RV infarction is a variant of acute MI in which there is extensive RV involvement. It usually accompanies inferior or inferoposterior MI, so there is almost always some LV involvement. This condition is important because it presents with a characteristic haemodynamic pattern and requires specific treatment.

Characteristics of RV infarction
- Inferior/inferoposterior MI pattern on ECG
- Impaired right ventricular function
    - ↑ RV end-diastolic pressure
    - ↑ RA pressure – elevated JVP, hepatic congestion
    - often RV dilatation and tricuspid regurgitation
- Hypotension due to ↓ left heart filling
- Cardiac enzymes elevated disproportionately to degree of LV dysfunction

Diagnosis

Patients usually present with inferior MI complicated by shock and signs of right heart failure. The JVP may have a prominent V wave and sharp y-descent. The following investigations are useful for confirming the diagnosis and guiding management.

ECG

- Inferior MI pattern, plus often ST depression/evolving R waves in V_{1-2} which signify posterior wall involvement
- V_4R to V_6R leads (correspond to V_4 to V_6, on right side of chest) show ST segment elevation.

Echo

- Dilated RV ± tricuspid regurgitation
- RV free wall motion reduced
- Variable LV involvement, often mild LV impairment only
- Excludes cardiac tamponade.

CXR

- Exclude pulmonary oedema.

Swan–Ganz catheterization (see below)

- Elevated RA pressure and RVEDP
- Normal or reduced RV and PA systolic pressure
- Low or normal PCWP.

Management

In the absence of clinical and X-ray signs of LV failure, the initial management is volume expansion to increase RV preload and output.

Volume expansion

Aliquots of 100–200 ml of plasma expander should be given and the patient examined frequently for signs of pulmonary congestion. Several litres of fluid may be required to drive RV output sufficiently to increase LV filling and to reverse shock. If after 1.5 l of fluid loading shock is not reversed, then Swan–Ganz catheterization should be considered (see Chapter 3). This helps guide whether further fluid loading is needed (PCWP <15 mmHg) or whether inotropes are needed to correct shock (see Cardiogenic shock, above).

 Warning: Do not treat patients with RV infarction and hypotension with diuretics or nitrates, despite signs of right heart failure, as they can cause a catastrophic fall in RV filling and blood pressure.

RV infarction with LV failure

This is a bad combination, associated with >80% mortality. Conversely, RV infarction associated with preserved LV function carries a better prognosis (~40% mortality). Initial treatment is with inotropes. Arterial vasodilators (e.g. hydralazine) help by reducing systemic vascular resistance, LVEDP and PA pressure. This in turn augments right-sided output. Swan–Ganz catheterization is mandatory in this situation as LV filling pressure may fall precipitously and volume expansion may then be required.

AV block and RV infarction

Atrial transport is critical for RV filling in RV infarction. High-grade second-degree AV block and complete heart block should be treated with temporary dual-chamber pacing to maintain AV synchrony.

Differential diagnosis of RV infarction

Two other conditions can mimic RV infarction, presenting with hypotension and signs of right heart failure after MI:

● Cardiac tamponade. This can be excluded using echo.
● Acute pulmonary embolism. Check for signs of systemic hypoxia, look for clinical signs of DVT and check arterial blood gases. If you are unsure about the diagnosis, heparinize and plan a lung perfusion scan or pulmonary angiography.

CHAPTER 6

CARDIAC FAILURE

ACUTE LEFT VENTRICULAR FAILURE

Acute LV failure can either occur *de novo* or on a background of chronic cardiac failure, i.e. acute-on-chronic cardiac failure. This is important because the aetiologies, clinical presentation and management are quite distinct.

CLASSIFICATION

Most cases of cardiac failure are associated with reduced systolic function and sometimes a low-output state. Diastolic dysfunction may also contribute to cardiac failure in patients with large infarct zones, cardiomyopathies, pericardial disease or mitral stenosis. In these cases reduced ventricular compliance limits diastolic filling, increases left and right atrial pressure and can limit cardiac output. Cardiac failure very occasionally occurs in the context of a high-output state (e.g. arteriovenous shunting).

> **Tip:** Pulmonary oedema and LV failure are not synonymous. Pulmonary oedema can occur because of altered loading conditions in the absence of cardiac disease, e.g. in acute renal failure. Also, non-cardiogenic pulmonary oedema can occur with major surgery, trauma or sepsis – this condition is probably inflammatory in origin and is known as the adult respiratory distress syndrome (ARDS).

AETIOLOGY

The following are common causes of acute cardiac failure.

Acute '*de novo*' cardiac failure
- Acute MI
- Acute native valve failure (e.g. chordal rupture, endocarditis) or acute VSD (see Chapter 4)
- Acute myocarditis
- Hypertensive crisis
    accelerated hypertension with background essential hypertension
    renovascular disease (e.g. renal artery stenosis)
    phaeochromocytoma
- Cardiac tamponade
- Profound bradycardia or tachycardia
- Myocardial depression due to drug toxicity
    tricyclic antidepressants
    β-blockers
    calcium channel antagonists.

Acute-on-chronic cardiac failure

- Non-compliance with or reduction in cardiac failure drug therapy (e.g. diuretic, ACE inhibitor) – a common precipitant
- Myocardial depressant drug or drugs that promote sodium/water retention (e.g. corticosteroids, NSAIDs)
- Intercurrent non-cardiac illness in a patient with chronic cardiac failure
- Progression of underlying cardiac disease
- Myocardial ischaemia/infarction
- Arrhythmias, especially atrial fibrillation
- Increased metabolic demand: anaemia, pregnancy, thyrotoxicosis.

CLINICAL PRESENTATION

Acute *de novo* LV failure usually presents with rapidly worsening fatigue, dyspnoea and limitation of effort tolerance. Orthopnoea, paroxysmal nocturnal dyspnoea and acute respiratory distress may supervene. There may also be prodromal symptoms which suggest an underlying aetiology, e.g. chest pain or palpitation. Physical signs of cardiac failure and underlying cardiac diseases are described more comprehensively in Chapter 1.

INVESTIGATION

- Laboratory tests
  - U&Es   – renal failure (predisposes to fluid retention)
  - – high or low K^+ predisposes to arrhythmias
  - ABGs   – systemic hypoxia
  - – acidosis (may be metabolic due to poor tissue perfusion, or mixed due to additional CO_2 retention)
  - virology – if viral myocarditis suspected (e.g. antecedent H_x of flu-like illness), serology may help identify the culprit organism
  - TFTs
  - FBC   – anaemia (exacerbates cardiac failure), ↑ WCC (infection)
- ECG
  - acute or previous MI
  - ischaemic features
  - arrhythmia, e.g. atrial fibrillation
- CXR
  - pulmonary oedema
  - pleural effusions, fluid in horizontal fissure
  - septal (Kerley B) lines
  - pulmonary pathology
  - cardiac size (cardiomegaly suggests long-standing pathology. *De novo* acute cardiac failure is often associated with normal heart size)
- Echo. This is essential to determine whether pulmonary oedema is due to systolic or diastolic dysfunction, or to non-cardiac factors such as volume overload.

- LV function (see Chapter 19)
- LVH (suggests hypertension, aortic stenosis or hypertrophic cardiomyopathy) – associated with diastolic dysfunction
- valve disease (see Chapter 19), e.g. mitral regurgitation, aortic stenosis
- pericardial effusion
- endocarditis

● Right heart catheterization. This is especially useful if cardiac failure occurs in the setting of an intercurrent illness, such as sepsis. Determination of left atrial pressure and systemic vascular resistance helps guide management in this difficult group of patients (see Chapter 3). It also helps in the diagnosis of left-to-right intracardiac shunts and adult

Key points: examination	
● General	– usually distressed or agitated
	– tachypnoea (reduced respiratory effort/rate suggest exhaustion and possible need for mechanical ventilation)
	– semiconscious or unconscious in severe/protracted cases
	– signs of sympathetic activation/low cardiac output
	pallor
	sweating
	cool peripheries
	peripheral cyanosis
	– cutaneous stigmata of endocarditis
	– signs of non-cardiac illness
	clinical anaemia
	fever
	thyroid signs
● Pulse	– usually tachycardic. Relative bradycardia can worsen cardiac failure by limiting cardiac output
	– may be irregular; suggests atrial fibrillation
	– may be low ($\downarrow$ output) or normal pulse volume
● Blood pressure	– hypotension heralds poor prognosis
	– hypertension may aggravate cardiac failure
	– check for pulsus paradoxus
● JVP	– often elevated, but not invariably so
● Precordium	– apex usually not displaced in *de novo* cardiac failure; may be dyskinetic in anterior MI
	– apex often displaced in chronic heart failure
	– murmur (may suggest valve pathology or acute VSD)
	– 'gallop' rhythm: $S_3 \pm S_4$
	– inspiratory crepitations
	– pleural effusions in chronic cardiac failure
● Other	– peripheral/sacral oedema, pulsatile hepatomegaly, ascites, right parasternal lift most often accompany chronic right-sided cardiac failure, but are uncommon in *de novo* cardiac failure.

respiratory distress syndrome (pulmonary oedema in the presence of low or normal left atrial pressure).

MANAGEMENT

Acute cardiac failure should be managed in a high-dependency or coronary care unit. Patients who are unable to maintain adequate systemic oxygenation or acid–base balance despite initial therapy need to be managed in an intensive care unit with ventilation facilities. ECG, blood pressure and O_2 saturation monitoring are mandatory.

Initial management
- IV access
- High-flow O_2 (60–100%)
- Nitrates – this is at least as important as diuretic R_X. Most patients with pulmonary oedema are not volume overloaded. Fluid volume needs to be redistributed into capacitance vessels. Venodilation with nitrates also acutely reduces left atrial pressure. Nitrate dose is usually titrated upwards every 10–20 min until either systolic BP <110 mmHg or until clinical improvement is observed
  - buccal **GTN** 2–5 mg   OR
  - IVI **GTN** 0.6–12 mg min^{-1} OR
  - IVI **isosorbide dinitrate** 2–10 mg h^{-1}
  - (IVI **sodium nitroprusside** 10–200 µg min^{-1} is useful in acute cardiac failure associated with hypertensive crisis (see Chapter 10) as it is a potent arteriolar dilator)
- Opiate – IV **morphine** 5–20 mg helps reduce sympathetic drive and helps reduce preload through venodilation. It also reduces anxiety and distress
- Loop diuretic – IV **frusemide** 50–100 mg bolus   OR
  – IVI **frusemide** 5–20 mg h^{-1}
  The acute effect of loop diuretic is venodilation; intravascular volume reduction occurs later
- Digoxin – useful for rate control in atrial fibrillation; role in cardiac failure in sinus rhythm controversial
  - oral dose: 0.5 mg, repeated after 6 hours
  - IVI: 0.5 mg over 20 min, repeated after 6 hours
- Treat identifiable triggers, e.g. aspirin and thrombolysis for acute MI.

An additional agent (e.g. ACE inhibitor) may be needed if nitrate therapy fails to control hypertension. Arrhythmias are often poorly tolerated. Atrial fibrillation can cause catastrophic haemodynamic collapse because of the loss of atrial contribution to ventricular filling. In these cases DC cardioversion ± **IVI amiodarone** via a central venous catheter (300 mg over 30 min, followed by 900 mg over 24 h) may be needed.

Management of resistant cardiac failure

Advanced haemodynamic support

Hypotensive patients with cardiac failure may benefit from inotropes. These agents are only suitable for short-term therapy because the gain in terms of cardiac output and perfusion is offset by an increase in heart rate, cardiac work and O_2 consumption. Inotropic agents also tend to be arrhythmogenic, especially in patients with myocardial ischaemia. Useful agents include:

• **Dobutamine** 5–20 µg kg^{-1} min^{-1}. This agent is useful because it has a moderate peripheral vasodilator effect (β_2 effect, ↓ afterload) but does not usually cause excessive tachycardia.
• **Dopamine** 2.5–5 µg kg^{-1} min^{-1}. At this dose dopamine has little inotropic effect but is useful because it causes renal vasodilatation; diuresis may be induced in oliguric patients. It can be used in conjunction with IV dobutamine. Higher dopamine doses (5–10 µg kg^{-1} min^{-1}) have more inotropic effect but tend to cause tachycardia and may cause renal and peripheral vasoconstriction.
• **Adrenaline** 1–12 µg min^{-1} has additional α-vasoconstrictor properties which render it more suitable for patients with low systemic vascular resistance, e.g. sepsis. It is more arrhythmogenic than dobutamine.
• **Noradrenaline** 1–12 µg min^{-1} is predominantly an α agonist and is mainly used in septic shock to increase systemic vascular resistance.

Phosphodiesterase inhibitors, e.g. **milrinone** (50 µg kg^{-1} IV over 10 min, followed by IVI 0.375–0.75 µg kg^{-1} min^{-1}), have both vasodilator and positive inotropic effects. Prolonged use is associated with increased mortality, but these agents may have a limited role in bridging patients with resistant cardiac failure to transplantation.

• **Intra-aortic balloon pumping** (see Chapter 3) may be needed to stabilize some patients, especially if myocardial ischaemia contributes to cardiac dysfunction. It reduces afterload and improves coronary perfusion pressure and is also a useful bridge to definitive treatment, e.g. CABG.

Renal failure

Patients with fluid overload in whom diuresis is not achieved may require extracorporeal haemofiltration. Although haemofiltration does not cause the large fluid shifts associated with haemodialysis, invasive monitoring with a Swan–Ganz catheter may help avoid excessive fluid removal. In extreme circumstances venesection is sometimes used in fluid-overloaded patients, although there is little evidence to support its efficacy.

Respiratory failure

If, despite medical management, the patient remains in a state of respiratory compromise, mechanical ventilation should be considered. Ominous signs are exhaustion, persistent arterial hypoxia (PaO_2 <8 kPa), worsening acidosis and hypercapnia (PCO_2 >6.5 kPa).

- **Intubation, paralysis and intermittent positive-pressure ventilation** reduce respiratory effort (and thus metabolic demand), increase alveolar pressure (mechanical clearing of alveolar oedema), improve oxygenation and acidosis and relieve hypercapnia. Cardiac output may be reduced because of increased intrathoracic pressure, but the benefits generally outweigh this.
- **Mask continuous positive airway pressure ventilation** avoids the need for general anaesthesia, is simple to use, delivers nearly 100% oxygen and can be applied in most high-dependency areas. It may help avoid the need for intubation and ventilation in borderline cases.

CHRONIC CARDIAC FAILURE

Chronic cardiac failure is a major public health problem in the UK, affecting between 1 and 2% of the general population. It is associated with a high morbidity and mortality and is a major cause of recurrent hospitalization. Chronic cardiac failure is characterized by diminished cardiac reserve and a complex series of maladaptive neurohumoral responses, principally involving the sympathetic and renin–angiotensin axes. The resultant increased peripheral vascular resistance and sodium and water retention serve to increase cardiac workload and worsen LV failure. Current drug therapies in chronic cardiac failure are directed at preventing sodium and water retention and antagonizing the humoral responses that cause peripheral vasoconstriction.

CLASSIFICATION

Cardiac failure is classified in several ways: acute and chronic, left and right, high output and low output, and systolic and diastolic dysfunction. All of these descriptive terms help in the classification of cardiac failure, although there is no single unifying system of classification. Cardiac failure *symptoms* are graded using the New York Heart Association system (see Chapter 1).

Diagnosis of *diastolic* heart failure requires:

- symptoms or signs of heart failure
- normal or mildly abnormal LV systolic function
- abnormal LV relaxation, filling or diastolic distensibility or stiffness.

AETIOLOGY

The main causes of chronic cardiac failure in western countries are:

- Ischaemic heart disease

- Hypertension
- Valvular heart disease
- Toxic: alcohol, adriamycin, cobalt
- Viral myocarditis: Coxsackie, HIV
- Other cardiomyopathies: hypertrophic, restrictive, dilated (sometimes familial)
- Infiltrative: amyloidosis, sarcoidosis
- Metabolic and nutritional: haemochromatosis, thyroid dysfunction, beri-beri.

CLINICAL PRESENTATION

The most common cause of chronic cardiac failure is IHD; cardiac failure usually follows presentation with an acute MI. In some cases myocardial ischaemia or infarction is silent and the first presentation may be with cardiac failure itself. Conversely, some patients with IHD have asymptomatic LV dysfunction. However, most patients with chronic cardiac failure present with exertional fatigue and breathlessness and/or symptoms of fluid retention (e.g. oedema), or with an episode of acute LV failure.

Patients with *compensated* cardiac failure are usually not symptomatic at rest. Resting indices of cardiac function (e.g. cardiac output, blood pressure, heart rate) are usually within the normal range. Symptoms occur because the heart cannot respond adequately when placed under physiological stress. In *decompensated* left-sided cardiac failure symptoms occur at rest because of pulmonary oedema – orthopnoea, paroxysmal nocturnal dyspnoea or dyspnoea at rest. Right-sided cardiac failure presents with fluid retention – hepatic congestion, ascites and peripheral oedema. Physical signs of heart failure are described in Chapter 1.

The 5-year mortality rate for patients with cardiac failure is high, at around 50%, and exceeds that of many cancers. The prognosis can be predicted from the severity of the symptoms: 1-year mortality for NYHA grade IV cardiac failure is ~60%, grades II–III ~25%, and grade I ~5%. The main modes of death are sudden arrhythmic death, progressive pump failure and recurrent myocardial infarction.

INVESTIGATIONS

- Laboratory tests

U&Es	– may be concomitant renal failure (due to renovascular disease, low cardiac output, or to diuretics, ACE inhibitor)
	– $\downarrow K^+$ because of diuretics
	– $\downarrow Na^+$ an ominous sign in advanced cardiac failure
glucose	– prognosis for diabetics with cardiac failure very poor
LFTs	– may be deranged because of liver congestion
TFTs	– hypo- and hyperthyroidism may exacerbate failure
FBC	– anaemia may exacerbate failure

cardiomyopathy screen — ferritin (haemochromatosis), Ca^{2+} (sarcoidosis), viral screen (Coxsackie, enterovirus, HIV)

autoantibody screen — probably disease marker rather than causative factor; anti-α- and β-myosin antibodies

blood group and tissue type — if transplantation being considered (see Chapter 13).

- ECG

  Rarely normal in cardiac failure. Look for:

  evidence of previous MI

  LVH (large voltages seen both with LVH and cardiac dilatation)

  conduction defects

  atrial fibrillation — other than in mitral valve disease, an ominous prognostic sign

  — loss of atrial contribution worsens cardiac output and cardiac failure.

- CXR

  cardiomegaly

  cardiac contour (e.g. left or right atrial enlargement) may give clue to aetiology

  upper lobe venous diversion, interstitial oedema, pleural effusions, Kerley B lines may be present.

- Echo. The single most helpful investigation. See Chapter 19 for echo assessment of systolic and diastolic ventricular function and valve function.

- Radionuclide ventriculography. A useful tool for assessing LV function in poor echo subjects (see Chapter 20).

- Stress testing. Revascularization can improve LV function in patients with ischaemic LV dysfunction who have 'hibernating' myocardium. Stress echo and myocardial perfusion scanning are useful for identifying this (see Chapters 19 and 20).

- Cardiac catheterization. In patients with cardiac failure due to IHD this is only needed if stress test is abnormal, or if revascularization is planned. Cardiac catheterization allows assessment of coronary anatomy, systolic and diastolic ventricular function and mitral and aortic regurgitation. Quantitative information about haemodynamics, intracardiac shunts and valve gradients can be derived from right heart catheterization (see Chapters 3 and 18). RV biopsy may help establish a diagnosis in patients with cardiomyopathies (see Chapter 18).

MANAGEMENT

Drug therapy

There are two objectives in treating patients with chronic cardiac failure: relief of symptoms and improvement of prognosis.

Diuretics

Loop diuretics, e.g. **frusemide** (typically 40–120 mg d^{-1}) or **bumetanide** (typically 1–4 mg d^{-1}), relieve symptoms caused by peripheral and pulmonary oedema. Therapy is titrated to the clinical response (e.g. symptom response, resolution of oedema, chest signs). Baseline U&Es and creatinine should be checked before initiating diuretic therapy and rechecked 1 week afterwards. Intravascular volume depletion may cause blood urea to increase; the diuretic dose should be reduced if this occurs. Hypokalaemia is common with loop diuretics and potassium-sparing diuretics can be co-prescribed, e.g. **amiloride** 5–10 mg d^{-1} *or* **spironolactone** (50–200 mg bd). The latter is useful in patients with diuretic-resistant oedema because it directly antagonizes the salt- and water-retaining effect of aldosterone. Recent data from the RALES trial show that low-dose spironolactone (25 mg d^{-1}) reduces mortality in patients with severe cardiac failure.

In patients with resistant cardiac failure the combination of a loop diuretic and thiazide diuretic, e.g. oral **metolazone** 2.5–5 mg once or twice weekly, or **hydrochlorthiazide** 25–50 mg once or twice weekly, can produce a profound diuresis. This potent combination has the potential to cause marked hypotension, hyponatraemia, hypokalaemia and renal failure and is often initiated in hospital.

Nitrates

Nitrates, e.g. oral **isosorbide mononitrate** (30–120 mg d^{-1}), dilate the capacitance vessels and have a minor effect on systemic vascular resistance. Nitrates can help relieve symptoms of cardiac failure, but there is no evidence (other than in combination with hydralazine) that they improve prognosis.

Vasodilators

● Oral ACE inhibitors, e.g. **captopril** 12.5–50 mg tid, **enalapril** 10–20 mg bd or **lisinopril** 10–20 mg d^{-1}, improve symptoms and prognosis in patients with cardiac failure. First-dose hypotension can be avoided by starting with a low dose (e.g. captopril 6.25 mg) taken in bed at night and by ensuring the patient is not hypovolaemic. Initiation of therapy in hospital should be considered in frail elderly patients with severe cardiac failure and in patients taking high diuretic doses. Their use after MI is summarized in Table 5.2. ACE inhibitors also reduce mortality in asymptomatic LV dysfunction if LV ejection fraction <35% (SOLVD prevention trial). Side effects, e.g. dry cough, loss of taste, angio-oedema and renal dysfunction (in patients with renovascular disease) can limit their use (see also Chapter 5).

 Warning: The combination of a potassium-sparing diuretic with an ACE inhibitor (or potassium supplement) can cause significant hyperkalaemia.

- Oral AT_1 receptor antagonists, e.g. **losartan** 50–100 mg d^{-1}, are less likely to cause side effects, although they have the same propensity to cause renal dysfunction. Definitive evidence of mortality reduction with these agents has yet to be established.
- In patients with renal dysfunction or intolerance of ACE inhibitors and AT_1 receptor antagonists, the combination of **hydralazine** and a nitrate is a suitable alternative. The regimen used in the VeHEFT-II trial was **hydralazine** 75 mg qid and **isosorbide dinitrate** 40 mg qid, although different dosing intervals and nitrate preparations can be used to improve compliance. Hydralazine can cause a reversible lupus-like syndrome, especially in slow acetylators and in patients receiving >200 mg hydralazine daily. A positive ANF is unhelpful as it is seen in around half of patients receiving long-term hydralazine treatment.

Inotropes

Inotropes improve cardiac failure symptoms but increase cardiac work in an already failing heart. Some inotropic agents increase mortality. Inotropes can induce arrhythmias and increase myocardial O_2 consumption. There are several classes of agents, such as adrenergic agonists (e.g. isoprenaline, ibopamine) and phosphodiesterase inhibitors (e.g. milrinone, enoximone). These are occasionally used in patients with severe uncontrollable symptoms. Intermittent ambulatory low-dose IV dobutamine therapy is sometimes used for symptom control in patients awaiting cardiac transplantation. The exception is **digoxin** (62.5–375 µg d^{-1}). Its role in cardiac failure in sinus rhythm remains controversial, but there is some evidence that it improves symptoms, reduces recurrent hospitalization and has at least a neutral effect on mortality.

β-Blockers

Although the use of a negative inotrope in cardiac failure seems counterintuitive, β-blockers have a significant role in its treatment. Used carefully, β-blockers can improve symptoms and long-term prognosis in heart failure (CIBIS I and II trials), because of their favourable effect on diastolic filling and reduction in sudden death. Dosing has to be carefully titrated, e.g. **bisoprolol** 1.25 mg d^{-1}, increasing gradually to 10 mg d^{-1} if tolerated, or **carvedilol** 3.125 mg bd, increasing gradually to 25 mg bd if tolerated. The drug may need to be reduced or withdrawn if the patient decompensates.

Antiarrhythmics

Chronic cardiac failure is associated with a high incidence of non-sustained asymptomatic ventricular tachycardia. Antiarrhythmic therapy has not been proved to improve prognosis unless the arrhythmia causes symptoms, and the adverse effects of these drugs on pump function probably offset the benefit of their antiarrhythmic effects. Atrial fibrillation is common in cardiac failure and should be controlled with digoxin if possible. DC cardioversion can be considered but arrhythmia recurrence is common, especially in patients with mitral valve disease or hypertensive heart failure.

Anticoagulants

This is indicated in certain patients to reduce the risk of stroke and peripheral embolism. Patients with atrial fibrillation should receive warfarin. Patients with dilated cardiomyopathy should receive warfarin regardless of the underlying rhythm. Anticoagulation should also be considered in patients with mural thrombus or LV aneurysm, regardless of rhythm. The target INR range should be 2.0–3.0.

> **Tip:** Treatment of diastolic heart failure can be problematic unless there is a remediable underlying cause. Diuretics and β-blockers are useful (the latter increasing diastolic filling time) and may provide significant symptomatic improvement. Overdiuresis is potentially harmful because it reduces ventricular filling pressures and cardiac output.

Surgery

Revascularization

Chronic cardiac failure due to IHD may improve with revascularization because of recovery of the 'hibernating myocardium'. Indeed, the patients who gain the greatest prognostic benefit from revascularization are those with LV impairment. Myocardial perfusion scanning or low-dose dobutamine stress echocardiography may reveal areas of viable non-contracting myocardium and help plan revascularization.

Valve replacement

Patients with cardiac failure due to valve disease will need to be considered for valve repair or replacement. Patients with mitral regurgitation are most difficult to assess because the mitral regurgitation may be secondary to LV dilatation rather than the primary cause. Moreover, when cardiac failure is advanced mitral regurgitation helps offload the LV; mitral valve replacement increases the resistance to LV contraction and may cause it to fail completely. Management of valve disease is discussed fully in Chapter 12.

Cardiac transplantation

Patients with end-stage heart failure may be considered for orthotopic cardiac transplantation. Indications and preoperative evaluation are discussed in Chapter 13.

CARDIOMYOPATHIES

The term 'cardiomyopathy' is sometimes misused because strictly it describes a primary disease of the myocardium. However, terms such as 'ischaemic cardiomyopathy' and 'hypertensive cardiomyopathy' are often used. This section deals with primary dilated, hypertrophic and restrictive cardiomyopathies.

DILATED CARDIOMYOPATHY

Dilated cardiomyopathy should be considered in patients with cardiac failure in whom there is no evidence of IHD, hypertension, valve disease or congenital heart disease. Dilated cardiomyopathy is the most common cardiomyopathy. Causes include:

- Idiopathic
- Toxins: alcohol, cobalt, adriamycin
- Familial (may account for 25% of cases)
- Myocarditis: infective, autoimmune
- Peripartum: presents between 3 months before and 6 months after delivery
- Metabolic and nutritional: haemochromatosis, thyrotoxicosis, phaeochromocytoma, thiamine deficiency (beri-beri)
- Chronic tachyarrhythmia ('tachycardiomyopathy').

Patients with idiopathic or viral cardiomyopathies tend to have one of three patterns of disease progression: progressive deterioration, a chronic stable course, or spontaneous recovery. The clinical presentation is usually one of progressive chronic cardiac failure (see earlier), or sometimes precipitous LV failure (see earlier). Because dilated cardiomyopathy is effectively a diagnosis of exclusion, investigations are mainly targeted at identifying IHD, valve disease or congenital heart disease. A careful 'alcohol history' is an important component of the evaluation: abstinence and thiamine therapy can substantially improve cardiac function. Viral myocarditis is a relatively common cause, although it may run a long subclinical course before symptoms develop. Ventricular biopsy is often unhelpful (see Chapter 18) but may demonstrate a lymphocytic infiltration, suggesting an acute viral myocarditis. If an inherited cause is suspected then family screening is indicated.

Management is as described for chronic cardiac failure (see earlier).

HYPERTROPHIC CARDIOMYOPATHY

Hypertrophic cardiomyopathy (HCM) is characterized by myocardial hypertrophy in the absence of an identifiable cause such as hypertension or aortic stenosis. The distribution of hypertrophy may be concentric, asymmetrical or apical. Asymmetrical septal hypertrophy (ASH) can lead to

LV outflow tract obstruction, in which case the term hypertrophic *obstructive* cardiomyopathy (HOCM) is used.

Histologically, HCM is characterized by myofibril disarray and myocardial fibrosis. HCM can be either sporadic or hereditary: in 50% of patients a familial predisposition can be identified. Inheritance is usually autosomal dominant. A very large number of gene defects have now been identified and HCM encompasses a wide range of myopathic conditions. These gene defects usually affect structural myocyte proteins such as β-myosin, myosin-binding proteins, α-tropomyosin and the troponin subunits. **Family members of an affected individual should always be screened for this condition.** If HCM is suspected as a diagnosis, ask about family history of HCM or sudden death. The annual mortality from HCM is around 3% in adults; 10–15% of patients ultimately develop LV failure and dilatation. Clinical markers of high risk of sudden death are: young age at presentation (<30 years), a family history of sudden death, and non-sustained VT on ambulatory monitoring.

Symptoms
Patients are often asymptomatic, reinforcing the need for family screening. Otherwise, symptoms are similar to those that occur with aortic stenosis:

- Reduced effort tolerance
- Breathlessness   – impaired diastolic filling
  - reduced cardiac output during exercise
  - may be associated mitral regurgitation
- Angina can occur with normal coronary arteries due to:
  - large, inefficient LV muscle mass
  - ↑ LV work against obstruction
  - relative O_2 supply–demand mismatch
- Syncope   – outflow obstruction during exercise
  - ventricular arrhythmias
  - atrial fibrillation (poorly tolerated because atrial contribution to ventricular filling is important when LV compliance poor)
- Sudden death   – ventricular arrhythmias
  - myocardial infarction
  - pre-excited atrial fibrillation (association with Wolff–Parkinson–White syndrome).

Examination
- Signs of ventricular hypertrophy   – forceful apical impulse
  - S_4
  - prominent *a*-wave in JVP
- Signs of LV outflow obstruction   – double apical impulse
  - 'jerky' pulse (low volume if obstruction severe)

– harsh ejection systolic murmur, starts mid-systole, augmented by Valsalva manoeuvre.

Investigations

- ECG
  - can be normal
  - voltage criteria for LVH, often with repolarization (ST/T) abnormalities
  - large septal voltages (V_2–V_4)
  - inferior Q waves
  - associated pre-excitation
- Ambulatory ECG
  - non-sustained VT common (25%) and marker of risk of sudden death
- CXR
  - often normal
  - ↑ heart size/pulmonary congestion in advanced cases
- Echo (details in Chapter 19)
  - may be symmetrical or asymmetrical hypertrophy with ↓ LV cavity size
  - abnormal systolic anterior mitral (SAM) valve motion
  - increased LV outflow velocity with obstruction
- Cardiac catheterization
  - (caution, as easy to provoke VT with catheter)
  - coronary anatomy if angina present
  - intracavity and LV outflow gradient (use end-hole catheter); gradient may be increased with GTN
  - identify mitral regurgitation
- Electrophysiological testing
  - helpful if pre-excitation suspected
  - role of programmed ventricular stimulation for risk assessment not proven.

Management

Almost half of sudden deaths in HCM patients occur during or after strenuous exertion; this risk is present in patients without severe outflow obstruction. Patients should be cautioned against competitive sport or strenuous exercise. Digoxin should be reserved for patients with atrial fibrillation or systolic LV failure. Diuretics should be used carefully as they can worsen LV outflow obstruction through vasodilatation and volume depletion. Otherwise, treatments are as follows.

β-Blockers

β-Blockers reduce LVOT obstruction during exercise, reduce myocardial O_2 demand, improve diastolic filling by reducing heart rate and have helpful antiarrhythmic properties. β-Blockers are often used as first-line therapy in HCM. **Atenolol** 25–100 mg d^{-1}, or **metoprolol** 25–100 mg bd, are often used.

Calcium channel antagonists

Rate-limiting calcium channel antagonists (e.g. **verapamil** (long-acting) 240–480 mg d^{-1}, or **diltiazem** (long-acting) 200–500 mg d^{-1}) are preferable as they reduce myocardial contractility (and thus outflow obstruction) and heart rate and cause less vasodilatation than dihydropyridines such as nifedipine. Either agent can be prescribed along with a β-blocker, but the dose should be carefully titrated in case excessive bradycardia or AV block occurs.

Antiarrhythmic drugs

Both amiodarone and sotalol are effective at preventing supraventricular and ventricular arrhythmias in HCM. However, empirical therapy in all HCM patients cannot be recommended as both drugs have the potential for proarrhythmia.

Dual-chamber pacing

This should be considered in patients who remain symptomatic despite drug therapy. A short A-V delay (<125 ms) is used so that RV pacing occurs at all times. The induced LBBB activation pattern reduces LV outflow obstruction by desynchronizing septal and posterior wall contraction. Trial temporary dual-chamber pacing does not predict the long-term response to permanent pacing and is not appropriate. Ambulatory monitoring or low-intensity treadmill testing can be used to confirm RV capture during periods of activity, when the patient's intrinsic AV nodal conduction becomes more rapid. The programmed A-V delay should not be shortened too much, otherwise diastolic filling may be compromised.

Chemical septal ablation

Alcohol is injected into the first septal perforator branch of the left anterior descending coronary artery at cardiac catheterization, to infarct the bulky basal septum and reduce LVOT obstruction. Initial trial results from this technique are encouraging.

Surgery

Exceptionally, septal myotomy-myectomy can be used to debulk the basal septum. Because the risk of AV block is high owing to the proximity of the His bundle and bundle branches, temporary dual-chamber pacing is mandatory in the perioperative period. The operative mortality is 5–10%. The procedure reduces LV outflow tract obstruction by reducing septal mass, and sometimes by inducing LBBB.

Cardiac transplantation may be indicated in patients who enter the dilated stage of HCM and who develop systolic heart failure, or in patients with intractable arrhythmias. AICD may be used as a bridge to transplantation in the latter.

RESTRICTIVE CARDIOMYOPATHY

Restrictive cardiomyopathies are characterized by impaired diastolic ventricular filling due to myocardial infiltration or fibrosis. Distinction of restrictive cardiomyopathy from constrictive pericarditis is important because the latter can be treated surgically (see Chapter 9). Restrictive cardiomyopathies can be caused by:

- Amyloidosis
- Sarcoidosis
- Haemochromatosis
- Glycogen storage diseases
- Scleroderma
- Endomyocardial fibrosis and the hypereosinophilic syndrome.

The clinical presentation is dominated by fatigue, breathlessness and symptoms of right-sided cardiac failure (see Chapter 1). In addition to general signs of cardiac failure, there may be a rapid x- and y-descent of the JVP and a loud $S_3 \pm S_4$. Restrictive cardiomyopathy should be considered in patients who have good LV and RV systolic function on echo, elevated venous pressure and peripheral oedema and absence of primary renal failure.

Investigations

- ECG
  - P-mitrale or P-pulmonale
  - atrial fibrillation
  - reduced voltages and poor R-wave progression in chest leads
- CXR
  - heart size can be normal or increased
  - interstitial congestion
  - pleural effusions
  - pericardial calcification (constrictive pericarditis)
- Echo (see Chapter 19)
  - often normal LV/RV systolic function
  - thickened, speckled or bright LV/RV myocardium
  - $\downarrow$ systolic function in advanced disease
  - thickened interatrial septum
  - biatrial enlargement
  - restrictive inflow pattern on Doppler tracing
- Laboratory tests
  - haemochromatosis ($\uparrow$ serum iron, $\uparrow$ serum ferritin, $\downarrow$ iron-binding capacity)
  - sarcoidosis
  - amyloidosis (rectal or abdominal fat biopsy)
- Cardiac catheterization
  - rapid early diastolic filling in LV and RV, with dip and plateau (square root sign) waveform
  - a difference in LVEDP and RVEDP >7 mmHg

at end-expiration suggests pericardial constriction unlikely
– RV biopsy may confirm diagnosis

- Technetium scintigraphy ^99mTc-labelled pyrophosphate binds to amyloid deposits and is useful for diagnosing amyloid infiltration.

Treatment is directed at the underlying aetiology and cardiac failure. Atrial fibrillation and systemic embolism are common and should be treated with digoxin and anticoagulation.

Warning: Digoxin should be avoided in amyloidosis as patients are very digoxin sensitive: serious arrhythmias may occur. Digoxin sensitivity may be mediated by digoxin binding to amyloid fibrils.

CHAPTER 7

ACUTE ARRHYTHMIAS

NARROW-COMPLEX TACHYCARDIAS

See also Chapters 2 (referrals) and 5 (acute MI).

Narrow-complex tachycardias are one of the commonest reasons for referral to the cardiology registrar. Most cases are straightforward, if dealt with systematically – repeated calls about acute management of atrial fibrillation can be avoided by using the opportunity to educate the referring team! This section is intended as a practical reference for managing acute tachycardias in hospital and focuses on the practical issues. A brief description of the mechanism of each arrhythmia is given. Details of SVT mechanisms are discussed in Chapters 12 and 16.

DEFINITION

Clinically, narrow-complex tachycardias are defined as any cardiac rhythm >100 bpm, with QRS duration of <0.12 s. *Electrophysiologically* most of these arrhythmias are *supraventricular* and involve either an automatic focus or a re-entry circuit with an atrial and/or AV nodal component. The management principles described below also apply to broad-complex tachycardias which are supraventricular in origin. (The term 'SVT' in this section refers to any arrhythmia originating above the ventricles and includes atrial flutter/fibrillation.)

> **Narrow-complex tachycardias are only rarely ventricular in origin** (e.g. VT originating near His bifurcation may have QRS duration <0.12 s).
>
> **Broad-complex tachycardias are often supraventricular in origin** (e.g. SVT with pre-existing bundle branch block, aberrant conduction, or conducting antegradely over an accessory pathway).

ASSESSMENT OF PATIENTS WITH NARROW-COMPLEX TACHYCARDIAS

Immediate assessment

- Check airway, breathing, circulation. Establish IV access.
- Attach ECG monitor, ideally with printout so you can document response to treatment.

History

- Assess *pattern* of arrhythmia; find out how tachycardia started (if symptomatic, ask if onset gradual or sudden; check pulse rate on chart). Gradual acceleration of rate indicates sinus tachycardia. Assess whether any prodromal symptoms (e.g. chest pain, dyspnoea – pulmonary embolism is a common cause of atrial fibrillation in hospital).
- Check H_x of arrhythmia and any current drug treatments.

Warning: If patient is compromised (e.g. systolic BP < 90 mmHg, or acute cardiac failure) *and arrhythmia is continuous*, consider immediate DC cardioversion.

- This is best done under general anaesthetic, as the patient will be fully unconscious and the airway properly managed. Failing this, give IV diazepam 10 mg bolus and wait until patient is well sedated before cardioversion.
- Use a synchronized DC shock: start at 50 J, increase to 100 J, 200 J, then 360 J.
- If no response, consider the possibility you may be dealing with sinus tachycardia in response to systemic compromise.
- If sinus rhythm is restored temporarily, and then SVT recurs, further cardioversion is unlikely to help. Focus on treating the underlying causes and consider an antiarrhythmic agent, e.g. IV amiodarone.

- Check cardiac H_x (valve disease, IHD, cardiac failure and hypertension all predispose to supraventricular arrhythmias).
- Check recent illnesses (pyrexia, electrolyte disturbance, chest pathology (mechanical irritation) may predispose).
- Look for acute triggers (alcohol (atrial fibrillation), fluid overload (iatrogenic, or renal failure), hypoxaemia, cardiac failure, drug toxicity (especially digoxin)).

Examination
- Assess briefly, look for signs of compromise (↓ BP, failure) and potential causes (fluid overload, electrolyte disturbance, sepsis).

Investigations
- Examine ECG in sinus rhythm, if available. Look for atrial ectopics, which can initiate SVT, short P-R interval, delta wave.
- Examine **12-lead ECG**, not just rhythm strip, during tachycardia. The features of individual SVTs are described below.

Management
- Unless there is acute haemodynamic compromise, treat correctable factors above.
- Assess whether tachycardia is regular or irregular. For irregular SVTs (usually atrial flutter or fibrillation), decide between rate control and cardioversion strategies (see Chapter 12).
- For regular SVTs use vagal manoeuvres/IV adenosine test (see below) for diagnosis; these may terminate AV nodal and accessory pathway tachycardias.

- Consider AV node blockers/antiarrhythmics if SVT persists.
- Consider need for long-term arrhythmia prophylaxis after acute treatment.

CATEGORIES OF NARROW-COMPLEX TACHYCARDIAS

Narrow-complex tachycardias can be divided into regular and irregular types. Tachycardias caused by a re-entry mechanism involving the AV node can usually be terminated by vagal manoeuvres or AV node-blocking drugs. For each tachycardia type the usual response to an IV adenosine challenge is shown below.

Irregular narrow-complex tachycardia

Atrial fibrillation
- **Cause: multiple micro-re-entry circuits within (often diseased) atrial tissue**, resulting in a chaotic ventricular rhythm, absent P waves, fibrillation waves. If you can't recognize this by now you are not ready to specialize!
- **IV adenosine**: transient slowing of ventricular response; may unmask fibrillation waves more clearly. Does not terminate tachycardia.

Atrial flutter (see Fig. 16.3)
- **Cause: rapid intra-atrial circus depolarization**, resulting in a regular atrial rhythm c 300 bpm. The ventricular rhythm is often less chaotic than in atrial fibrillation, with regular spells due to runs of fixed AV block (usually 2:1, rate 150 bpm, or 4:1, rate 75 bpm). The atrial rate of 300 min^{-1} is easily recognized by flutter waves every large square (200 ms) on a standard ECG.
- **IV adenosine**: transient slowing of ventricular response, unmasking flutter waves. Does not terminate tachycardia.

Multifocal atrial tachycardia
- **Cause: firing of multiple atrial ectopic foci**. The rhythm is irregular and has multiple P-wave morphologies. It often is a precursor to atrial fibrillation.
- **IV adenosine**: may cause intermittent failure of P waves to conduct. Does not terminate tachycardia.

Regular narrow-complex tachycardia

Sinus tachycardia (physiological or pathological)
- **Cause: autonomic imbalance or sinus node re-entry**. The P-wave axis is the same as in sinus rhythm. Pathological (or inappropriate) sinus tachycardia can occur with many non-cardiac conditions (e.g. thyrotoxicosis, phaeochromocytoma), or may result from sinus node dysfunction (e.g. sinus node re-entry).
- **IV adenosine**: may cause sinus bradycardia, or occasionally an adenosine-

mediated sinus tachycardia. At higher doses AV block occurs but does not terminate tachycardia.

Atrial flutter with regular AV block
● Easily recognized by underlying flutter waves at c 300 min^{-1}, but can mimic sinus tachycardia if 2:1 AV block occurs; every second flutter wave may be masked inside the QRS complex.
● **IV adenosine**: usually not necessary as arrhythmia very obvious. Does not terminate tachycardia.

> A regular narrow-complex tachycardia with a heart rate of 150 bpm is likely to be **atrial flutter with 2:1 AV block**. Check for underlying flutter waves using carotid sinus massage or IV adenosine test.

AV node re-entry tachycardia (AVNRT) (see Fig. 16.4)
● **Cause: dual AV nodal conduction**. In 'typical' AVNRT antegrade AV conduction goes down a 'slow' conducting low right atrial pathway, into the AV node; retrograde conduction goes up a 'fast' conducting pathway at the same time as the ventricles are activated. This causes a 'short R-P, long P-R' tachycardia, rate 130–250 bpm. Often P waves are masked by the QRS complexes. In 'atypical' AVNRT antegrade conduction is down the fast pathway, giving rise to a 'long R-P, short P-R' tachycardia.
● **IV adenosine**: termination of tachycardia may be followed by a few sinus beats without AV conduction.

Accessory pathway (atrioventricular) re-entry tachycardia (see Fig. 16.4)
● **Cause: accessory atrioventricular connection**, usually rapidly conducting, which inserts into ventricular myocardium. In sinus rhythm there is often the short P-R interval and delta wave of Wolff–Parkinson–White syndrome. During tachycardia antegrade AV conduction is usually via the AV node (*orthodromic* tachycardia) and retrograde conduction via the accessory pathway; the delta wave is absent and heart rate is typically 170–220 bpm. The less common *antidromic* tachycardia is caused by antegrade accessory pathway conduction and retrograde AV nodal conduction; the delta wave is present during tachycardia.
● **IV adenosine**: termination of tachycardia may be followed by a few sinus beats without AV conduction.

Ectopic atrial tachycardia (see Fig. 16.1)
● **Cause: repetitive firing of ectopic atrial focus**, due to either increased automaticity or intra-atrial re-entry circuit, often in diseased atrium. The P-wave axis is usually abnormal (often with inverted P waves in inferior leads, owing to retrograde atrial activation) and the ventricular rate can range from 120 to 250 bpm.

- **IV adenosine**: may cause intermittent failure of P waves to conduct to ventricles. Does not terminate tachycardia.

ACUTE MANAGEMENT OF REGULAR NARROW-COMPLEX TACHYCARDIA ('SVT')

- Check airway, breathing, circulation.
- Ensure ECG monitor is attached, ideally with printout so you can document response to vagal manoeuvres or to IV adenosine test.
- Correct potentially treatable causes.
- Try vagal manoeuvres. These may terminate the tachycardia or give one of the responses listed above, which will help with your diagnosis.
- If no response to vagal manoeuvres, try IV adenosine test.

How to do vagal manoeuvres	
Carotid sinus pressure:	Do not try if carotid bruits present. Apply firm pressure over carotid artery, at level of upper thyroid cartilage, for 5 seconds. Try both sides, but **not at the same time**.
Valsalva manoeuvre:	Ask patient to exhale forcefully with mouth and nose sealed, for about 15 seconds.
Diving reflex:	Immerse patient's face in ice-cold water.
Eyeball pressure:	**Do not use. This is a very painful manoeuvre.**

How to do an IV adenosine challenge
1. Check patient is not asthmatic: adenosine can cause bronchospasm.
2. Warn patient about chest tightness/pain, flushing, headache, or a feeling of panic. Reassure that this only lasts about 20 seconds.
3. Run a continuous rhythm strip on ECG (lead II is good for P waves) so you can examine it in more detail afterwards.
4. Use a large vein for access; give each dose rapidly, followed by a flush of 10 ml IV 0.9% saline.
5. Start with **3 mg IV adenosine**. If no effect on rhythm within 30 seconds, increase to **6 mg, 9 mg then 12 mg** until AV block occurs on ECG. Patients usually develop symptoms once an effective dose is reached.
6. Adenosine will either terminate the tachycardia OR cause transient AV block, which will help you to diagnose the underlying atrial rhythm.
7. Start with very low dose (0.5–1 mg) in patients with cardiac transplant or dipyridamole.

- In patients with asthma, or if adenosine is ineffective at 12 mg, use **IV verapamil 5–10 mg** over 2 min. **Do not use in patients taking oral β-blockers, or in broad-complex tachycardias.**
- If above agents do not terminate tachycardia, or have a transient effect, consider short-term use of AV nodal blocker (e.g. **oral or IV digoxin**),

antiarrhythmic (e.g. **IV amiodarone**), or cardioversion. Rate control and antiarrhythmic strategies are discussed in Chapter 12.
- **Overdrive atrial pacing** (see Chapter 3) can be used to terminate tachycardia and for the suppression of further episodes.
- Consider whether long-term prophylaxis is needed. If there is an identifiable, treatable trigger (e.g. alcohol, fluid overload) no prophylaxis is needed. If recurrent symptomatic spontaneous episodes have occurred, consider the strategies listed in Chapter 3.

BROAD-COMPLEX TACHYCARDIAS

Broad-complex tachycardias are a common source of uncertainty because VT can be difficult to distinguish from SVT. SVTs can have broad complexes because of a pre-existing conduction defect (e.g. LBBB or RBBB), aberrant conduction (due to rapid rate, or to ischaemia), or antegrade conduction through an accessory pathway. Accurate diagnosis is important because it helps with prognostic assessment and guides treatment later on. Details of VT mechanisms are discussed in Chapters 12 and 16.

DEFINITION

Clinically, broad-complex tachycardias encompass any cardiac rhythm >100 bpm, with QRS duration of ≥ 0.12 s. *Electrophysiologically* most of these arrhythmias are *ventricular* in origin, involving an automatic focus or re-entry circuit within the ventricles. This section describes how to differentiate VT from broad-complex SVT. The treatments described focus on VT management, as the treatment of broad-complex SVTs follows the same principles as narrow-complex SVTs (see earlier).

Consider the patient's previous medical history when trying to determine whether VT or SVT is the most likely diagnosis.

ACUTE MANAGEMENT

Immediate assessment
- Check airway, breathing, circulation. Establish IV access.
- Attach ECG monitor, ideally with printout so you can document response to treatment.

History
- Assess *pattern* of current arrhythmia (if arrhythmia comes and goes, cardioversion won't have a lasting effect). Assess whether there are any prodromal symptoms (e.g. chest pain) to suggest a trigger.

Warning: IF PATIENT IS COMPROMISED (E.G. SYSTOLIC BP <90 MMHG, OR ACUTE CARDIAC FAILURE), *AND ARRHYTHMIA IS CONTINUOUS*, CONSIDER IMMEDIATE DC CARDIOVERSION.

- This is best done under general anaesthetic, to ensure that the patient is fully unconscious and the airway properly managed. Failing this, give IV diazepam 10 mg bolus and wait until patient is well sedated before cardioversion.
- Use a synchronized DC shock; start at 100 J, increase to 200 J, then 360 J.
- If no response to cardioversion, consider antiarrhythmic drug (e.g. IV amiodarone, or overdrive pacing).
- If sinus rhythm is restored and VT quickly recurs, further cardioversion is unlikely to help. Treat underlying causes and consider antiarrhythmic drug, e.g. IV amiodarone.

Key drugs which cause or aggravate ventricular arrhythmias

● sympathomimetics	– inotropic agents, noradrenaline, IV or nebulized salbutamol, theophyllines (potentiate catecholamine release).
● antiarrhythmics	– especially class Ic and class III (e.g. flecainide, sotalol).
● cardiac glycosides	– check level in any patient on digoxin with new tachyarrhythmia.
● antidepressants	– tricyclics, especially with amiodarone.
● antihistamines	– especially astemizole and terfenadine.
● motility stimulants	– cisapride (can cause QT prolongation).
● antibiotics	– IV erythromycin causes QT prolongation if co-prescribed with amiodarone/other QT prolonging agent
● antimalarials	– quinine and related drugs

- Check H_x of arrhythmia, proarrhythmic drugs.
- Check cardiac H_x (patients with previous MI or cardiomyopathies, previous VT, are at risk of VT). H_x of cardiac failure/LV impairment will influence choice of antiarrhythmic drug.
- Check recent illnesses (e.g. acute renal failure (K^+ ↑), acute coronary syndromes, LVF may predispose).
- Look for acute triggers (new MI, hypo/hyperkalaemia, hypoxaemia, cardiac failure, drug toxicity, illegal drugs (especially amphetamines, 'Ecstasy', cocaine), mechanical irritation (e.g. central line irritating tricuspid valve/RV)).

Examination
- Brief assessment focusing on signs of compromise (↓ BP, failure) and potential cause (e.g. hypoxaemia, fluid overload, sepsis).

Investigations
● Examine 12-lead ECG (in sinus rhythm, if available).

Clues from sinus rhythm ECG in assessing broad-complex tachycardia

● **LBBB or RBBB**? If QRS morphology same as in tachycardia, SVT is most likely diagnosis.
● **Examine any ventricular ectopic complexes**. If QRS morphology same as tachycardia complex morphology, VT is most likely diagnosis.
● **Is there evidence of pre-excitation?** Accessory pathways cause broad-complex tachycardias for several reasons:
  – atrial fibrillation with pre-excitation: irregular, very rapid tachycardia, often >300 bpm, with variably broad complexes.*
  – atrial flutter with pre-excitation: usually regular with broad complexes similar to morphology when pre-excited in sinus rhythm. Rate usually either 150 bpm (2:1 AV block) or 300 bpm (1:1 AV conduction).*
  – antidromic re-entry tachycardia (antegrade conduction goes down accessory pathway, giving delta wave during tachycardia).
● **QT interval prolonged?** QT_c >0.42 s is prolonged and may predispose to polymorphic VT, especially *torsade* (see below).
● **Evidence of pathology which predisposes to VT?** (e.g. LVH, Q waves of previous MI).

* Pre-excited atrial fibrillation and atrial flutter with 1:1 AV conduction almost always causes haemodynamic compromise and necessitates **immediate cardioversion**. Do not give adenosine, verapamil or digoxin.

● Examine **12-lead ECG**, not just rhythm strip, during tachycardia. There is no 100% reliable way of diagnosing the rhythm, but certain features favour VT or SVT. See Figures 16.7–16.9 for examples of rhythm strips.
● CXR – look for signs of cardiac enlargement/failure.
● Bloods – check $K^=$, Mg^{2+}, Ca^{2+} have been ordered. Consider ABGs to assess for hypoxia, acidosis.
● Echo – not essential during acute management, but may show evidence of previous MI/cardiomyopathy (predispose to VT), or valve disease/atrial enlargement (predispose to SVTs).

Management
● Unless patient is acutely compromised, start by treating correctable factors.
● If unsure whether VT or SVT, try vagal manoeuvres or IV adenosine test (see earlier).
● If **episodes are brief and self-terminating**, acute antiarrhythmic treatment is not needed.
● If **not compromised** and LV not impaired, give **IV lignocaine** 100 mg

VT or not VT?

Favours VT

- AV dissociation   – almost diagnostic of VT
- VA relationship   – atrial rate is a fraction of ventricular rate, e.g. 2:1 retrograde VA block

(P waves may be difficult to see on surface ECG, so the above are often not obvious)

- Fusion beats   – hybrid of sinus and tachycardia QRS complex caused by simultaneous ventricular activation via His bundle and VT focus
- Capture beats   – sinus morphology complexes embedded in tachycardia caused by intermittent successful transmission of atrial impulses via AV node/His bundle
- Extreme left or right axis deviation
- QRS duration >0.14 S
- Concordance   – QRS complexes in the chest leads all either +ve or -ve.

Favours SVT

- Slowed/terminated by vagal manoeuvres/adenosine
- Short VA time   – R-P interval <0.1 s signifies accessory pathway
- Initiated by atrial ectopic beat
- VA relationship   – atrial rate is a multiple of ventricular rate, e.g. 2:1 antegrade AV block

(50 mg if <50 kg) over 2 min, then infuse at 4 mg min^{-1} for 30 min, 2 mg min^{-1} for 2 h, 1 mg min^{-1} for up to 24 h.

- If **evidence of cardiac failure or poor lV function**, give **IV amiodarone** 5 mg kg^{-1} over 30–120 min via central line.
- If above agents fail, consider the following options:
  second-line drug (see box)
  DC cardioversion
  overdrive ventricular pacing (see Chapter 3).
- Consider whether long-term prophylaxis is needed. If there is an identifiable treatable trigger (e.g. acute MI, electrolyte disturbance, mechanical irritation), no prophylaxis is needed. If recurrent episodes occur, or if no cause is identified, further assessment is needed as described at the end of this section.

TORSADES DE POINTES VT

This form of polymorphic VT occurs when ventricular repolarization is delayed. The QT interval is prolonged in sinus rhythm. The ECG shows progressive movement of the axis and the complexes appear to twist around the baseline. The arrhythmia is usually non-sustained and repetitive, but can degenerate into VF.

Other drug options for acute VT

All of these agents can cause hypotension and aggravate cardiac failure.

β-**Blockers** may be useful if hyperadrenergic state implicated.

Flecainide 2 mg kg^{-1} IV over 20 min (max. 150 mg). Avoid in cardiac failure, AV block. Can cause rise in temporary/permanent pacemaker threshold.

Mexiletine 100–250 mg IV over 10 min, then 250 mg h^{-1} for 1 h, 125 mg h^{-1} for 2 h, 30 mg h^{-1} thereafter. Do not use in cardiogenic shock. Can aggravate arrhythmias (e.g. *torsade*) and cause neuropsychiatric disturbance.

Procainamide 500–600 mg IV over 30 min, then 2–6 mg min^{-1}.
Can cause *torsade*, lupus-like syndrome.

Disopyramide 2 mg kg^{-1} IV over 5–10 min, then 200 mg orally tid
Most effective in post-MI VT. Can cause VF and *torsade*.

Bretylium tosylate 5–10 mg kg^{-1} IV over 15–30 min, repeat every 1–2 h to maximum of 30 mg kg^{-1}. Do not give with sympathomimetic amines (antagonize bretylium). Can exacerbate digoxin-induced arrhythmias.

Causes of *torsades de pointes* VT

Antiarrhythmic drugs	especially sotalol, amiodarone, quinidine, disopyramide
Bradycardia	sinus node disease, complete AV block
Electrolyte disturbance	$\downarrow K^+, \downarrow Mg^{2+}, \downarrow Ca^{2+}$
QT-prolonging drugs	see Key drugs box, carrier
Congenital long QT syndrome	Romano–Ward syndrome (autosomal dominant), Jervell and Lange–Nielsen syndrome (autosomal recessive, congenital deafness)

Treatment is mainly directed at removing the cause. Overdrive atrial pacing or, if AV block, ventricular pacing, at 100 bpm will usually suppress *torsade*. IV **isoprenaline** 0.5–10 μg min^{-1} (make up 1 mg in 500 ml 5% glucose, infuse at 15–300 ml h^{-1}) can be used as temporizing measure if pacing is not immediately available. IV **magnesium** (8 mmols over 15 min then 72 mmols over 24 h) should be given in all cases.

INVESTIGATION AND LONG-TERM MANAGEMENT OF VENTRICULAR ARRHYTHMIAS

Further investigation is needed if the cause of the arrhythmia is not transient or reversible, or is not identified. The key aim of investigation is to identify underlying structural or ischaemic heart disease. Since IHD is the most common cause of ventricular arrhythmias, investigations are first directed at this pathology. Details of investigations and management are given in Chapter 12.

Pulseless VT and VF

Survival from out-of-hospital ventricular arrhythmias is becoming increasingly common because of emergency services' defibrillation initiatives. A comprehensive appraisal of the likely cause of cardiac arrest is crucial when planning investigations and management, as the patient's risk of further cardiac arrest determines the line of investigation. Ischaemic heart disease is the cause in over 90% of out-of-hospital cardiac arrest survivors. Several mechanisms exist in these patients:

● **Acute MI** is the commonest cause. Patients who survive MI complicated by early (<48 h) VT or VF arrest are not at significantly greater risk of cardiac arrest after discharge than those who have uncomplicated MI, and treatment does not differ.

● **Ischaemic heart disease with LV dysfunction** is also a common substrate for VF. It is often difficult to tell whether the arrhythmia relates to ischaemia or to an infarct-zone focus (e.g. left ventricular aneurysm). These patients are at high risk of further cardiac arrest and need comprehensive evaluation.

● **Acute ischaemia without infarction**, in the setting of good LV function, is a less common cause of VT/VF.

● **Other causes, such as aortic stenosis**, mitral valve prolapse, HOCM or non-cardiac triggers (e.g. hyperkalaemia), will have been identified during the index admission.

Three phases of assessment and treatment are needed:

1. *Is the patient's prognosis seriously limited by coexisting illness?* If so, then invasive I_x and R_x may not be appropriate. Empirical drug treatment with oral **amiodarone 200–400 mg d^{-1}** is effective.
2. *Is acute ischaemia considered to be a likely substrate?* (Was arrest preceded by ischaemic symptoms, or by exertion? Was a critical, likely culprit lesion seen at angiography?) If so, revascularization should be undertaken if technically possible. The benefit of this approach was shown in the CABG-PATCH trial. The effectiveness of revascularization at preventing inducibility should be assessed afterwards with stress testing ± electrophysiological testing.
3. *In patients without an ischaemic trigger, or in whom revascularization is not possible, the optimal choice of treatment is controversial.* The options are empirical drug therapy (e.g. amiodarone), drug treatment guided by electrophysiological study, or implantation of an AICD.

● **Empirical drug therapy**. This means treatment with a drug, without efficacy testing using electrophysiological study. Although this may seem a haphazard approach it is effective. **Amiodarone** is the commonest drug used, based on its effectiveness in the CASCADE study and its tolerability in patients with LV impairment.

● **EP-guided drug therapy**. This involves testing of the effectiveness of a drug by its ability to prevent arrhythmia induction during EPS. Drugs may be tested either by administration during EPS, or arrhythmia inducibility tested before and after a period of oral drug therapy. This approach has not been shown in trials to be superior to empirical amiodarone therapy.

● **Implantable defibrillators** are an expensive but effective treatment option. The AVID and MADIT trials indicate that AICD therapy reduces mortality significantly over antiarrhythmic drug therapy in patients with symptomatic ventricular arrhythmias or resuscitated cardiac arrest. Local health budgets will probably determine whether AICDs are used in patients whose prognosis is also limited by ventricular impairment and heart failure.

BRADYCARDIAS AND AV BLOCK

See also Chapters 3 (temporary pacing), 11 (dizziness and syncope), 5 (acute MI) and 17 (pacing indications).

Bradycardias are often an unnecessary cause of alarm in hospitals and can result in a panic call to you about, for example, an asymptomatic sinus bradycardia. Conversely, potentially dangerous rhythms such as complete heart block may be overlooked or considered benign. There are many causes of bradycardia and the key to their management is to identify the cause. This determines what treatment, if any, is needed. This section deals with management of acute bradycardias as they present in hospital or the emergency room.

DEFINITION

The textbook definition of bradycardia being a rhythm with ventricular rate <60 bpm is not clinically useful. Many healthy individuals fall into this category and many patients with heart disease (appropriately) have heart rate <60 bpm as a result of medication. Also, some patients with heart rate >60 bpm are inappropriately bradycardic for their clinical state (e.g. heart failure or cardiogenic shock). A more useful definition of a pathological bradycardia is one that causes symptoms, haemodynamic compromise, or places the patient at risk of syncope or cardiac arrest.

> **Tip:** Asymptomatic bradycardias, other than complete heart block, do not require emergency intervention.

ACUTE MANAGEMENT OF BRADYCARDIAS

Immediate assessment

● Check airway, breathing, circulation. Establish IV access.
● Attach ECG monitor, ideally with printout so you can document response to treatment.

Warning: For asystole or pulseless bradycardia, follow the guidelines for cardiac arrest (Chapter 4).

- Follow the *Peri-arrest arrhythmias* algorithm of the UK Resuscitation Council (Chapter 4).

Key causes of bradycardia

- Physiological (e.g. athletes, sleep)
- Parasympathetic response
  vasovagal faint (e.g. situational syncope)
  malignant vasovagal syndrome
  other vagal response (e.g. to vomiting, instrumentation of viscera)
  carotid sinus hypersensitivity
- Sinus node disease ('sick sinus syndrome')
- AV node disease
- Myocardial ischaemia/infarction (may cause sinus or AV node ischaemia, or vagal response)
- Drugs (β-blockers, especially with verapamil or diltiazem, digoxin, most antiarrhythmic drugs. Don't forget β-blocker eye drops)
- Raised intracranial pressure (e.g. subarachnoid haemorrhage)
- Hypothyroidism
- Hypothermia
- Cholestatic jaundice

History

- Assess *context* in which bradycardia occurred:
  situational triggers (e.g. instrumentation or procedures in hospital) usually denote a transient vasovagal response and do not merit long-term R_x
  check for symptoms of MI/ischaemia. Bradycardias associated with MI are discussed in Chapter 5
  history of cold exposure?
  drug toxicity/overdosage?
  did symptoms occur when moving neck? (carotid sinus hypersensitivity)
- Check previous H_x of dizziness, syncope, atrial arrhythmias (may denote sinus node disease), rate-slowing drugs
- Check past cardiac H_x (IHD predisposes to SA and AV node failure. Aortic valve disease/replacement/endocarditis can cause AV block because of the proximity of the valve to the AV node). Myocarditis can cause CHB.

Investigations

- Examine ECG during bradycardia. A long rhythm strip (>20 s) helps determine the AV relationship; on short recordings, in CHB, atrial and ventricular rates may be similar, giving the illusion of AV node conduction (*'isorhythmic complete heart block'*).

    – HR during bradycardia

    – are P waves visible? (if not, consider junctional bradycardia or atrial fibrillation with CHB. Fibrillation waves are often present in the latter)

    – are P waves associated with QRS complex (if not, consider AV dissociation or CHB – see box)?

    – if P waves are associated, do they occur in or after QRS complex? (if so, junctional bradycardia or idioventricular rhythm)

    – if P waves absent, or CHB present, is QRS width normal or broad? Broad-complex escape rhythms are more liable to degenerate to asystole, as they usually originate from a 'low' (ventricular) origin with no 'fallback' focus should the rhythm fail.

Examination

Key points in examination: Bradycardias

- Vital signs ($\downarrow$ BP?, conscious level, hypothermia?)
- Evidence of cardiac failure (may be precipitated by bradycardia)
- Signs of aortic valve disease
- Jaundice
- Raised intracranial pressure (VIth nerve palsy, papilloedema, depressed consciousness)
- Signs of hypothyroidism (goitre, hoarse voice, dry skin and hair, delayed relaxation of tendon reflexes, vitiligo)

Complete heart block and AV dissociation are not the same thing! (See Figs 16.12, 16.13)

Discriminating complete heart block (CHB) and AV dissociation is important because AV dissociation in itself is benign, but CHB can predispose to asystole.

- **AV dissociation** means that atria and ventricles activate independently of each other. This can occur when the AV node fails, in CHB. It also occurs when the intrinsic ventricular rate speeds up above the sinus rate (e.g. accelerated idioventricular rhythm), or when the sinus rate slows below the intrinsic junctional or ventricular rate (e.g. extreme sinus bradycardia). **AV dissociation can occur without CHB.**
- In **CHB** the atrial rate usually exceeds ventricular escape rate. Because of AV node failure, P waves and QRS complexes are dissociated. **In CHB there is always AV dissociation**.
- On the ECG, compare atrial and ventricular rates. In AV dissociation without CHB atrial rate is slowest. P waves do not conduct to the ventricles because they occur when the AV node is refractory. However, occasionally the P wave falls after the AV node refractory period and conduct, triggering an early QRS complex. **The ventricular rhythm is not regular in AV dissociation without CHB**.

● If bradycardia intermittent or resolves, examine **12-lead ECG in sinus rhythm**. If bradycardia constant, look at previous ECGs for clues:
  – heart rate; is patient normally bradycardic?
  – atrial fibrillation or atrial ectopic beats (sinus node disease)
  – evidence of first- or second-degree AV block (predispose to CHB)
  – intraventricular block (LBBB, RBBB, bifascicular, trifascicular block – see Chapter 16)
  – ST changes of MI or ischaemia
  – long QT interval (can denote class III antiarrhythmic drug toxicity)
  – J waves/shiver waves – occur in hypothermia.

● Consider ECG during carotid sinus massage (see earlier) if you suspect carotid hypersensitivity. See Chapter 11 for diagnosis of syndrome.

● Ambulatory monitoring helps if no rhythm strip is recorded during bradycardia and to determine the nature, frequency and duration of bradycardias.

● CXR: check for cardiac enlargement/pulmonary oedema.

● Bloods: check TFTs, digoxin level, cardiac enzymes (exclusion of MI is mandatory in CHB. In MI, CHB usually resolves and most patients do not require permanent pacing).

● Echo: look for wall motion defects (suggest IHD), aortic valve disease/vegetations.

Long-term management

● The need for long-term treatment in patients with acute bradycardias is determined by the cause. After initial resuscitative management, start by treating correctable factors (e.g. stop rate-limiting drugs).

● Digoxin and β-blocker toxicities are discussed in Chapter 4.

● If long-term management is needed, this usually consists of implantation of a permanent pacemaker. Indications for temporary pacing are discussed in Chapter 3 and indications for permanent pacing are discussed in Chapter 17.

INFECTIVE ENDOCARDITIS

NATIVE ENDOCARDITIS

Infective endocarditis has an annual incidence of approximately 1500 cases in the UK. Symptoms are often non-specific and consequently the diagnosis may not be made for some time. The overall mortality from native endocarditis is high at approximately 15%, but the chance of death in an individual patient depends on the infecting organism and the site of infection. Whereas previously endocarditis was most common in patients with prior rheumatic fever, other factors such as a more elderly population (with a high prevalence of degenerate valves), survivors of corrected congenital heart disease, an increasing population with prosthetic valves and an IV drug abuser population, have served to change the types of patient (and organism) now seen.

AETIOLOGY

Native endocarditis usually affects abnormal or diseased valves. However, occasionally it can affect apparently normal valves, especially right-sided valves in IV drug abusers. Endocarditis can also occur at sites of vascular or myocardial anomalies; the feature which is common to 'high-risk' lesions is the presence of a jet between high- and low-pressure chambers. This may cause endothelial damage and inflammation and form a bed on which infective organisms can multiply.

TABLE 8.1 Risk stratification for susceptibility to endocarditis

High-risk lesions	Intermediate risk lesions	Low-risk lesions
Mixed mitral valve disease	AV fistula	ASD
Rheumatic aortic valve	Mural thrombus	Pulmonary stenosis
Mitral regurgitation due to structural disease (e.g. prolapse)	Mitral regurgitation in previously normal valve (e.g. due to LV dilatation)	Mitral valve prolapse without significant regurgitation
Prosthetic heart valves	Subaortic membrane	Permanent pacemaker
Aortic coarctation	HOCM	Closed PDA
Cyanotic congenital heart condition	Bicuspid aortic valve	
PDA	Isolated mitral stenosis	

The infecting organism is usually bacterial, but other pathogens may be seen:

- *Streptococcus viridans* (α-haemolytic): 55% of cases

oral origin	– *Strep. mitior, Strep. mutans,* *Strep. milleri, Strep. sanguis*
digestive origin	– *Streptococcus bovis, Enterococcus faecalis*
● Staph.	– 15–20% of cases
	– *Staph. aureus*
	– coagulase –ve staphylococci (*Staph. epidermidis*)
● Gram-negative bacilli	– 5% of cases
● Fungi and other organisms	– 15–20% of cases

Rarer organisms include *Chlamydia* and *Coxiella* spp., which may present with culture-negative endocarditis.

PREVENTION

There is no definitive evidence that antibiotic prophylaxis reduces the risk of infective endocarditis. However, it is considered sensible to give prophylactic antibiotics in patients at risk of endocarditis who undergo the following procedures:

● Dental work
● All surgical procedures
● Endoscopic GI biopsy
● Urinary tract instrumentation
● Permanent pacemaker insertion.

Antibiotic regimens are given in Chapter 12. The role of antibiotic prophylaxis for endoscopy, sigmoidoscopy and vaginal delivery is not clear. Many centres administer antibiotics in these situations.

CLINICAL PRESENTATION

Many patients present with a rather non-specific history, typically of malaise, intermittent fever, sweating and anorexia. The portal of entry or index episode of bacteraemia is usually not identified. Three-quarters of patients have a history of cardiac or valvular abnormalities and nowadays one-fifth have a history of IV drug abuse. The triad of fever, murmur and haematuria is the most common sign in patients with endocarditis (80–90%). Splenomegaly, neurological abnormalities, embolic signs and cutaneous manifestations of endocarditis are seen in a minority of patients. A new murmur, or a change in the character of an existing murmur, may indicate valve damage and is significant. See also Chapter 1 for physical signs in endocarditis and valve lesions.

INVESTIGATIONS

● **Blood cultures**. At least three (preferably six) samples should be taken from

Clinical criteria for endocarditis can be divided into major and minor. A diagnosis can be on the basis of two major criteria OR one major and three minor criteria OR five minor criteria.

Major criteria
- Positive blood culture   – typical organism from two blood cultures
                            – persistent positive blood cultures taken >12 h apart
                            – >3 positive blood cultures taken over more than 1 h
- Endocardial   – positive echo findings (vegetation, abscess)
  involvement   – new valvular regurgitation or dehiscence of
                            prosthesis

Minor criteria
- Predisposing valvular or cardiac abnormality
- IV drug abuser
- Pyrexia >38°C
- Embolic phenomenon
- Vasculitic phenomenon
- Blood cultures suggestive – organism grown but not achieving major criteria
- Suggestive echo findings, not meeting major criteria above

different sites over several hours. Sampling during a temperature peak does not improve the sensitivity of blood cultures. If the patient is stable it is appropriate to delay antibiotic treatment to allow comprehensive sampling, which will increase the likelihood of isolating the culprit organism. If cultures are negative, samples can be taken in special media which allows the growth of fastidious organisms (e.g. HACEK group, *Brucella*, *Legionella* spp.).

- **Laboratory tests**

  ESR, C-reactive protein – provide an index of activity of infection and can be used to assess response to R_x. Should be measured and can be used to follow subsequent response (measure once or twice weekly)

  immune complex titres – further evidence of active infection
  FBC   – normochromic normocytic anaemia (80–90%)
                          – neutrophilia
  U&Es   – renal and hepatic impairment may occur
  urine microscopy   – haematuria an early manifestation
  microbiology   – culture any suspected entry site (e.g. CVP line)

- **ECG** (weekly) – new PR interval prolongation or AV block suggests aortic root or septal abscess and is an indication for temporary pacing

- **CXR** (weekly) – progressive cardiomegaly suggests cardiac dilatation or pericardial effusion
                    – pulmonary congestion
                    – lung abscesses in IV drug abusers

- **Echo** (weekly) Transthoracic echo can detect most vegetations, although transoesophageal is more sensitive (65% vs 95%), particularly for mitral and prosthetic valve lesions. Transoesophageal echo is more sensitive at detecting aortic root and septal abscesses and leaflet perforations
- **Dental X-rays** – e.g. oral pantomogram, to identify source.

Cardiac catheterization is usually not indicated, especially with aortic valve endocarditis, because of the risk of coronary or systemic embolization and perforation.

MANAGEMENT

Antibiotic therapy
After completing blood cultures high-dose IV antibiotics should be started immediately. A tunnelled central venous line is useful because it allows the administration of IV antibiotics over several weeks without the need for repeated cannula or central line changes, which are uncomfortable and risk introducing secondary infection.

Depending on the suspected organism, appropriate antibiotics should be commenced for at least 4 weeks as follows:

Streptococcus – IV benzyl penicillin 2 g 4 hourly
– IV gentamicin 80 mg 12 hourly
Staphylococcus – IV flucloxacillin 3 g 6 hourly
– IV gentamicin 80 mg 12 hourly
– (IV fusidic acid 500 mg 8 hourly)

If the patient is allergic to penicillin then either IV **vancomycin** (1 g bd) or IV **teicoplanin** (400 mg bd for 3 days, thereafter daily) can be used as monotherapy. In responsive *Strep. viridans* endocarditis antibiotics can be changed to oral amoxicillin after 2 weeks and gentamicin withdrawn. Close liaison with a senior microbiologist is essential to guide antibiotic therapy and dosing.

Gentamicin and vancomycin plasma concentrations need to be monitored every 48–72 hours because of the risk of ototoxicity and nephrotoxicity.

TABLE 8.2 Target peak and trough plasma concentrations for gentamicin and vancomycin therapy

	Trough concentration (pre dose)	Peak concentration (2 h post dose)
Gentamicin	<2 mg l^{-1}	6–10 mg l^{-1}
Vancomycin	<10 mg l^{-1}	18–26 mg l^{-1}

Once the infecting organism is identified and its sensitivities known, the antimicrobial regimen can be adjusted to target that organism.

Culture-negative endocarditis

In some cases of endocarditis blood cultures do not identify a culprit organism. There are several possible reasons for this:

- Patient has recently received antibiotics
- Failure to isolate the organism
- Atypical endocarditis or fastidious organism, e.g. fungal infection or *Coxiella*
- Non-infective endocarditis (e.g. Libman–Sacks or marantic endocarditis)
- Incorrect diagnosis.

If the patient is stable, antibiotics may need to be stopped and blood cultures repeated using specific media for fungal or fastidious pathogens. Serology for *Brucella*, *Coxiella*, *Bartonella*, *Legionella* and *Chlamydia* spp. may be helpful. Marantic and Libman–Sacks endocarditis rarely cause significant valvular dysfunction. Such vegetations are usually an incidental finding at autopsy.

Response to therapy

Minimum inhibitory concentrations (MIC) of antibiotics help guide dosing, usually with guidance from the microbiology laboratory. The aim of therapy is to achieve trough plasma concentrations which are at least 10 times greater than the MIC. Titration with the patient's own plasma may help establish whether blood antibiotic concentrations are adequate.

The response to therapy is monitored in three ways:

- **Clinical status**: patients often respond dramatically to antibiotic therapy, with resolution of symptoms, fever and haematuria. Failure to respond clinically does not necessarily indicate the use of an inappropriate antibiotic regimen: large vegetations or abscesses may take some time to resolve, or may not resolve with medication.
- **Echo** (weekly): assess resolution or progression of vegetations, the development of aortic root abscess and new valve lesions.
- **Inflammatory markers**: ESR and serum C-reactive protein.

If fever or symptoms do not improve within 5–7 days of initiating therapy, check the sensitivity of the organism, MICs and consider transoesophageal echo to identify aortic root or septal abscess. Repeat CXR and consider an abdominal CT scan to identify other sources of sepsis. It may be necessary to add another antibiotic, or to consider surgery in patients who do not respond to appropriate antibiotic treatment. Remember that a persistent temperature and rash sometimes occur because of a reaction to antibiotics, rather than failure of therapy! Treatment usually continues for between 4 and 8 weeks. Discontinuation depends upon the organism and the clinical response.

Surgery

Surgery is indicated in patients with:

- Moderate to severe cardiac failure due to valve compromise
- Uncontrolled infection despite antimicrobial therapy
- Relapse after optimal medical therapy
- Threatened or actual systemic embolism
- *Staph. aureus*, *Coxiella burnetii* and fungal infections
- Paravalvar infection, e.g. aortic root abscess
- Sinus of Valsalva aneurysm
- Valve obstruction.

It is often difficult to judge how long to persevere with antimicrobial therapy before submitting the patient to surgery. The risk of surgery is high if the patient is septic, but is similarly high if the patient is haemodynamically compromised beforehand. Each case has to be assessed individually.

PROSTHETIC ENDOCARDITIS

Prosthetic endocarditis accounts for approximately 20% of cases nowadays and affects between 0.5 and 1% of patients after valve replacement. It is most common in the immediate postoperative period, but thereafter has an annual incidence of 4 per 1000 patients. The mortality is high from this condition (50%), partly because of the prevalence of staphylococcal infections. Prosthetic endocarditis most often affects valves, but can also affect vascular grafts or endocardial pacing electrodes.

AETIOLOGY

Prosthetic endocarditis is caused by similar organisms to native endocarditis, with a slightly different frequency:

- *Streptococcus viridans* (α-haemolytic) 35%
- Staphylococci 30%
    (*Staph. epidermidis* 15%)
    (*Staph. aureus* 15%)
- Other organisms: as native endocarditis 35%.

Staphylococci (>50%), Gram-negative bacilli (10%) and fungi (10%) predominate when prosthetic endocarditis occurs in the immediate postoperative period.

CLINICAL PRESENTATION

The clinical presentation and diagnostic criteria are the same as with native valve endocarditis. Complications may be more serious: in the immediate postoperative period valve infection often extends into the adjacent ring and tissues, causing abscesses, fistulae and valve dehiscence, especially with aortic valves. Bioprostheses may also undergo rapid leaflet destruction and paraprosthetic regurgitation is common. These complications are more common when the indication for valve replacement is native valve endocarditis.

INVESTIGATIONS
See earlier.

MANAGEMENT
See earlier.

> **Tip:** As the infective organism is more likely to be Staphylococcus, flucloxacillin and gentamicin should be used as first-line therapy. If methicillin resistance is suspected or confirmed, IV vancomycin 30 mg kg^{-1} d^{-1} should also be given, in two divided doses.

Many patients with prosthetic endocarditis require surgical intervention. Prosthetic dehiscence or paraprosthetic regurgitation is common and, unless the area of dehiscence is limited, is an indication for surgery. Around half of patients with prosthetic endocarditis develop cardiac failure because of valve dysfunction. The mortality from *Staph. aureus* prosthetic endocarditis exceeds 80%. Invasive aortic root infections, and endocarditis within prosthetic graft material, require technically demanding and extensive reconstructive surgery.

Endocarditis affecting endocardial pacing systems requires that the system, including pacing wires, be removed. If the patient is pacemaker dependent temporary pacing will be needed during antimicrobial therapy. The permanent pacing system should not be replaced until the infection has been eradicated (see Chapter 17).

Warning: If there are signs of haemodynamic decompensation assess the prosthesis immediately using echo or fluoroscopy. Valve dehiscence is characterized by abnormally free motion of the valve ring: it often appears to rock in its seating. Restricted leaflet movement occurs if there is valve thrombosis or an obstructive vegetation, although this can also occur in old valves where there is encroachment of myxomatous material (pannus).

PERICARDIAL DISEASE

ACUTE PERICARDITIS

This is caused by primary or secondary inflammation of the parietal and visceral pericardium and is a common cause of chest pain in young adults, more so in men than in women. The most common presenting symptom is chest pain. It is an important condition because it is sometimes mistaken for acute MI and because a proportion of patients develop a haemodynamically significant pericardial effusion or chronic pericardial constriction.

AETIOLOGY

Most cases are thought to be viral in origin, although the culprit virus is often not identified. The major causes are:

- Viral
    Coxsackie A and B
    echovirus, adenovirus
    Epstein–Barr virus, zoster
    mumps virus
- Bacterial
    pneumococcus
    staphylococcus, streptococcus
    gonococcus
- Tuberculosis
- Fungal
    histoplasmosis, coccidiomycosis
- Uraemia
- Neoplasia
- Autoimmune
    acute rheumatic fever
    SLE, rheumatoid arthritis, scleroderma
    sarcoidosis
- Trauma
    chest trauma, post pericardiotomy
- Acute MI
    immediate (due to local infarct-related myopericarditis)
    delayed (Dressler syndrome – Chapter 5)
- Idiopathic.

CLINICAL PRESENTATION

The diagnosis is supported by a recent history of flu-like illness; this usually suggests an acute viral pericarditis.

Symptoms
- Chest pain   – retrosternal or left-sided, sharp character

      – radiates to trapezius ridge or neck
      – often worse on inspiration, coughing, swallowing or lying flat
● Breathlessness   – shallow breathing because of pleuritic pain
      – due to pericardial effusion.

Signs

● **Pericardial friction rub**. This is a 'scratchy' sound, often confused with a pleural rub or a murmur. It can be transient, intermittent and positional. Usually best heard during inspiration or full expiration, with the patient leaning forward. It classically consists of three components:
    presystole (atrial systole): 70% of cases with rub
    systole (ventricular systole): 100%
    diastole (rapid ventricular filling): rare
● **Signs of tamponade**. These are described in Chapter 4.

INVESTIGATIONS

ECG

ECG abnormalities may not develop for several hours or days after the onset of pain. The characteristic ECG pattern is of 'concave upwards' or 'saddle' ST segment elevation, affecting all leads except aVR and lead I. Other features are:

● PR segment depression
● ST segment axis: 30–60° in pericarditis, 100–120° in acute MI
● Upright T waves, although can invert if there is associated myocarditis.

CXR

● Cardiomegaly may suggest pericardial effusion.
● May show intrathoracic pathology, e.g. neoplasm, TB.

Suggested laboratory tests

● FBC   – ↑ WCC
● U&Es, creatinine
● Inflammatory markers – ESR, C-reactive protein may be abnormal, haematology (raised white cell count) and serology
● Cardiac enzymes – elevated if myocardial involvement and in MI
● Microbiology/virology – acute and convalescent (2 weeks) viral titres
      – throat swab/ASO titre
      – (urine and faeces needed for comprehensive screen).

Further tests can be performed according to the suspected aetiology, e.g. connective tissue screen, blood cultures.

Echo (see Chapter 19)

- Identify pericardial effusion, site, size.
- Assess LV function; may deteriorate if associated myocarditis.
- Helps differentiate pericarditis from acute MI.

MANAGEMENT

All patients should be admitted for observation and the exclusion of myocardial infarction. Serial echocardiograms need to be performed to detect and observe the development of pericardial effusions. In one series tamponade occurred in as many as 1 in 10 patients with acute pericarditis.

The underlying cause should be treated and, where appropriate, this may include pericardial drainage and prolonged antibiotic therapy. However, conservative management is all that is usually necessary with high-dose non-steroidal analgesics to treat the associated discomfort. Rarely, high-dose steroids (oral **prednisolone** 60 mg d^{-1}) may be necessary in patients with resistant painful pericarditis. Anticoagulation should be avoided because of the risk of haemopericardium.

CHRONIC CONSTRICTIVE PERICARDITIS

This is a result of chronic pericardial inflammation causing fibrotic thickening of the pericardium, usually associated with fusion of the visceral and parietal pericardium which obliterates the pericardial space.

AETIOLOGY

- Idiopathic – presumed postviral pericarditis
- Post pericardiotomy
- Tuberculosis
- Radiation therapy
- Malignancy
- Prior purulent pericardial effusion
- Miscellaneous: uraemia, rheumatoid arthritis, systemic lupus erythematosus, drugs.

CLINICAL PRESENTATION

Patients present with symptoms and signs of chronic heart failure (see Chapter 6). However, in addition patients may remark upon platypnoea (dyspnoea when sitting upright). Examination reveals a high JVP which classically demonstrates Kussmaul's sign. A pericardial knock may also be audible and should be distinguished from a gallop rhythm, the opening snap of mitral stenosis and the concurrent split second sound. Volume overload with pleural effusions, hepatic engorgement, ascites and marked peripheral oedema is common.

Investigations

● **CXR** – pericardial calcification is seen in half of patients, especially when related to tuberculosis.

● **ECG** – generalized T-wave flattening and low-voltage QRS complexes.

● **Echocardiogram** – flattened left ventricular diastolic wall motion, abnormal septal motion and deranged spectral Doppler signals (see Chapter 19) are seen. Marked respiratory changes occur in transvalvular spectral Doppler velocities. Spontaneous echo contrast may be seen in the right atrium.

● **CT scanning** and **magnetic resonance imaging** – assess thickening and calcification of the pericardium.

● **Cardiac catheterization** – equalization of end-diastolic pressures in all four chambers.

The differentiation from restrictive cardiomyopathy (see Chapter 6) and cardiac tamponade may be difficult (Table 9.1).

TABLE 9.1 Distinguishing features of constriction, restriction and cardiac tamponade

	Constrictive pericarditis	Cardiac tamponade	Restrictive cardiomyopathy
Pericardial knock	+	–	–
Pericardial calcification	+	–	–
Pulsus paradoxus	+/–	++	+/–
Kussmaul's sign	+	–	–
Square root sign	+	–	+
End-diastolic pressures	LV = RV = LA = RA	LV = RV = LA = RA	LV > RV
Pericardial thickening (CT or MRI)	+	–	–
Myocardial thickening (echocardiography)	–	–	+
Pericardial effusion	+/–	++	+/–
Respiratory variation of spectral Doppler	++	+/–	–
Endomyocardial biopsy	–	–	+

MANAGEMENT

Curative treatment of constrictive pericarditis requires resection of the pericardium. This is successful in the majority of patients and is associated with an improvement in symptoms and prognosis. Poor outcomes of surgery are seen in patients with myocardial involvement (atrophy and fibrosis) and radiation pericarditis.

Diuretic therapy may alleviate the symptoms of dyspnoea and fluid retention. The associated sinus tachycardia is compensatory and negatively chronotropic drugs should be avoided.

CHAPTER 10

ACCELERATED HYPERTENSION AND PULMONARY EMBOLISM

ACCELERATED HYPERTENSION

Accelerated hypertension occurs most commonly in patients with essential hypertension. The risk of complications is more closely linked with the rate of rise in blood pressure than the absolute blood pressure level, because patients autoregulate to compensate for chronic hypertension. When blood pressure rises rapidly, cerebral, retinal and renal damage may ensue and the patient may develop acute LV failure. Accelerated hypertension is uncommon, affecting 1% of patients with essential hypertension. It carries a high mortality risk: untreated, 1-year survival is approximately 25%; with treatment, 1-year survival is around 90%. Although it usually occurs on a background of essential hypertension, other secondary causes should be considered:

- Renovascular disease (e.g. renal artery stenosis)
- Phaeochromocytoma
- Acute glomerulonephritis
- Collagen vascular disorders (e.g. systemic sclerosis)
- Pregnancy
- Food/drug interaction with monoamine oxidase inhibitor.

Different terminologies are used. Accelerated hypertension is defined as hypertension causing retinal haemorrhage or exudates, whereas malignant hypertension is characterized by papilloedema. They are, however, essentially the same and carry the same prognosis.

CLINICAL PRESENTATION

Patients may present with headache, irritability, visual disturbance, confusion, drowsiness or seizures. Nausea and vomiting are common. Sometimes the first presentation is with acute LV failure.

Signs
- **Blood pressure**. Diastolic BP often exceeds 130 mmHg; when this is the case renal, retinal and cerebral vascular damage is very likely. Systolic BP often exceeds 200 mmHg
- **Pulse**   – usually tachycardia. Atrial fibrillation may occur
- **Cardiovascular** – may be displaced or forceful apical impulse (if chronic hypertension)
                          – may be signs of acute LV failure
                          – check for unequal limb pulses (coarctation, aortic dissection)
                          – systolic murmur (coarctation)
                          – renal bruit (renal artery stenosis)
- **Retinal signs**   – papilloedema
                          – retinal haemorrhages/exudates.

INVESTIGATIONS

Essential

- Urinalysis/microscopy – haematuria, proteinuria imply renal damage or underlying glomerulonephritis (also casts)
- U&Es, creatinine – renal failure common
  – hypokalaemia may accompany secondary hyperaldosteronism or phaeochromocytoma
- Coagulation screen – check for disseminated intravascular coagulation
- FBC – microangiopathic haemolytic anaemia may accompany DIC (anaemia, thrombocytopenia, fragmented red cells)
- CXR – cardiomegaly if chronic hypertension
  – pulmonary oedema due to pressure overload
- ECG – LVH ± atrial fibrillation in chronic hypertension
  – ischaemia/MI may occur during hypertensive crisis.

The following should also be considered:

- 24-hour urine collection – assess creatinine clearance
  – screen for phaeochromocytoma (metadrenalines)
- Haemolysis screen – free haemoglobin
  – ↓ haptoglobin
  – Coomb's negative
- Echo – LVH if background chronic hypertension
  – monitor LV systolic function and dilatation
- Renal ultrasound – detect urinary tract obstruction, kidney size
  – unilateral small kidney suggests renal artery stenosis
  – bilateral small kidneys suggest chronic hypertensive or ischaemic nephropathy; can accompany bilateral renal artery stenosis
- CT head scan – if intracranial haemorrhage or cerebral infarction suspected.

MANAGEMENT

Rapid control of escalating blood pressure is essential, but this has to be achieved by a slow, sustained reduction. Reduction of blood pressure to 180–200 mmHg (systolic) and 90–110 mmHg (diastolic) is appropriate in the first 24 hours.

Warning: Aggressive blood pressure reduction can cause tissue and cerebral ischaemia and infarction, because in most cases the tissues have autoregulated to require a greater than normal perfusion pressure.

Antihypertensive drugs
- IVI **labetalol** (2 mg min^{-1}, to total dose of 50–200 mg) is useful first-line therapy, as its combination of α- (vasodilatation) and β-blockade render it effective.
- IVI **esmolol** (500 µg kg^{-1} min^{-1} for 4 min, then 150–300 µg kg^{-1} min^{-1}) has a more rapid onset of action and is rapidly metabolized if relative hypotension occurs. It does not share the α-blocking properties of labetalol.
- IVI **sodium nitroprusside** (0.5–6.0 µg kg^{-1} min^{-1}) is effective but must be titrated carefully, as it can cause a precipitous fall in BP. In the presence of renal failure thiocyanates accumulate rapidly and treatment for >24 h should be avoided.
- IVI **hydralazine** (initially 200–300 µg min^{-1}, maintained at 50–150 µg min^{-1}) is useful, but contraindicated if there is associated aortic dissection.
- IV **phentolamine** (2–5 mg, repeated if necessary) or **phenoxybenzamine** (1 mg kg^{-1} daily in 200 ml 0.9% saline over 2–4 h) are powerful α blockers which are used, in combination with a β-blocker, in hypertensive crises due to phaeochromocytoma.
- IVI **glyceryl trinitrate** (10–200 µg min^{-1}) is a relatively weak arteriolar dilator and should not be used as first-line therapy for hypertensive crisis. It is useful when hypertension is complicated by LV failure.
- Oral or sublingual **nifedipine** (10–20 mg) can be used to correct transient increases in blood pressure.

Because of pressure natriuresis patients may be in a state of intravascular volume depletion and relatively hyponatraemic. Intravenous saline should therefore be given to prevent prerenal exacerbation of renal failure. Renal replacement therapy may be necessary if renal failure deteriorates. ACE inhibitors and AT$_1$ receptor antagonists should be avoided in the early phase because of the risk of renal decompensation and because abrupt hypotension can occur in patients with high-renin states.

Once blood pressure has been controlled for at least 48 hours using one of the IV regimens above, patients can be converted to oral antihypertensive agents. Antihypertensive therapy is discussed further in Chapter 12.

PULMONARY EMBOLISM

Pulmonary embolism (PE) is included in this book for two reasons: first, it is relatively common in patients with heart disease; and secondly, because these patients may be admitted to a cardiac care facility for cardiac and haemodynamic monitoring, for administration of thrombolysis and sometimes for mechanical interventions. PE is increasingly common because of the increasing elderly population, who are at relatively high risk of the condition.

AETIOLOGY/PATHOPHYSIOLOGY

Virchow's triad – damage to the vessel wall, stasis and increased coagulability

– describes the conditions that increase the likelihood of intravascular thrombosis and pulmonary embolism. It is now recognized that many patients with venous thromboembolic disease are genetically predisposed to it, through mutations or deletions in coagulation factor genes.

Increased coagulability

Many systemic factors increase blood coagulability, e.g. sepsis, dehydration and polycythaemia. Malignant disease is often accompanied by an inflammatory response which increases the tendency to coagulation and venous thromboembolic disease is very common in these patients. The combined oral contraceptive pill also increases the risk of DVT and PE. Also, deficiencies in the concentrations or function of certain coagulation inhibitors can lead to *thrombophilia*, or increased propensity to thrombosis, in some patients:

- Protein C and protein S deficiencies (relatively rare)
- Resistance to activated protein – Factor V Leiden mutation (relatively common: 3% population frequency)
- Antithrombin III deficiency (relatively rare).

Concentrations of these proteins can be measured in patients with recurrent thrombotic or embolic events.

> **Tip:** Heparin lowers antithrombin III concentration and warfarin can lower protein C and protein S concentration.

Stasis

Stasis can be caused by several factors:

- Reduced cardiac output and slow circulation time
- Immobility (lack of use of 'muscle pump' in deep veins of legs)
- Obstruction to venous return, e.g. by extrinsic compression of leg veins or IVC.

Venous thromboembolism is more common in elderly and immobile patients, especially those with heart failure. Immobility also occurs during admission to hospital with, for example, acute MI, or after surgery (especially hip surgery and pelvic surgery). Prophylactic regimens for these patients are described later in this section.

Vessel wall damage

This is not a common cause of venous thrombosis, but instrumentation, e.g. temporary pacemaker or Swan–Ganz catheter insertion via the femoral route, predisposes to DVT and PE, especially if the insertion site becomes infected.

CLINICAL PRESENTATION

Symptoms

Around 60–70% of patients with PE present with the 'classic' symptoms of pleuritic chest pain and breathlessness, often accompanied by sweating and apprehension. The remainder present with more subtle symptoms and the diagnosis is often missed in these cases:

- Leg pain or swelling – only present in ~25% of patients with PE
- Haemoptysis
- Palpitation (due to sinus tachycardia or atrial fibrillation)
- Angina ('right heart' angina due to increased RV work ± hypoxia)
- Syncope (due to transient fall in cardiac output).

> **Tip:** Look for clinical, ECG and echocardiographic signs of right heart strain in patients with recurrent syncope: recurrent pulmonary embolism is an underdiagnosed cause.

Signs

Physical signs are often absent or subtle in patients with PE (see box).

Physical signs in acute pulmonary embolism

- Restlessness
- Tachypnoea
- Tachycardia
- Central cyanosis
- Sweating
- Loud P_2 (due to pulmonary hypertension)
- Fourth heart sound
- Elevated JVP
- Crepitations or pleural rub
- Hypotension, systolic BP <90 mmHg } massive PE
- Depressed conscious level
- Clinical signs of DVT (only 25–30% of patients)

DIAGNOSIS AND INVESTIGATIONS

In patients with suspected PE there are several non-invasive investigations that can be performed to help support or refute the diagnosis and to help elicit a cause.

Laboratory tests

- ABGs: ↓ Po_2 <10.5 kPa, ↓ Pco_2 (due to hyperventilation) ± metabolic acidosis

- **Plasma D-dimer** (a fibrin degradation product produced by endogenous fibrinolysis in presence of clot): very sensitive, but non-specific. Patients with heart disease may have elevated D-dimer for other reasons, e.g. recent MI. However, a normal D-dimer virtually excludes PE
- **FBC**: check for ↑ haematocrit
- **U&Es**: ↑ urea may suggest dehydration.

ECG

The most common ECG abnormality is sinus tachycardia; the following may also be seen if PE is large and right heart strain ensues:

- Atrial fibrillation
- RSR' pattern in lead V_1
- S wave >1.5 mm leads I and aVL
- Q waves in leads III, aVF
- T-wave inversion V_1–V_4 ± leads III and aVF.

CXR

This is often normal early after PE. Oligaemia (lack of vascular markings) may be seen in lobes or segments affected by large emboli. Atelectasis, segmental collapse, elevation of hemidiaphragm and a reactive pleural effusion may be seen if pulmonary infarction occurs. Infectious changes may be seen after PE. In patients with chronic recurrent PE thromboembolic pulmonary hypertension may be associated with cardiomegaly and 'pruning' of the pulmonary vasculature.

Echo

Large or recurrent PE causes right heart dilatation, if pulmonary hypertension occurs. Echo findings may be:

- RV dilatation with hypokinesis of the free wall
- Flattening of interventricular septum due to ↑ RV pressure
- Tricuspid incompetence
- Dilatation of PA with pulmonary incompetence (more common in chronic thromboembolic pulmonary hypertension)
- Thrombus 'in transit', i.e. clot seen in RA or RV.

Specific diagnostic tests for pulmonary embolism

Radionuclide lung perfusion scan

γ-Labelled microspheres or albumin are administered by IV injection; these lodge in the pulmonary capillaries and so are trapped preferentially in areas of lung with good perfusion. A γ camera is used to image the lungs from different angles, to detect perfusion defects in the major segments. A separate ventilation scan can be used to determine whether the perfusion defect corresponds with a region of lung collapse. Lung perfusion scans can be abnormal in patients with chronic lung disease, pleural effusions or pulmonary oedema. Scans are graded as normal, low (<20%), intermediate or high (>80%) probability of PE, depending on the number and the size of perfusion defects seen.

> **Tip:** Bayesian theory applies (see Chapter 16). Perfusion scans must be interpreted in the light of clinical suspicion of PE. A good clinical history and a low-probability scan corresponds with **up to 40%** chance of PE.

Pulmonary angiography
This invasive test involves right heart catheterization and placement of a pigtail catheter in each of the main pulmonary arteries. Although it carries the risk of instrumenting the heart and hypotensive reaction to contrast, it does have some advantages over other diagnostic tests:

- Allows measurement of PA pressure
- Helps differentiate thromboembolic pulmonary hypertension from primary pulmonary hypertension
- Allows mechanical fragmentation of pulmonary artery clot.

Branch vessel occlusion or intravascular filling defects may be seen in acute PE, whereas PA dilatation with small distal vessels is seen in chronic thromboembolic pulmonary hypertension. A good knowledge of pulmonary arterial anatomy is required to detect small, segmental emboli.

CT pulmonary angiography
This is a newer, non-invasive technique involving the peripheral injection of contrast followed by a timed, rapid spiral CT lung scan. It is good for the detection of central pulmonary artery embolism, although small peripheral emboli may be missed.

MRI scanning
Allows the detection of central pulmonary emboli without the need for contrast injection. Requires considerable operator expertise and is not currently a first-line investigation.

PROPHYLAXIS
Measures should be taken to minimize the risk of DVT and PE in all patients admitted to hospital. This includes avoiding dehydration, early mobilization when safe and practical and the use of graduated compression stockings in patients undergoing elective surgery. After MI, low- or high-dose subcutaneous heparin regimens can be used as prophylaxis for DVT and PE:

- Low dose: **unfractionated heparin** 5000 U SC bd until ambulant

- High dose: **unfractionated heparin** 12 500 U SC bd (reduces incidence of mural thrombus, but greater bleeding risk).

In other settings, e.g. elective surgery, low molecular weight heparins have been proved at least as effective as unfractionated heparin, with no greater risk of bleeding.

- **Dalteparin** 2500 units SC 1–2 h before surgery, then 2500 units SC d^{-1} for 5–7 days (5000 units SC d^{-1} in high cases, e.g. hip surgery)
- **Enoxaparin** 20 mg (2000 units) SC 2 h before surgery, then 20 mg SC d^{-1} for 7 days (40 mg d^{-1} in high-risk cases).

Laboratory monitoring of anticoagulation is not needed with these regimens unless bleeding occurs. **Protamine** only partially reverses the effects of low molecular weight heparins.

MANAGEMENT OF PULMONARY EMBOLISM

Management strategies for pulmonary embolism depend on the facilities available at the admitting centres and the patient's mode of presentation.

Acute massive pulmonary embolism
Patients who present with massive pulmonary embolism (i.e. with hypotension or profound systemic hypoxaemia) may benefit from prompt intervention to alleviate right heart strain and improve cardiac output. Several strategies can be used.

Thrombolysis
Thrombolysis has not been shown to reduce mortality after PE but does resolve emboli and associated haemodynamic compromise more rapidly and the incidence of recurrence is lower (possibly because of dissolution of the clot source). The 'window' during which these benefits are seen is several days after initial presentation, although thrombolysis is best reserved for acutely ill patients. IV heparin is given after thrombolysis until oral anticoagulation has been established.

Pulmonary embolism without haemodynamic compromise
Treatment is directed at preventing further pulmonary embolism and at shifting the endogenous thrombosis – thrombolysis balance in favour of thrombolysis: in other words, allowing the clot to break down. There is no evidence in this group of patients that thrombolysis is helpful. Opiate analgesia is helpful to relieve pain/distress. Inhaled O_2 should be given to hypoxic patients.

Heparin therapy
This is the mainstay of initial therapy for pulmonary embolism. IVI unfractionated heparin has traditionally been used, but certain SC low

molecular weight heparins are as effective and do not tie the patient to a heparin infusion device. Example regimens are:

- IV bolus **unfractionated heparin** 5000 units, followed by IVI 1000 units h^{-1}, adjusted according to aPTT. (Target aPTT ratio 1.5–2.5.) Continued aPTT monitoring required.
- SC **tinzaparin** 175 units kg^{-1} daily. aPTT monitoring not required.

Oral anticoagulation with warfarin is normally started at the same time; heparin is continued for 5–7 days. The target INR for DVT or PE is 2.0–3.0; and 3.0–4.5 for recurrent DVT or PE. Anticoagulation is continued for 6 months, or indefinitely if DVT or PE is recurrent.

Inferior vena caval interruption
Patients with recurrent or life-threatening PE despite adequate anticoagulation can have wire filters implanted percutaneously into the IVC, below the renal veins. Benefit in terms of mortality reduction has not been established.

Further management
Investigations are directed at identifying a source of PE and any underlying pathology. Lower limb venography or Doppler ultrasound helps identify residual *in situ* venous thrombosis. A thrombophilia screen is essential in patients with recurrent DVT or PE. Pelvic and abdominal ultrasound and CT scanning may help identify underlying malignant pathology which predisposes to these problems.

MANAGEMENT OF OUTPATIENT CARDIAC PROBLEMS

CHAPTER 11

NEW PATIENT CONSULTATIONS

HOW TO DO OUTPATIENT CLINICS

For many patients outpatient clinics are the first point of contact with the cardiologist and serve as the focus for initiating investigations and treatment. Clinics tend to be busy and very time constrained. A typical review clinic appointment lasts 15 minutes; new patients need to be assessed in as little as 30 minutes. Because time is precious it is helpful to spend a short time before the clinic starts reviewing the records of the patients you are going to see and getting ready.

Saving time in outpatient clinics

- Read the last clinic letter, find out the patients' current problems; look at recent discharge summaries.
- Check whether risk factor assessment has been documented recently.
- Chase up any results you need and which are missing.
- Prepare any request forms in advance; label blood tubes.
- Complex cases: are you capable of evaluating the patient's condition? If not, read up about it and ask for senior advice beforehand.
- Is there another doctor in the clinic who has seen the patient before? A lot of time is wasted by yet another doctor retaking the patient's history.
- Dictate a structured clinic letter (see end of section). This saves a lot of time at the next visit.

Frustration is not conducive to good doctor–patient relationships. Always be punctual for clinics: if you run late, acknowledge this and apologize to the patient. If you run very late, call for extra help: it is easy to fall behind if your patient is ill and needs admission from the clinic. Most patients will understand if you explain that there is not always enough time allocated to tackle complex problems and that it is preferable to run a little late for the sake of being thorough.

HISTORY TAKING

Especially in review clinics it is impossible to take a comprehensive history every time. Reading the notes beforehand allows you to focus on the main issues. In new patient clinics obtaining a good description of the presenting symptom is the key to making a diagnosis. This chapter, on new referrals, is therefore symptom-based. In review clinics the diagnosis is often made already and therefore Chapter 12, review consultations, is diagnosis based.

EXAMINATION

By necessity, examination also has to be focused. Remember that you don't have to do a full examination on every patient (see Chapter 1). For example, patients may attend specifically for you to assess their response to new

Key points: history taking in outpatient clinics

- Start by asking open-ended questions: How have you been since the last visit? How have you been managing since your heart attack?
- Focus by asking about the key symptoms relating to the patient's condition (e.g. in aortic stenosis, ask specifically about syncope, dizziness, dyspnoea, angina, palpitation).
- Assess how symptoms affect daily activities (housework, job, recreation).
- For angina and heart failure, grade symptoms (see Chapter 1).
- Ask about potential side effects of medication.
- Address patient-modifiable risk factors in a non-confrontational manner (smoking, obesity, physical activity).
- Don't forget that depression and anxiety commonly accompany heart disease: ask about patients' and families' anxieties regarding health and prognosis, and about mood.

medication, or to monitor risk factors, or to explain the results of tests. Don't waste time examining if it's better spent explaining!

EXPLAINING DIAGNOSES AND RESULTS

Effective communication helps the patient understand their condition and why tests and treatments are being done. Speak in plain language: most patients don't know what a *coronary artery* or a *ventricle* is. It often helps to use a diagram or heart model to explain concepts such as a stenosed artery or heart valve. If you plan any tests, explain the reason for these to the patient, the waiting time and when to expect the result. For invasive investigations or treatments, explain the risks but be reassuring (see also Chapters 17 (pacing complications), 16 (RF ablation complications) and 18 (cardiac catheterization/PTCA complications). Informing patients about risk is a medicolegal requirement but it is easy to raise their anxiety level by tactless explanation. Explain that there may be a risk in leaving their condition without proper investigation, as this might preclude optimal treatment. Give written information about diagnosis, tests and treatment (e.g. British Heart Foundation booklets) to reinforce your explanation.

If you are unsure about how to proceed with a difficult case, ask a senior colleague. If no-one is available, explain that you need to take advice and that you will call the patient later. If necessary, arrange another appointment.

CONCLUDING THE CONSULTATION

Try not to deluge the patient with information or nothing will be retained. It helps to conclude by reinforcement and giving patient-specific targets (e.g. 'You have made a very good recovery from your heart attack. You managed well on the treadmill, so you should be able to start work again now. Try to increase your walking to half an hour four times a week. You have done well to cut down to five cigarettes a day but you should set a date to stop completely within the next month.'). Give ample time for the patient to ask questions. Finally, decide whether a further appointment is needed, or whether discharge is appropriate. Discharge is appropriate not only for patients who are well: some with chronic intractable cardiac problems are better seen on an 'as required' basis, as an appointment may serve no purpose if symptoms are stable.

ANGRY PATIENTS AND RELATIVES

There are many reasons why anger may be directed at you in the clinic:

- You may have made a mistake – forgotten to request an investigation, or been late seeing the patient.
- Anxiety or fear may be expressed as hostility.
- The patient or relative may feel you are not doing enough. Especially in chronic illness (e.g. heart failure or inoperable coronary disease) the patient may feel out of control and deprived of effective treatment. Also, you may not have explained *why* a further angioplasty won't help.
- Waiting lists are a bad source of frustration, especially if symptoms are worsening. If so, write to the surgeon and explain the change in symptoms. Ask the patient to direct a written complaint if they are still dissatisfied.

Do not trivialize patients' complaints and do not respond to hostility with hostility. Establish what are their main concerns/complaints. If you have made an error, acknowledge this, apologize and do your best to rectify the situation. Otherwise, spend time talking about the illness, tests and treatments. Fear of the unknown often underlies angry or overcritical behaviour. If the patient remains dissatisfied, offer to make them an appointment with a senior colleague.

THE STRUCTURED CLINIC LETTER

The letters you dictate during clinics serve two purposes. They are a form of communication with the patient's GP and should not be long-winded. The important diagnoses, tests and recommendations should be highlighted. Secondly, they are part of the patient's record and are a key to continuity for you and any other doctor who subsequently sees the patient. A structured clinic letter ensures that you are comprehensive, succinct and clear. An example is given below; the main headings are in **bold**.

- Summarize the extent of coronary disease, if known (see example below).
- Detail any bypass grafts (e.g. LIMA to LAD, vein grafts to RCA and OM_1).
- Detail valve type and size (e.g. 23 mm ATS aortic valve replacement); this is important information when interpreting echo.
- Document varicose veins on diagnosis list – relevant if CABG planned

John R Smith   D.O.B. 01/01/28

Diagnoses

Ischaemic heart disease	– 2-vessel disease (LAD, Cx)
	– PTCA to LAD 08/98
	– mild left ventricular impairment
	– CCS class II angina
Hypertension	– controlled with β-blocker since 1992
Depression	– quiescent

Current treatment

aspirin 150 mg d^{-1} atenolol 50 mg d^{-1}

GTN spray as needed

Progress

Mr Smith's angina has improved since his recent angioplasty. His exercise tolerance is unlimited on the flat, but he still has chest tightness on hills and stairs. This is associated with dyspnoea. He has no other symptoms and has returned to his work as an insurance clerk. He tolerates his medication well and has no major side effects.

Examination

Pulse was 86, regular; BP 162/82. There was no clinical evidence of heart failure, heart sounds were normal with no murmurs and the chest was clear. Fundoscopy was normal.

Investigations

The ECG showed sinus rhythm and inverted inferior T waves, as before. Echo showed good left ventricular function, no LVH and normal valves. An ETT was performed and he managed 8 minutes of the Bruce protocol before developing inferior T-wave inversion which resolved within 2 minutes of stopping. His blood pressure response was normal.

Summary

Mr Smith's angina has improved significantly since his angioplasty. He has good effort tolerance and has some ischaemia at high workloads, which probably reflects residual circumflex disease. This does not merit intervention. His resting heart rate is high and his β-blocker should be increased because of his residual angina.

Recommendations

1. Increase atenolol to 100 mg daily.
2. Please recheck heart rate and BP in 2 weeks.

Follow-up

Professor Branch-Block's clinic, 2 months.

CHEST PAIN

Chest pain or discomfort is the most common presenting symptom seen in cardiology clinics. Evaluation is initially directed at establishing or excluding a diagnosis of ischaemic heart disease and at risk-stratifying patients in whom this diagnosis is confirmed. A new diagnosis of angina is associated with up to 1 in 3 risk of having a major adverse cardiac event in the next 1–2 years.

AETIOLOGY

The differential diagnosis of chest pain is very large! Consider Table 11.1:

TABLE 11.1 Main differential diagnoses of chest pain

Cardiovascular	Respiratory/chest
Classic angina	Pulmonary embolism
Myocardial infarction	Pneumonia (usually lobar)
Variant (vasospastic) angina	Pneumothorax
Syndrome X (microvascular angina)	Acute asthma
Aortic dissection	Pneumomediastinum
Thoracic aortic aneurysm	
(Myo)pericarditis	

GI	Other
Oesophagitis	Chest wall/musculoskeletal pain
Oesophageal spasm	Psychogenic chest pain
Hiatus hernia	Costochondritis
Peptic ulcer disease	Cervical spondylosis
Biliary colic	
Pancreatitis	

HISTORY TAKING

Establishing a correct diagnosis depends heavily on the clinical history: this alone is sufficient to make a diagnosis in most cases. Of patients referred to cardiology clinics, 80–90% have either ischaemic heart disease or musculo-skeletal chest pain. As with any symptom, focus on the timecourse (first episode, number of episodes, onset, duration, precipitating and relieving factors, character and severity of discomfort, associated symptoms). Watch the patient's hands! As he describes symptoms, ischaemic pain is often demonstrated by making a fist over the chest; dyspeptic pain is often shown as retrosternal, pointing with fingertips. Musculoskeletal pain is often pinpointed to a specific spot. Note cardiovascular risk factors (Chapter 12) as this will have a large bearing on the likelihood of a cardiac diagnosis (see Table 11.2).

TABLE 11.2 Distinguishing characteristics of cardiac and non-cardiac chest pain

	Cardiac origin	Non-cardiac origin
Pain	Heaviness Band Gripping Dull ache	Dull ache Sharp, shooting 'Knife-like' Pleuritic
Localization	Central Radiation to left arm, neck or teeth	Left submammary
Precipitants	Exertion Stress Cold weather	Specific body motion Tender to palpation

EXAMINATION

Examination is often normal in patients with ischaemic chest pain. Focus on the following:

Key examination points

- General – anxious? anaemic? cyanosed? cachectic?
  - abnormal posture? (suggests musculoskeletal/locomotor origin)
  - signs of joint pathology (cervical spondylosis, rheumatoid disease)
  - cervical nodes (intrathoracic malignancy)
- Musculoskeletal – trunk torsion, neck flexion and chest wall pressure help elicit musculoskeletal pain
- Pulse – tachycardia/atrial fibrillation may exacerbate angina
  - asymmetric pulses (aortic dissection OR atherosclerotic disease)
- BP – ↑ BP increases risk of IHD and aortic pathology
- Precordial examination – signs of aortic stenosis (angina)
  - abnormal pulsations (thoracic aneurysm or cardiac chamber enlargement)
- Respiratory – Focal chest signs indicate pulmonary/mediastinal pathology
- Abdomen – epigastric tenderness, abdominal aneurysm

INVESTIGATIONS

Investigations are helpful in establishing a diagnosis in cases in which history and examination have failed. However, investigations are more often used for risk-stratification of patients with a high suspicion of IHD from the history and for identifying possible precipitating/exacerbating factors.

ECG

- Resting rhythm
- Evidence of previous MI/ischaemia
- Pericarditic features (see Chapter 9)
- LVH (associated with hypertension/aortic stenosis)
- Evidence of right heart strain, e.g. p-pulmonale, dominant R-wave lead V_1, RBBB, right axis deviation (associated with chronic lung disease or recurrent pulmonary embolism/pulmonary hypertension)

CXR

- Pulmonary/mediastinal masses
- Pleural pathology
- Focal lung disease (e.g. collapsed segment)
- Evidence of pulmonary hypertension ('pruning' of pulmonary vessels, large main pulmonary artery)

- Cardiomegaly/chamber enlargement
- Abnormal aortic contour (thoracic aneurysm/chronic dissection).

Optional investigations
- Laboratory tests – FBC, TFTs if anaemia/thyroid disease suspected as exacerbating ichaemic chest pain
  – lipid profile, glucose **if IHD suspected**
- Lateral cervical spine X-ray – if restricted neck movements
- Echo – if structural heart disease suspected
- Cardiac catheterization – usually only indicated in patients with suspected IHD after stress testing
- CT/MRI chest – if pulmonary/mediastinal/aortic pathology suspected
- Barium studies/upper GI endoscopy/abdominal USS.

> **Tip:** Stress testing (e.g. ETT) is only indicated in certain patient subgroups. Stress testing in inappropriate patients often leads to a false positive diagnosis of IHD, can lead to risky invasive investigation and generates unnecessary anxiety. **Stress testing in patients with unstable chest pain is dangerous**. See Chapter 16 for indications for ETT.

MANAGEMENT

Ischaemic heart disease
Risk-stratification and management of unstable and stable angina are described in Chapters 5 and 12. Patients with unstable chest pain require in-hospital treatment, stabilization and investigation. Patients who have clinical markers of high risk of subsequent MI or death should undergo cardiac catheterization (see Chapter 18). A normal stress test does not exclude ischaemic heart disease but is a marker of good prognosis, allowing you to reassure the patient that future cardiac events are unlikely.

Occasionally patients attend recurrently with continuing chest pain and inconclusive or negative non-invasive tests. Under these circumstances cardiac catheterization can assist the future management and treatment (e.g. allaying the patient's fears of IHD, decision about secondary prevention) of this difficult group of patients, but patients should always appreciate the risk of invasive testing where there is no firm indication for this.

Musculoskeletal pain
Reassurance and analgesia are usually all that is required. Occasionally further investigation may be necessary. Consider referral to a rheumatologist

or orthopaedic surgeon if you suspect significant arthropathy or cervical spine pathology.

Other causes of chest discomfort

The management of pericarditis (see Chapter 9) and aortic pathology (Chapter 12) are described elsewhere. It is beyond the scope of this book to describe the management of GI and other non-cardiovascular pathologies.

PALPITATION (see also Chapter 7, arrhythmias)

Palpitation accounts for around 20% of new referrals to cardiology clinics in the UK. The symptom is distressing, often not because of discomfort or incapacity, but because of the fear it raises about collapse, 'heart attack' or the heart stopping. Patients' descriptions of palpitation vary widely, reflecting both cardiac and non-cardiac pathology.

Main causes of palpitation

Intermittent tachycardias
- SVTs, e.g. AV nodal re-entry tachycardia, accessory pathway tachycardias, atrial tachycardia
- VT, often associated with dizziness and sometimes syncope
- atrial fibrillation and flutter

Intermittent bradycardias
- sinus node disease
- intermittent AV block

Extrasystoles

Augmented stroke volume
- anaemia
- thyrotoxicosis
- pyrexia
- aortic regurgitation

Non-cardiovascular
- increased awareness of normal rhythm
- anxiety/panic attacks
- hyperventilation syndrome
- diaphragmatic flutter

HISTORY TAKING

A detailed description of symptoms helps greatly with diagnosis. The following points should be checked:

- **Character of palpitation.** Pauses and thumps suggest extrasystoles with postextrasystolic (compensatory) pauses, or sinus node disease. Continuous palpitation suggests paroxysmal tachy- or bradyarrhythmia. Flutters suggest atrial fibrillation, frequent extrasystoles or a non-cardiac aetiology.

● **Regular or irregular**? Irregular palpitation suggests atrial fibrillation or frequent extrasystoles.

● **How fast is heart rhythm**? Ask the patient to tap rhythm out on desk. A slow, forceful rhythm suggests bradycardia or bigeminy rhythm with compensatory pauses. A normal rate suggests increased stroke volume or awareness of normal rhythm.

● **Frequency and duration of episodes**. This determines whether drugs or RF ablation are justified once arrhythmia is diagnosed and on embolic risk in intermittent atrial fibrillation.

● **Associated symptoms**. With tachycardias dizziness is common and not necessarily ominous. Presyncope and syncope suggest serious haemodynamic compromise due to VT. With bradycardias, dizziness and syncope strengthen any argument for pacemaker implantation. Chest discomfort during palpitation does not necessarily represent myocardial ischaemia. Severe dyspnoea may signify myocardial ischaemia or arrhythmic cardiac failure.

● **Precipitants**. Ask about relationship of symptoms to:
  – exertion (e.g. exercise can induce VT or RV outflow tract tachycardia, but may suppress extrasystoles)
  – posture (vasovagal syndrome)
  – emotional stress (often sinus tachycardia)
  – alcohol (atrial fibrillation)
  – caffeine (questionable relationship to extrasystoles).

● **Medication**. See Chapter 7 for main classes of proarrhythmic drugs.

> **Tip:** Phaeochromocytoma is rare but easy to miss. Consider this diagnosis in patients with rapid palpitation associated with headache, flushing or hypertension.

EXAMINATION

The examination should focus on identifying underlying IHD, valvular and myocardial disease, as the treatment of arrhythmias is targeted at the underlying cause.

INVESTIGATIONS

The key to diagnosis is in obtaining an ECG recording during symptoms. Because a **12-lead ECG** yields the most diagnostic information, ask the patient to attend for an ECG *during symptoms*, if episodes are sufficiently prolonged to allow this. Exertional symptoms should be investigated by exercise stress testing.

Key examination points

- General examination – anxious?
  - anaemic?
  - thyroid status
- Pulse rhythm – extrasystoles? irregular – atrial fibrillation?
- BP – hypertension associated with IHD, LVH, phaeochromocytoma → arrhythmia
- Precordial examination – displaced apex beat
  - murmurs (especially mitral)
  - signs of cardiac failure (increased risk of atrial fibrillation and VT)

ECG

- Resting rhythm
- Evidence of previous MI (↑ risk of VT)
- LVH (↑ risk of VT)
- AV or intraventricular block
- Short PR interval/delta wave (pre-excitation)
- Large/bifid P waves (↑ risk of AF/SVT).

Ambulatory ECG

- 24- or 48-hour recorder if symptoms frequent (e.g. daily).
- Repeated recordings or a patient-activated system if symptoms infrequent.

It is essential to correlate rhythm disturbances with symptoms. Asymptomatic 'abnormalities' are common in otherwise healthy individuals.

- Extrasystoles are common and usually benign.
- Type I second-degree AV block may occur at night if vagal tone is high (e.g. athletes).
- Other common benign findings are:
  - atrial fibrillation <5 beats (elderly)
  - nocturnal sinus bradycardia
  - junctional bradycardia
  - sinus arrhythmia
  - sinus pause up to 2 s (young, high vagal tone)

Echo

As with syncope the prognosis is dictated partly by the presence or absence of structural heart disease. See later for key echo points.

Laboratory tests
- Haemoglobin
- Thyroid function
- (24-hour urine collection for metadrenalines).

Optional investigations
- Exercise ECG – useful if ischaemia-related or cathecholamine-dependent arrhythmia suspected.
- Electrophysiological studies only indicated if malignant arrhythmia is suspected and non-invasive studies fail to establish a diagnosis.
- Implantable event recorder – occasionally helpful for patients with infrequent episodes but significant compromise; conventional recorders are unlikely to capture the episode. Implantable event recorders resemble a small pacemaker, without an external electrode, and can monitor the cardiac rhythm over a period of months.

 Warning: For patients with suspected exercise-induced arrhythmia, establish IV access and check resuscitation equipment is to hand before starting ETT.

BREATHLESSNESS

Breathlessness is usually caused by disorders of the respiratory or cardiac system. Breathless patients are likely to be referred to a cardiology clinic if the suspected underlying diagnosis is cardiac failure. It is worth noting that, because of common aetiological factors (e.g. smoking), cardiac and respiratory diseases often coexist.

AETIOLOGY

- Cardiovascular – LV systolic failure (including cardiomyopathies)
  - LV diastolic failure (underdiagnosed – can accompany LVH, any cause of systolic failure, restrictive cardiomyopathy)
  - right heart failure and other low-output states
  - myocardial ischaemia (LV dysfunction)
  - valvular heart disease
  - intracardiac and extracardiac shunts
  - pericardial disease
  - intermittent arrhythmias
- Respiratory – obstructive lung disease (e.g. asthma, COPD)
  - upper respiratory tract obstruction (e.g. tracheal compression)

- interstitial lung disease
- respiratory infection
- intrathoracic malignancy
- (recurrent) pulmonary embolism
- pleural effusions
- primary and secondary pulmonary hypertension

● Other
- anaemia
- metabolic acidosis
- hyperventilation syndrome.

HISTORY TAKING

It is quite difficult to make a diagnosis based on symptoms alone. Ask about precipitants. Orthopnoea or paroxysmal nocturnal dyspnoea, especially if recent in onset, suggest cardiac failure. Exertional dyspnoea is common to both cardiac and respiratory causes, but accompanying chest discomfort suggests an ischaemic aetiology. Ask about exposure history/allergens (e.g. house dust, cats, dogs) and other atopic symptoms (hayfever, eczema) which may suggest allergic asthma.

Check for items in the previous medical history which might make a cardiovascular diagnosis more likely, e.g. previous MI, hypertension, rheumatic fever. Ask also about smoking history and about episodes of winter bronchitis, which would indicate COPD. To identify other respiratory aetiologies, ask specifically about:

● Cough (productive? haemoptysis? NB: cough also accompanies cardiac failure)
● Pleuritic pain (infection, pulmonary embolism)
● Weight loss/anorexia (malignancy).

Some patients feel breathless because of hyperventilation. Anxiety does not always accompany this. Common associated symptoms are light-headedness, perioral and peripheral paraesthesia.

EXAMINATION

Watch the patient's breathing pattern as they come into the consulting room: there may be a marked reduction in effort tolerance. Also, anxious patients may hyperventilate during consultation but breathe normally at other times.

INVESTIGATIONS

These are usually directed towards cardiovascular or respiratory pathology, depending on the history and examination findings. A full blood count, chest X-ray, ECG and echo should be done as a basic work-up.

Key examination points/refresher on respiratory examination

- General – anxious? cyanosed? anaemic?
  - cachectic? digital clubbing? hoarse voice? (recurrent laryngeal nerve compression)
  - Horner syndrome/upper limb weakness (apical tumour)
  - peak flow rate, if airway obstruction suspected
- Cardiovascular – pulse irregular? (atrial fibrillation common in breathless, elderly patients)
  - hypertension
  - signs of cardiac enlargement/failure
  - murmurs
- General respiratory – neck (lymphadenopathy, masses/upper airway obstruction)
  - resting respiratory rate
  - breathing pattern (prolonged expiratory phase, pursed-lip breathing denote airways obstruction)
  - hyperinflation ($\downarrow$ cricosternal distance (<2 fingerbreadths), $\uparrow$ AP diameter, 'barrel' shape)
- Chest expansion – symmetrically $\downarrow$ – restrictive or obstructive lung disease
  - asymmetric $\downarrow$ – unilateral/focal collapse/consolidation
- Percussion – hyperresonance (emphysema, pneumothorax)
  - dullness (effusion, consolidation, elevated hemidiaphragm (common after cardiac surgery – phrenic nerve trauma))
- Auscultation – wheeze (lower airway obstruction), stridor (upper airway obstruction)
  - crepitations (fine – fibrosis ('dry'), congestion ('wet', may clear with coughing); coarse – mucus or infection)
  - other focal signs (e.g. of effusion, consolidation)

ECG

It is vanishingly rare for the ECG to be normal if there is cardiac failure.

- Resting rhythm (atrial fibrillation a common cause of breathlessness in the elderly)
- Previous MI?
- LVH (aortic stenosis, hypertension, HCM)
- Evidence of right heart 'strain' (e.g. RVH, p-pulmonale, RBBB, T-wave changes in V_1, V_2).

CXR

- Cardiomegaly/chamber enlargement
- Interstitial oedema/septal lines/fluid in horizontal fissure
- Pulmonary/mediastinal masses
- Pleural pathology/effusion
- Focal lung disease (e.g. collapsed segment)
- Evidence of pulmonary hypertension ('pruning' of pulmonary vessels, large main pulmonary artery).

Echo

- Assess LV systolic *and diastolic* function (easy to miss restrictive/constrictive physiology unless it is looked for; see Chapter 19)
- RV dilatation/impairment (suggests pulmonary hypertension or intracardiac shunt)
- Valve disease
- Pericardial effusion.

Optional investigations

- ABGs – essential if recurrent pulmonary emboli or intrinsic lung disease suspected
- Lung function tests – check FEV_1, FVC, ratio and response to inhaled β_2-agonist if airways obstruction suspected
    - CO transfer factor in suspected interstitial lung disease
    - consider testing for exercise-induced bronchoconstriction/hyperventilation
- Exercise tolerance testing, with either ECG (ischaemia) or pulse oximetry (respiratory disease), can be useful if there is doubt about the diagnosis or functional severity of exertional dyspnoea.
- Cardiac catheterization is not usually needed. Right heart catheterization helps identify pulmonary hypertension, left-to-right shunts and restrictive/constrictive physiology (see Chapters 3 and 18). Left heart catheterization helps assess coronary anatomy, aortic and mitral valves (see Chapter 18).

MANAGEMENT

This depends on the cause. Breathlessness can be multifactorial, especially in the elderly, for example some patients with cardiac failure cope well until decompensated by the development of atrial fibrillation or a chest infection.

Sometimes the cause of breathlessness is difficult to determine. If there is evidence of pulmonary hypertension without significant ventricular dysfunction or valve disease, consider intrinsic lung disease (hypoxic) or left-to-right shunting (usually normoxic). If there are clinical or radiological signs of cardiac failure, but apparently good LV and RV function, consider constrictive or restrictive physiology (see Chapters 6 and 9), diastolic cardiac failure, or cardiac failure due to high-output state, pressure or volume overload (see Chapter 6).

It is beyond the scope of this book to cover the management of respiratory disease. If the diagnosis or management is unclear, consider seeking advice from a respiratory specialist.

DIZZINESS AND SYNCOPE (see also Chapters 7 and 12)

Dizziness affects around a third of people aged over 65: it is one of the most common complaints for which the elderly consult their GP. Syncope affects >20% of the population during their lifetime and constitutes 5% of medical admissions. Recurrent symptoms affect the ability to work and to drive, increase susceptibility to falls and reduce independence in the elderly. In the Framingham study, 11% of cases of syncope were thought to be cardiac. The incidence of sudden death over 5 years in this group was 30%, versus 9% for patients with non-cardiac syncope.

Main mechanisms of syncope

- **Cardiac syncope** affects patients with structural or conducting system disease. Reduced cardiac output results from arrhythmia, outflow obstruction (aortic stenosis or HOCM) or ventricular impairment.
- **Inappropriate vasodilatation** is the most common cause of recurrent syncope when the heart is normal. This includes situational syncope, vasovagal faints and the vasovagal syndrome.
- **Neurogenic syncope** includes epilepsy and cerebrovascular ischaemia.
- **Metabolic disturbance**, notably hypoglycaemia.

Tip: In the elderly dizziness and syncope are often multifactorial, e.g. cardiac impairment, vasodilator medication and coexisting cerebrovascular disease.

HISTORY TAKING

A diagnosis can usually be established without needing extensive, expensive investigations. The aim of history taking is to obtain a clear description of the symptoms and to identify precipitants and any pattern. It helps to ask the patient or carer to keep a diary of symptoms to elucidate any diurnal pattern or relationship between symptoms and physical activity or meals. A description of the episode from the patient *and* a witness helps distinguish between *neurogenic* and *cardiac* syncope. Ask about current medications, especially diuretics, vasodilators and drugs with proarrhythmic potential (see Chapter 7).

Warning symptoms

Light-headedness, chest discomfort, palpitation and dyspnoea suggest a cardiovascular aetiology. Headache, confusion, hyperexcitability, olfactory hallucination or an 'aura' sensation suggest a neurogenic aetiology. Try to identify precipitants: exertion (e.g. aortic stenosis, HOCM or exercise-induced arrhythmia), standing (orthostatic hypotension, vasovagal syncope), cough/micturition (↓ vasomotor response), or neck extension (vertebrobasilar insufficiency, carotid hypersensitivity).

Syncope

Syncope is likely to be cardiovascular in origin if colour drains from the face, unconsciousness is brief (<1 min) and recovery is rapid without confusion. Prolonged syncope, seizure activity, tongue biting and urinary incontinence indicate epilepsy or a neurogenic cause.

> **Tip:** The chicken and egg scenario! Seizures can be triggered by low cerebral perfusion during arrhythmia and cardiac arrhythmias may occur during a motor seizure.

Recovery

This is usually quick after cardiac syncope, although nausea and malaise may last a few minutes after vasovagal attacks. Prolonged recovery time (>5 min), drowsiness, headache and focal neurological signs suggest neurogenic syncope.

EXAMINATION

Examination is directed mainly at establishing the presence or absence of structural heart disease. This determines subsequent investigations and is prognostically important.

Key examination points

- General – clinical anaemia
  - central cyanosis (pulmonary embolism)
- Pulse rate and rhythm – evidence of arrhythmia
- Erect and supine BP – orthostatic hypotension = systolic postural drop >20 mmHg
- Precordial examination – displaced apex beat
  - murmurs
  - signs of cardiac failure
- Neurological – carotid bruits
  - focal neurological signs

The technique for assessing carotid sinus hypersensitivity is detailed below.

> **Tip:** The absence of postural hypotension during examination does not exclude orthostatic hypotension, which is influenced by diurnal and environmental factors.

INVESTIGATIONS

Investigations for recurrent dizziness and syncope are dictated by the history and examination findings. Broadly, the algorithm in Figure 11.1 should be followed:

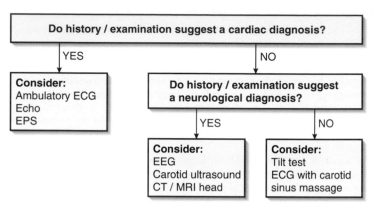

Fig. 11.1 Algorithm for investigating recurrent dizziness or syncope.

ECG
(Abnormal in 50% of patients with recurrent syncope.)

- Evidence of previous MI
- LVH (↑ propensity to arrhythmia, may accompany aortic stenosis, HOCM)
- AV or intraventricular block
- Pre-excitation.

Exercise ECG
Echo should be done before exercise to rule out LV outflow obstruction. If exercise-induced arrhythmia is suspected, establish IV access and ensure resuscitation equipment is at hand.

- Myocardial ischaemia
- Hypotension
- Exercise-induced arrhythmia.

Ambulatory ECG
- Always check recorded rhythm disturbances against reported symptoms, as asymptomatic 'bystander' arrhythmias are common, especially in the elderly (see Chapter 12 for a summary of these).
- 24- or 48-hour recorder if symptoms frequent (e.g. daily).
- Repeated recordings or a patient-activated system if symptoms are infrequent.
- Implantable event recorders are now available for very infrequent symptoms.

Echo
This is the key investigation for identifying structural heart disease.

- LV function (regional (IHD), global (cardiomyopathy))
- LVH (look for accompanying evidence of HOCM; see Chapter 19)
- Valve disease (especially aortic stenosis).

Tilt testing (see Chapter 13)
Tilt testing is used for diagnosing vasovagal syndrome. It involves studying the haemodynamic response to prolonged upright posture. As with ambulatory recording it is critical to correlate symptoms with abnormalities during the test.

Electrophysiological studies
Not usually needed, but in patients with structural heart disease and recurrent symptoms it may be helpful as symptoms and prognosis may be improved by antiarrhythmic therapy.

Electroencephalogram
Although useful, the EEG is normal in up to 40% of epileptic patients. Sensitivity is increased with photic stimulation, sleep deprivation and hyperventilation. Ambulatory EEG is now available and simultaneous EEG and ECG are available in some centres. This can help identify the initiating pathology in some cases.

CARDIOVASCULAR CAUSES OF DIZZY SPELLS AND SYNCOPE

Bradycardia
- **Sinus node disease**. Permanent pacing is indicated for symptomatic bradycardia or pauses, but is usually not needed for pauses <3 s.
- **AV block**. Other than nocturnal Wenckebach, second- and third-degree AV block generally necessitates permanent pacing unless a reversible cause is found.

Tachycardia
- **SVTs** (including atrial fibrillation) rarely cause syncope but may cause dizziness, especially in elderly patients with ventricular dysfunction (see Chapter 12).
- **VT** causes dizziness and syncope (see Chapter 12).

Myocardial ischaemia
- **Severe global ischaemia** and **regional ischaemia** with pre-existing LV impairment can cause symptoms from reduced cardiac output.
- **Ischaemia-induced arrhythmias.**
- **GTN syncope** due to excessive vasodilatation.

Vasovagal syndrome
Neurally mediated inappropriate vasodilatation, usually in response to upright posture. For detailed description and management, see Chapter 13.

- **Cardioinhibitory** (bradycardic) response
- **Vasodepressor** (hypotensive) response
- **Mixed response.**

Situational syncope is caused by parasympathetic activation due to an identifiable trigger, e.g. micturition and cough syncope, vasovagal faint due to emotion or noxious stimulus.

Carotid sinus hypersensitivity (CSH). Caused by hypersensitive carotid artery baroreceptors. This results in parasympathetic activation, then bradycardia and/or vasodilatation. Patients may describe symptoms when pressure is applied to the neck (e.g. wearing a tight collar). Diagnosis is by ECG monitoring and carotid sinus massage (CSM).

Testing for carotid sinus hypersensitivity

- Listen over carotid arteries for bruits.
- Do not attempt CSM if bruits heard, or there is known cerebrovascular or carotid vascular disease.
- Massage (don't compress) carotid artery with neck slightly extended for a maximum of 5 s. Test each side in turn.
- **Never attempt bilateral carotid sinus massage!**
- Positive cardioinhibitory response = sinus pause >3 s.
- Positive vasodepressor response = fall in systolic blood pressure >50 mmHg.
- A positive response is seen in 10% of the general elderly population; less than one-quarter of these suffer spontaneous syncope. Do not diagnose CSH unless symptoms are reproduced during CSM and the history supports this diagnosis.
- Treatment is permanent dual-chamber pacing (see Chapter 17 for details of appropriate pacing modes).

Postural hypotension

This involves the failure of normal postural compensatory mechanisms. Hypovolaemia, sympathetic degeneration (e.g. diabetes, Parkinson's, advanced age) and drugs (e.g. vasodilators, neuroleptics) cause or aggravate the condition. Treatment involves removing causative factors, the use of graduated elastic stockings (to reduce venous pooling) and sometimes fludrocortisone (expands blood volume). Advise patients to avoid prolonged standing and to rise slowly.

LV outflow obstruction

- Severe aortic stenosis
- HOCM.

Both conditions cause syncope, because of restriction of cardiac output with exercise and ventricular arrhythmias. Aortic stenosis is sometimes associated with AV block.

Miscellaneous

● **Recurrent pulmonary embolism** is an underdiagnosed cause of syncope.
● **Atrial myxoma/ball valve thrombus** are rare causes of syncope due to
impaired ventricular filling.

NEW MURMURS

Cardiac murmurs are common at the extremes of life. Up to a third of children
have a detectable murmur, usually a pulmonary flow murmur. In the elderly,
valve problems due to ischaemic, rheumatic or degenerative disease are
common. All adults with an unexplained murmur should be investigated.

CLASSIFICATION AND AETIOLOGY

TABLE 11.3 Classification of murmurs

Systole	Midsystolic	Mitral regurgitation, especially mitral valve prolapse* Physiological Flow
	Pansystolic†	Mitral regurgitation Tricuspid regurgitation Ventricular septal defect
	Ejection systolic	Aortic stenosis Outflow tract obstruction, such as subvalvular stenosis Aortic sclerosis Pulmonary stenosis
Diastole	Early diastolic	Aortic regurgitation Pulmonary regurgitation Graham–Steell (pulmonary regurgitation)
	Mid-diastolic	Mitral stenosis* Tricuspid stenosis Austin–Flint (functional mitral stenosis due to aortic regurgitation) Myxoma
	Presystolic	Mitral stenosis, when in sinus rhythm
Continuous		Patent ductus arteriosus Arteriovenous fistulae – coronary, pulmonary Ruptured sinus of Valsalva Venous hums

*Associated with an opening click or snap.
† May be early rather than a truly pansystolic murmur.

HISTORY TAKING

Murmurs are often asymptomatic and discovered during routine medical
examination. New murmurs associated with fever or signs of infection

may merit inpatient investigation in case of endocarditis (see Chapter 8). Check for points that suggest an underlying aetiology or associated structural disease:

- History of rheumatic fever
- History of thyroid disease/anaemia/haemodialysis shunts/arteriovenous malformations/chronic liver disease/pregnancy – associated with flow murmurs
- Previous MI. Mitral regurgitation is common in this group.
- History of congenital disease/syndrome may be associated with valve stenosis and endocardial cushion defects (see Chapter 14).
- Dizziness/syncope may indicate LV outflow obstruction (e.g. HOCM or aortic stenosis).
- Angina is associated with aortic stenosis and IHD with functional (LV dilatation) or dynamic (papillary muscle dysfunction) mitral regurgitation.
- Cardiac failure symptoms imply that the murmur is not benign.

Innocent murmurs are usually ejection in character and are not associated with a precordial thrill, added heart sounds or signs of cardiac enlargement. They can be associated with hyperdynamic circulation (e.g. pregnancy, anaemia, anxiety).

EXAMINATION

This should focus on defining the nature of the murmur and identifying associated atrial fibrillation, structural heart disease and cardiac failure. Also, check for signs of aortic coarctation (radioradial/radiofemoral delay or drop in BP, murmur radiates to back).

INVESTIGATIONS

Echo

This is clearly the single most important investigation. If there is no obvious valve lesion to explain the murmur, recheck the following:

- Peak valve flow velocities (if all ↑, hyperdynamic circulation)
- LV outflow velocity (↑ with LVOT obstruction)
- Pulmonary flow (↑ relative to aortic flow with pulmonary stenosis and left-to-right shunts)
- Descending aorta velocity from suprasternal notch (↑ in coarctation)
- Consider contrast echo if ASD suspected
- Consider transoesophageal echo if images inadequate or if diagnosis not established in patient with *symptomatic* murmur.

ECG

- Atrial fibrillation (common with mitral, less common with aortic valve disease)

- P-mitrale/pulmonale (atrial enlargement associated with mitral and tricuspid valve disease)
- Conduction defects (associated with ASD; see Chapter 14)
- AV block (endocardial cushion defects, aortic valve disease)
- LVH (HOCM, aortic stenosis).

CXR
- Heart size, chamber enlargement
- Aortic contour (aortic root widened with aortic stenosis (poststenotic dilatation) and regurgitation (aortoannular ectasia, Marfan syndrome, syphilis), absent or double aortic knuckle ± rib notching (coarctation))
- Pulmonary masses (arteriovenous malformation)
- Associated signs of cardiac failure.

Laboratory tests
- FBC: anaemia
- TFTs: thyrotoxicosis.

MANAGEMENT

Benign (innocent) murmurs are those for which no structural cause is found. They do not require follow-up. It may help to give the patient a letter stating that the murmur has been fully investigated, as this may have implications for some jobs and for obtaining certain types of insurance.

The management of valve disease is described in Chapters 12 and 13.

REVIEW CONSULTATIONS

RISK FACTOR MANAGEMENT– GENERAL (see also Chapter 12, hypertension and hyperlipidaemia)

This short section accompanies the review clinic consultations and serves as an overview of risk factor management. The future risk of adverse coronary events can be estimated using risk prediction charts (Fig. 12.1). Some specific risk factors are discussed in more detail in individual sections on hypertension, hyperlipidaemia and cardiac rehabilitation.

MODIFIABLE RISK FACTORS

Smoking
Smoking is the most important treatable risk factor. Around 70% of smokers do want to stop completely, but there is no easy method. Counsel about the hazard of smoking (reinfarction rate is two to three times higher among those who continue than in those who quit), set a target (e.g. a date for stopping, or a target reduction in consumption) and follow up to motivate adherence to goals. Often other family members who smoke are the patient's Achilles heel! Behaviour therapy programmes, which involve substituting healthy behaviour for smoking, are helpful but usually not available. Some swear by interventions such as acupuncture and hypnotherapy: trial evidence is scarce, but they may provide a motivation for stopping. Nicotine substitutes (e.g. patches) can help in patients with withdrawal symptoms within 48 hours of smoking cessation, but not for those who lapse after a longer time (psychological factors, not nicotine, are the culprit here). They should be avoided in patients with severe angina or uncontrolled hypertension and for the first 8 weeks afther MI.

Diabetes
Check the notes: abnormal glucose levels are common during MI, but if random glucose was >6.0 mM then fasting glucose should be measured. Insulin is the preferred treatment after MI for diabetic patients in whom diet does not control glucose level (see Chapter 5).

Blood pressure
Do not label with hypertension unless you have at least three abnormal readings spaced a week apart. Treatment threshold is lower in patients with CAD than in those without (systolic >160 mmHg, diastolic >90 mmHg). If possible, increase the dose of β-blocker to avoid polypharmacy. If there is coexisting LV impairment, adjusting ACE inhibitor dose (or, if not tolerated, losartan) upwards is the best approach. Chapter 12 covers hypertension in detail.

Lipids
After MI the reassessment of lipids should be delayed for at least 8 weeks, as

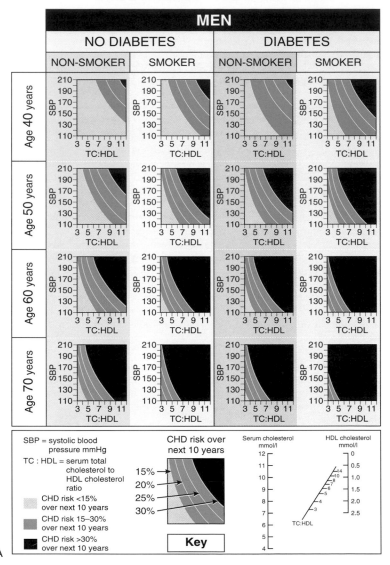

Fig. 12.1 Coronary risk prediction charts. (Adapted from *Heart* 1998;80 (Suppl.2) with permission.)

CORONARY RISK PREDICTION CHART

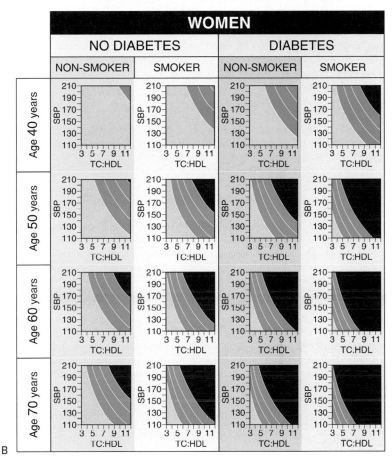

Fig. 12.1 (cont'd)

total cholesterol and especially HDL are lowered by the metabolic effects of MI. The target level for total cholesterol has steadily decreased as more trial data have become available. For secondary prevention, most centres now use threshold total cholesterol levels of 5.2 mmol l^{-1} (based on the 4S trial, using **simvastatin** 20–40 mg at night) or 4.8 mmol l^{-1} (based on the CARE trial, using **pravastatin** 40 mg at night) after a trial of dietary modification for initiation or titration of lipid-lowering medication. Simvastatin, pravastatin and atorvastatin are the agents with the greatest evidence base for reducing coronary risk. Recent evidence is that statins may lower the relative risk of coronary events by around 30%, regardless of the starting cholesterol level (LIPID trial, **pravastatin** 40 mg at night). Fibrates (e.g. **bezafibrate** 400 mg d^{-1}) can be used if statins are not tolerated, and in mixed hyperlipidaemias. The effect of a new lipid-lowering agent or dose adjustment should be assessed after approximately 8 weeks. Primary and secondary prevention is discussed in detail in Chapter 12.

Obesity
This is diagnosed from body mass index (BMI): weight (kg)/height(m)^2. Grade 1 obesity = BMI 25–30 kg/m^2. Grade 2 = 30–40 kg/m^2. Grade 3 = >40 kg/m^2. Obesity is arguably an independent risk factor, but its association with diabetes, hyperlipidaemia, hypertension and reduced effort tolerance renders this argument academic.

Sedentary lifestyle
Although it is debatable whether physical exercise is an *independent* modifier of coronary risk, there is no doubt that sedentary individuals are at higher risk of CAD. Exercise serves to reduce weight, total cholesterol and blood pressure and increases HDL cholesterol. The result is that individuals with a sedentary lifestyle have roughly twice the risk of death from CAD as those with a physically active lifestyle. Most exercise programmes recommend at least three sessions of aerobic exercise (e.g. brisk walking, jogging, swimming, aerobics class) of 30 minutes per week. Clearly the level of exercise has to be tailored to the individual's ability and the type of exercise should be one that the individual enjoys, otherwise it is unlikely they will keep it going. In patients with established CAD it is sensible to base recommendations for exercise on stress test results. Exercise will be discussed in more detail in Chapter 15 (cardiac rehabilitation).

NON-MODIFIABLE RISK FACTORS

Family history
First-degree relatives of MI sufferers aged <70 years have a relative risk of CAD 2.2 times higher than normal. It is sensible that they pay close attention to modifiable risk factors to minimize this risk. There is no role for stress testing in this group unless symptoms are present.

Age
Around 80% of fatal MIs occur in patients aged over 65. As these patients' absolute risk of coronary events is high, correction of modifiable risk factors will have proportionately more effect in this group and advanced age is not an excuse for less rigorous attention to risk factor management. In the presence

of comorbidity the benefits of risk factor modification should be weighed against the patient's overall life expectancy.

Gender

Coronary events and coronary deaths are approximately twice as common in men as in women, although the risk in women increases more steeply after the menopause. Once coronary disease is clinically manifest, however, women have a similar or slightly worse prognosis than men. Although male gender is a risk factor, management of modifiable risk factors does not generally differ between males and females.

Hormone replacement therapy (HRT) is a controversial issue in cardiology. HRT increases HDL cholesterol and may prevent oxidation of LDL. There is evidence that HRT may prevent the development of coronary atheroma and coronary events in postmenopausal women when given over a long period; a meta-analysis of primary prevention studies suggests a relative risk of 0.6 for the development of symptomatic coronary disease in postmenopausal oestrogen users. This needs to be weighed against a potential early prothrombotic effect and an increased risk of endometrial cancer (which may be partly offset by combined oestrogen/progestogen therapy) and breast cancer (in patients with a past history or family history of breast cancer). There is currently little information about the effects of HRT in secondary prevention. The American College of Physicians currently advocates the use of HRT in postmenopausal women at high risk of CAD or osteoporosis and who are not at high risk of breast cancer.

POST-MI FOLLOW-UP

This is a key consultation which assesses patients' progress, risk and long-term management. Patients are usually seen 4–8 weeks after the MI, when they may be discharged if well, so it is critical to pay attention to detail. Begin with open-ended questions to give the patient the freedom to voice concerns, and then focus on the key points below.

Objectives of review

- Assess recovery and progress
  physical
  social (return to work, social and sexual activities)
  psychological (anxiety, depression, understanding of condition)
- Assess and treat symptoms
- Assess and (if necessary) modify coronary risk factors
- Assess risk of future coronary events
- Plan revascularization if appropriate
- Explain, set goals, plan discharge or subsequent management.

BEFORE CONSULTATION

Ensure that you are familiar with:

- Territory and extent of MI
- ECG, CXR and echo results from admission
- Risk factor profile
- Patient's previous level of activity
- Patient's occupation
- Discharge medications.

CONSULTATION

History

Assess recovery and progress

- Ask about physical recovery: 'Are you getting back to your normal activities?'
- Ask about effort tolerance.
- If progress is slow, ask why. The patient may be afraid to exercise, or be restricted by a well-meaning but overprotective spouse, rather than by physical symptoms.
- Ask about interests and activities and whether these have been resumed.
- Return to work depends on the type of work and the completeness of recovery. With less physical jobs, 4–6 weeks off work is advisable. For some it is more stressful to be off work for weeks than to return early, so don't be too dogmatic. With physical jobs (e.g. manual work, heavy lifting, or with a lot of walking/climbing stairs), defer the return to work until after stress testing.
- Many patients do not resume social activities because of loss of confidence or self-esteem, physical symptoms, fear of a heart attack or the social environment (smoking and drinking.) Sexual activity is a difficult issue: most patients will not broach it at all. Fear of sex provoking a heart attack is common, as is male impotence after MI. Your approach needs care: older patients, and those of the opposite sex to you, may find questions offensive or embarrassing.

> **Tip:** Depression affects one in five patients after MI. Depressed patients are up to five times more likely to die in the first 6 months.

- Anxiety is common: fear of death, further MI, inability to work and chronic illness are common triggers. A useful aid is the Hospital Anxiety and Depression (HAD) questionnaire, which is quick to use and will identify most cases. Anxiety may arise from misunderstanding of the illness or the implications of having a heart attack, so take time to address this in plain language.

Assessing symptoms

Postinfarct angina

- This is prognostically important: patients have a twofold higher mortality and rate of MI.
- Ensure compliance.
- Advise to use GTN before exercise.
- Ensure adequate β-blockade: aim for a resting heart rate 50–60 bpm.
- Add: long-acting nitrate (e.g. **isosorbide mononitrate** 60 mg od) OR long-acting calcium channel blocker (e.g. if β-blocked, **amlodipine** 5–10 mg od, OR, if not β-blocked, **diltiazem** LA 200–300 mg od), OR potassium channel opener (e.g. **nicorandil** 10 mg bd).

Post-MI chest discomfort can be caused by post-MI (Dressler) syndrome (see Chapter 5), or may be anxiety related.

Breathlessness

- On exertion usually reflects ischaemic LV dysfunction.
- Was echo done before discharge? Is ACE inhibitor indicated?
- Examination and CXR will identify congestion requiring a diuretic.
- If symptoms, examination findings and echo don't add up (e.g. marked dyspnoea and mild LV impairment), consider:
    ischaemic LV dysfunction
    mitral incompetence (papillary muscle infarction)
    bronchospasm (due to β-blocker)
    anaemia.

Palpitation

- May reflect heightened awareness of a normal heartbeart or extrasystoles (see Chapter 1).
- Ask about relation to exercise (may reflect ischaemic or catecholamine-driven VT).
- Presyncope or syncope are ominous and often reflect malignant arrhythmia.
- Ambulatory monitoring and stress testing (make sure you have IV access before you start!) are helpful in establishing a diagnosis.

Fatigue

- Very common after MI.
- May reflect:
    a slow but normal recovery
    loss of general physical fitness

Warning: If patient has unstable post-MI angina (see Chapter 5), admission to hospital for stabilization is mandatory.

LV impairment
depression
side effect of medication (especially β-blockers and diltiazem)
- Check haemoglobin!

Examination
This should focus on identifying signs of cardiac enlargement, heart failure, new murmurs (e.g. mitral regurgitation), atrial fibrillation and hypertension.

MANAGEMENT

Risk assessment
This means the risk of death or further MI. The usual screening method is a treadmill ETT (see Chapter 16). If patient can't manage, or the baseline ECG precludes interpretation, a stress myocardial perfusion scan or stress echo are useful. For patients over 70, in whom the risk of invasive assessment is higher, it is reasonable to guide management by clinical assessment alone.

If ETT shows early ischaemia (flat or downsloping ST depression ≥ 2 mm in lead group at workload <6 METs, or persistent ST/T-wave changes >5 min in recovery, or fall in systolic BP >10 mmHg), this indicates a high risk and angiography should be considered. For stress perfusion scanning or stress echo, multiple reversible perfusion/wall motion defects signify multivessel coronary disease and angiography should be considered.

Risk factor assessment
Coronary risk factors need to be dealt with and explained. See Chapter 12.

Basic investigations
- **ECG. Always compare with predischarge ECG.** Look for new atrial fibrillation, evidence of infarct extension (if so, ask if further episode of infarct-type pain), persistent ST segment elevation to suggest LV aneurysm.
- **CXR. Always compare with previous CXR.** Look for pulmonary congestion, pleural effusions, increasing heart size, prominent LV border (? LV aneurysm).
- **Echo.** Indicated if echo was not performed during admission, or if there is new heart failure or reduced effort tolerance. Look for:
  – wall motion defects
  – LV dilatation
  – LV aneurysm
  – new mitral regurgitation.
- **Bloods.** Check U&Es and creatinine in patients on diuretics/ACE inhibitors. Lipids and glucose are discussed in Chapter 12, risk factors.

Making a management plan
Be honest with the patient and set realistic goals (see also Chapter 15,

components of rehabilitation). Patients with severe cardiac impairment after MI need to know that they may not get much better, so that they can plan work, finances, housing and social activities. It isn't easy to break such news, but subsequent management is easier because the patient has no unrealistic expectations. Conversely, a positive approach helps with patients who are slow to progress but who have a satisfactory assessment.

- **If clinical assessment and stress test are satisfactory** the patient can be discharged. Ensure he/she knows the prognosis is good, the reason for and duration of treatment with medications and has targets to work towards for risk factor modification. Aspirin is continued indefinitely. β-Blockers confer the most benefit in the first year and should be continued indefinitely if tolerated. ACE inhibitors for LV dysfunction are continued indefinitely.
- **At discharge**, make the management plan clear to the GP.
- **Postinfarct angina** can be managed medically if ETT is reassuring, but a follow-up visit should be scheduled. If symptoms persist despite medical treatment angiography may be needed despite the ETT result.
- **If stress test is positive** angiography may be needed. Explain this is to allow planning of future management. Explain the risks of the procedure, but also that not investigating may carry a risk by depriving the patient of optimal treatment.
- **Slow recovery** may necessitate referral for rehabilitation. A staged exercise programme may help and psychological input may be needed if anxiety is a prominent factor.

UNSTABLE ANGINA FOLLOW-UP

This roughly follows the principles of post-MI management (see previous section). For patients treated conservatively follow-up should be 2–3 weeks after discharge. For patients treated with PTCA, follow-up should be at 6–8 weeks (if restenosis occurs this tends to be in first 2 months), with an option of an earlier visit if symptoms are a concern.

Objectives of review
- Assess recovery
- Assess and treat symptoms
- Assess and (if necessary) modify coronary risk factors
- Assess risk of future coronary events
- Plan revascularization if appropriate
- Educate patient: advise about impact of condition on lifestyle, work, physical and social activities.

BEFORE CONSULTATION

Ensure that you are familiar with:

- Territory of ischaemia during previous admission
- ECG (± CXR and echo) results from admission
- Risk factor profile
- Patient's previous level of activity
- Patient's occupation
- Discharge medications.

CONSULTATION

History

Assess recovery
- Assess physical and psychological recovery.
- Assess effort tolerance.
- Identify activities that bring on angina, if any.
- As with MI, return to work depends on the type of work and symptoms. A rough guide is:
    - if angina is well controlled, for less physical jobs 2–4 weeks off work
    - for physical jobs defer return to work until after stress testing, unless a definitive procedure (e.g. PTCA) was done during admission.
- Psychological reaction to UA may be similar to that in post-MI patient, although depression is less common. Ask about mood and anxieties regarding health and, if suspicious, screen with HAD questionnaire.

Assess symptoms

Chest pain
- **Recurrent angina** is prognostically important. In patients treated conservatively the decision about angiography depends on the severity of symptoms and stress testing.
- **Occasional or mild angina** is treated by increasing antianginal medication (maximize existing medication, especially β-blocker, rather than adding to regimen). Assess with ETT or stress myocardial perfusion scan/stress echo.
- **Episodic rest angina** in an otherwise stable patient suggests intermittent coronary spasm. A long-acting nitrate (e.g. **isosorbide mononitrate** 60 mg d^{-1}) or calcium channel antagonist (e.g. **amlodipine** 5–10 mg d^{-1}) may help.
- **Frequent or severe** typical angina probably merits assessment with angiography, regardless of the ETT result.
- **Atypical** symptoms are harder to assess and stress testing should determine whether angiography is warranted.
- **In patients initially treated with PTCA** limiting angina normally warrants

Warning: If any severe or prolonged episode of 'angina' since discharge, look for evidence of MI on ECG ± echo.

repeat angiography to identify restenosis at site. ETT/stress perfusion scan/stress echo is helpful to confirm that the ischaemic territory matches the site of the presumed 'culprit' stenosis.

> **Tip:** Keep an open mind about the original diagnosis of unstable angina, especially if symptoms are atypical or if there are no accompanying ECG features.

Breathlessness
- May reflect:
    ischaemic LV dysfunction (i.e. 'angina equivalent')
    LV impairment, reflecting MI since discharge.
- Consider ETT and echo to assess for these.

> **Tip:** Examination should focus on identifying signs of heart failure, new murmurs (e.g. mitral regurgitation), atrial fibrillation and hypertension.

MANAGEMENT

Risk assessment
- For patients treated conservatively during admission who have not had a predischarge stress test, an ETT or pharmacological stress test is required (see Chapter 16).
- The need for stress testing is questionable in patients who have had angioplasty and/or stenting, because angiography will already have shown whether a high-risk pattern of disease (necessitating CABG) is present. If not, the only reason to proceed to repeat angiography is on the basis of recurrent symptoms. The exception to this is in patients who hold a vocational licence (e.g. heavy goods vehicle).

Risk factor assessment
Risk factors should be the main focus of the consultation (see earlier).

Basic investigations
- **ECG. Always compare with predischarge ECG.** Look for new atrial fibrillation, new Q waves or T-wave inversion to suggest infarction since discharge (ask about any severe or prolonged episodes of 'angina').
- **CXR** is not necessary unless you suspect either MI or the development of heart failure since discharge.
- **Echo** is indicated if breathlessness is a prominent symptom, or if you suspect MI has occurred from the history or ECG. Look for wall motion defects, LV dilatation, new mitral regurgitation, unsuspected aortic stenosis.
- **Laboratory tests**. Fasting blood glucose may need checking if level high

during admission. Assuming they were assessed and any necessary treatment was started during admission, lipids do not need to be rechecked unless 2 months have elapsed (see hyperlipidaemia section for details).

Making a management plan

This should have several components:

- Decision about the need to proceed to angiography, based on symptoms and stress testing.
- Adjustment of any pharmacological treatment for coronary risk factors (e.g. intensifying lipid-lowering or antihypertensive therapy).
- Advice about lifestyle modification if needed (smoking, diet, exercise, alcohol).
- Individual attention to circumstances. Clearly, the decision whether to proceed to invasive management is partly dictated by circumstance. A young manual labourer and an elderly, sedentary man will have different perceptions of health, given the same symptom limitation.
- You may see patients who are on maximum medication whose coronary disease is not amenable to invasive treatment. These patients need to know, so that they can reappraise their lives. Again, be honest and realistic: it is much easier if the patient does not have unrealistic expectations of you and of their treatment. Be positive and focus on what they *can* achieve.
- **If clinical assessment and stress test are satisfactory** the patient can be discharged. Aspirin should be continued indefinitely. Antianginal treatment is there for symptom control; advise that the GP be informed prior to any attempt to reduce medication. At discharge, make the management plan clear to the GP and advise on risk factors that need monitoring.
- **If stress test is positive** angiography may be needed to plan management. Explain the risks of angiography, but also that not investigating may carry a risk by depriving the patient of optimal treatment.

> Tip: The balance of risk and benefit for angiography is not the same in all patients with a positive ETT. Angiography is sensible in a symptomatic but otherwise fit patient with an early positive ETT, because the prognosis and symptoms may be altered by CABG. The same is not true for an older, asymptomatic patient with chronic lung disease because CABG may not be an option anyway.

Explain:

- Your management plan (in terms of risk and benefit)
- About the importance of managing risk factors
- About the advisability and timing of return to work
- About medications, their purpose and the common side effects.

STABLE ANGINA FOLLOW-UP

Angina is the most common symptom of IHD. It affects 6% of men and 4% of women aged between 45 and 59 years. This figure rises to 20% of men and women aged between 65 and 74 years. Thirty percent of patients with recent-onset angina have a significant cardiac event within 1–2 years. Treatment should be directed at the control of symptoms and improvement of prognosis. This can involve drug therapy, risk factor modification and revascularization. Patients with stable angina who have adequately controlled symptoms and who are assessed as having a low risk of coronary events do not require regular review.

Objectives of review
- Assess and treat symptoms
- Assess and (if necessary) modify coronary risk factors
- Assess risk of future coronary events
- Plan revascularization if appropriate
- Educate patient; advise about impact of condition on lifestyle, work, physical and social activities.

BEFORE CONSULTATION

Ensure that you are familiar with:

- Previous ECG
- Previous risk assessment (e.g. ETT, angiogram results)
- Risk factor profile
- Patient's usual level of activity
- Current medication.

CONSULTATION

History

Assess symptoms
- Frequency and severity of anginal episodes
- Effort tolerance
- Associated symptoms (e.g. breathlessness, palpitation, syncope)
- Impact of these on daily activities, work and social activity
- Check for pattern of crescendo or unstable angina – may require admission.

Examination
This should focus on identifying hypertension, signs of heart failure, murmurs (e.g. aortic stenosis), adequacy of heart rate control if taking β-blocker, and atrial fibrillation.

MANAGEMENT

Secondary prevention

Antiplatelet therapy
A meta-analysis of antiplatelet trials by the Antiplatelet Trialists Collaboration has shown that **aspirin** 75–325 mg d^{-1} significantly reduces the risk of coronary events in patients with established coronary disease. For patients who are intolerant of aspirin, **clopidrogel** 75 mg d^{-1} is an effective alternative.

Risk factor assessment
Risk factors should be the main focus of the consultation (see earlier).

Symptom control

There are four major classes of antianginal drugs: β-blockers, nitrates, calcium channel antagonists and potassium channel activators. All are effective at controlling symptoms. β-Blockers are usually used as first-line treatment. The introduction of a second drug improves symptoms but the benefit is modest. There is little evidence that addition of a third or fourth drug is helpful. Once-daily or sustained-release preparations should be used wherever possible to aid compliance.

β-Blockers
There is no randomized trial evidence that β-blockers improve *survival* in patients with isolated stable angina. However, risk *is* reduced in patients with hypertension or acute MI, and for this reason, β-blockers are used as a first-line treatment. Some third generation cardioselective β-blockers (e.g. carvedilol, bisoprolol) have also been shown to improve survival in patients with associated LV dysfunction. For patients with angina and normal LV function, proprietary β-blockers such as atenolol or metoprolol are also suitable first-line agents.

> **Tip:** Because of receptor upregulation caused by β-blockade, patients should not be withdrawn from β-blockers suddenly. This can cause a rebound tachycardia or hypertension and may aggravate angina.

Nitrates
Sublingual or buccal nitrates produce rapid and effective relief of angina. All patients should be shown how to use a sublingual nitrate preparation. Buccal preparations give more protracted release of the nitrate and are appropriate for prolonged activities that might induce angina.

Long-acting nitrates (e.g. **isosorbide mononitrate** LA 60–120 mg d^{-1}) are effective prophylaxis against angina. Nitrate tolerance can develop and a nitrate-free period of at least 8 hours is necessary to prevent this.

Calcium channel antagonists

Patients who are intolerant of a β-blocker should be prescribed a rate-limiting calcium channel antagonist, e.g. **diltiazem** (LA 300 mg od) or **verapamil** (SR 240 mg od). There is some evidence that these agents improve outcome after non-Q wave MI in the absence of heart failure. There is some concern that calcium channel antagonists can aggravate heart failure. **Amlodipine** (5–10 mg d^{-1}) is known to be relatively safe in these patients (PRAISE study).

Potassium channel activators

These novel antianginal agents are coronary vasodilators and may have added cardioprotective actions (related to ischaemic preconditioning). Currently, nicorandil is the only preparation of this class in clinical use. It is effective in the treatment of angina and has both nitrate and potassium channel opening properties.

RISK STRATIFICATION AND CONSIDERATION FOR REVASCULARIZATION

Patients with a new diagnosis of angina merit risk assessment to determine whether revascularization would improve their prognosis. Also, patients with previously stable angina who deteriorate, or patients in whom medical therapy fails to control symptoms, should be considered for angiography (see Chapter 18).

Risk stratification initially involves the assessment of clinical risk predictors (e.g. recent MI, LV dysfunction) and non-invasive stress testing. For most patients treadmill stress testing is used (see Chapter 16), although a stress myocardial perfusion scan is helpful if the ECG is difficult to interpret, or if the patient cannot manage the exercise protocol (see Chapter 20). Stress echo (see Chapter 19) is also a useful alternative. In addition, low-dose dobutamine stress echo can help identify viable non-contracting myocardium in patients with LV dysfunction.

INDICATIONS FOR ANGIOGRAPHY

Indications for angiography are covered in Chapter 18. However, guidelines cannot cover all clinical situations and each case needs to be considered individually. There are some patients who suffer ischaemic-type chest pain in whom non-invasive investigations are negative. These patients may be recurrently admitted to hospital because of their symptoms. In this setting a coronary angiogram can be helpful in excluding obstructive coronary artery disease, removing uncertainty about the diagnosis, reassuring the patient and reducing the consumption of health-care resources.

LEFT-SIDED VALVULAR HEART DISEASE

Patients with minor valve disease (e.g. mild mitral or aortic regurgitation, tricuspid regurgitation) do not require regular review. Some valve pathologies are associated with disease progression and patients should be reviewed every 2–3 years (e.g. small VSD, bicuspid aortic valve, mild pulmonary stenosis). Patients with significant mitral or aortic valve disease should be seen on at least an annual basis.

Objectives of review

- Identify disease progression through H_x, examination and screening tests
- Educate patient about potential symptoms of disease progression
- Educate patient about dental hygiene and antibiotic prophylaxis
- Prescribe medication (e.g. digoxin, warfarin) if appropriate
- Assess need for valve repair/replacement

BEFORE CONSULTATION

Ensure that you are familiar with:
- Nature of the valve lesions
- Symptoms and signs at last consultation
- Cardiac rhythm at last consultation
- Previous CXR and echo findings
- Maintenance medications.

CONSULTATION

History

- Effort tolerance: absolute level and any change from last review?
- Breathlessness: on exertion, orthopnoea, nocturnal
- Fatigue
- Dizziness/syncope: ominous signs in aortic valve disease
- Chest pain
- Palpitation: may indicate atrial fibrillation (especially mitral valve disease) or ventricular arrhythmia (especially aortic valve disease)
- Systemic embolism: e.g. TIAs, amaurosis fugax.

Examination

This should focus on identifying pulmonary congestion, atrial fibrillation, altered or new murmurs (e.g. aortic stenosis), signs of pulmonary hypertension and right-sided cardiac failure.

Investigations

The following investigations are helpful at each key review assessment:

- **ECG**
    - new atrial fibrillation, rate control
    - AV block (aortic valve disease)

- signs of atrial enlargement (P-pulmonale, P-mitrale)
- LVH (aortic valve disease), RVH (mitral/pulmonary valve disease)
- **CXR** Always compare with previous CXR, if possible with those taken several years previously, as subtle changes in cardiac size and contour may be more apparent.
  - increase in cardiothoracic ratio?
  - chamber enlargement?
  - pulmonary congestion?
- **Echo** (see Chapter 19 for echo assessment of valve disease)
  - identify progression of valve disease
  - identify sequelae of valve disease (LV, RV dysfunction, atrial enlargement, pulmonary hypertension)
- **Cardiac catheterization** Indications for cardiac catheterization are given under 'Management'. Cardiac catheterization provides useful quantitative information about the severity of valve lesions, LV dysfunction and pulmonary hypertension (see Chapter 18). It also documents coronary anatomy in case concurrent CABG is indicated. It is contraindicated in patients with aortic valve endocarditis because of the risk of coronary and systemic embolism.

MANAGEMENT

Aortic stenosis

The frequency of surveillance depends on the severity of stenosis. Asymptomatic patients with mild aortic stenosis (peak gradient <30 mmHg) require only yearly or 2-yearly assessment, focusing on echo estimation of valve gradient. Patients with severe (peak gradient ≥ 60 mmHg) aortic stenosis may require 6-monthly assessment. Patients with moderate or severe aortic stenosis should be advised to avoid strenuous physical activity (especially explosive activity, e.g. heavy lifting) and competitive sport. Associated hypertension should be treated either with a β-blocker or a diuretic. Vasodilators should be avoided if possible.

If symptoms (e.g. breathlessness, chest pain or syncope) develop then the patient should be reviewed immediately. If the patient is otherwise suitable for valve surgery, he or she should promptly undergo cardiac catheterization with a view to this.

> **Tip:** Don't forget to tell the patient about antibiotic prophylaxis in valvular heart disease (see Chapter 19).

Aortic or mitral regurgitation

Stable patients should be reviewed annually, with CXR and echo. There is limited evidence that vasodilators (e.g. ACE inhibitors or nifedipine) improve symptoms and prevent LV dilatation by reducing afterload and regurgitant volume. Symptomatic patients, or asymptomatic patients with evidence of LV dilatation (progressive cardiomegaly on CXR, or LV end-systolic dimension >55 mm, or LVEF <55%), should be considered for cardiac catheterization with a view to valve replacement or, in some cases of mitral regurgitation, valve repair.

Mitral stenosis

Asymptomatic patients should be reviewed annually to monitor valve area and to identify pulmonary hypertension (by assessing tricuspid regurgitant flow; see Chapter 19). Intervention should be considered in patients with limiting symptoms or mitral valve area <1.0 cm^2. Patients with atrial fibrillation should receive warfarin, aiming for INR 2.0–3.0. Patients with significant mitral stenosis *in sinus rhythm* should receive warfarin if there is evidence of systemic embolism, spontaneous contrast in the left atrium, or a low-output state and right heart failure. Patients with a mitral valve orifice area <1.5 cm^2 can be reviewed every 6 months to identify disease progression early.

Valve surgery

Emergency valve replacement should be considered in patients with:

- Critical aortic stenosis with pulmonary oedema, syncope or angina
- Severe acute mitral or aortic regurgitation – usually associated with chordal rupture (see Chapter 4) or endocarditis (see Chapter 8).

Elective valve replacement should be considered in patients with:

- Limiting symptoms due to valve disease
- Asymptomatic or minimally symptomatic valve disease and evidence of LV dilatation/compromise, pulmonary hypertension or critical aortic stenosis.

Mitral valve repair should be considered in preference to valve replacement, as the operative risk is lower and LV function better preserved after surgery. TOE provides a detailed assessment of leaflet anatomy and helps the surgeon decide whether repair is possible (see Chapter 19). Patients with mitral valve prolapse are particularly suitable for valve repair.

Percutaneous balloon mitral valvuloplasty can be used to treat patients with symptomatic mitral stenosis in whom the valve is not heavily calcified and when there is no significant mitral regurgitation. Valvuloplasty is hazardous if there is evidence of atrial thrombus or systemic embolism; TOE helps delineate valve anatomy and identifies thrombus in the left atrial appendage. Thickened or rigid valve leaflets, or chordal fusion, are associated with a poorer outcome from valvuloplasty, with a significant risk of iatrogenic severe mitral regurgitation and the need for emergency valve replacement (see Chapter 19).

> **Tip:** Patients being considered for valve replacement should be reviewed by a
> dentist and appropriate dental work undertaken before valve surgery is
> performed.

RIGHT-SIDED VALVULAR HEART DISEASE

Right-sided valvular disease is often overlooked as right-sided valve stenoses
are relatively rare and tricuspid and pulmonary regurgitation usually
asymptomatic. However, patients with rheumatic heart disease may have
right-sided valve lesions contributing to symptoms and right heart
endocarditis is increasingly common in IV drug abusers. A systematic clinical
approach and attention to the right heart during echo are essential to detect
these lesions.

TRICUSPID INCOMPETENCE (TI)

The most common cause is tricuspid annular dilatation due to right heart
failure and pulmonary hypertension. In this situation severe TI can aggravate
heart failure by diminishing right-sided output against increased pulmonary
vascular resistance.

Other causes of tricuspid incompetence
Rheumatic heart disease
Infective endocarditis
Ebstein's anomaly (see below)
Congenital (often cleft valve)
SLE
Carcinoid syndrome
Marfan's syndrome
Papillary muscle dysfunction
Cardiac tumours

Symptoms
- Fatigue/↓ effort tolerance
- Neck pulsation, headache
- Abdominal and lower limb swelling.

Signs
- (Often) weight loss, muscle wasting – cardiac cachexia
- JVP with prominent systolic wave, sharp y-descent
- Atrial fibrillation; if sinus rhythm, a-wave in JVP may be prominent
- Parasternal heave and loud P_2 signify pulmonary hypertension
- (Sometimes) PSM at left sternal border, accentuated by inspiration

- (Sometimes) jaundice, hepatomegaly
- Ascites
- Peripheral oedema.

Echo (see Chapter 19)
- Use short-axis view (aortic root level) and four-chamber view
- TI jet velocity mirrors PA pressure
- Look for Ebstein's anomaly, RV dilatation, prolapse, vegetations, valve stenosis.

Management
Antibiotic prophylaxis is only needed if there is structural (e.g. rheumatic) valve disease.

Surgery is not usually needed. Loop diuretics, spironolactone and digoxin can be used for right heart failure and atrial fibrillation. Tricuspid annuloplasty is the preferred surgical treatment, in which a rigid ring is used to support a dilated annulus. Alternatively a large bioprosthesis can be implanted. For tricuspid endocarditis leaflet excision is surprisingly well tolerated, allowing several weeks of antimicrobial therapy prior to insertion of a prosthesis.

EBSTEIN'S ANOMALY

In this congenital tricuspid valve defect the tricuspid leaflet attachments are sited within the RV. The valve tissue is abnormal and the cusps adhere to the RV wall, leading to TI. A segment of the RV is 'atrialized' and lies above the tricuspid valve. Sometimes asymptomatic, it usually presents between infancy (poor prognosis) and early adulthood. There is a wide spectrum of clinical presentations. Ebstein's anomaly is associated with:

- Other cardiac lesions
    PFO or secundum ASD
    pulmonary stenosis/atresia
    cushion defect (primum ASD, VSD)
    congenitally corrected great vessel transposition
    right-sided accessory pathways
- Right-sided cardiac failure
- Arrhythmias: SVTs and right ventricular tachycardia.

ECG
- RBBB with first-degree AV block and P-pulmonale
- Type B (LBBB pattern) Wolff–Parkinson–White syndrome.

Echo
- Inferior displacement of tricuspid leaflet attachments, relative to mitral valve

- Delayed tricuspid valve closure (relative to mitral)
- TI and right ventricular dilatation.

Cardiac catheterization
Rarely needed to confirm diagnosis; ventricular arrhythmias often induced.

Management
Antibiotic prophylaxis against endocarditis indicated.

In adulthood tricuspid annuloplasty and valve reconstruction can be considered, along with ASD closure (if present) and plication of atrialized RV free wall tissue. This is recommended for symptomatic patients and patients with progressive cardiomegaly.

TRICUSPID STENOSIS (TS)

Almost always rheumatic, TS is invariably associated with TI. Functionally significant TS is evident in about 5% of patients with rheumatic heart disease. The ECG shows signs of right atrial (P-pulmonale) or biatrial (tall, bifid P waves) dilatation, or atrial fibrillation. CXR shows cardiomegaly with prominent right heart border and prominent SVC.

Symptoms
- Similar to TI; heart failure due to RV inflow obstruction rather than RV volume overload.

Signs
- Right heart failure, cardiac cachexia, as with TI.
- JVP – prominent a-wave in sinus rhythm, slow y-descent.
- Opening snap, MDM at lower LSE; often drowned out by louder mitral sounds.
- Murmur louder on inspiration and after exertion.

Echo (see Chapter 19)
- **2D**: thickened leaflets, doming in diastole, reduced diastolic separation
- **Doppler**: ↑ pressure half time and peak diastolic velocity.

Cardiac catheterization
- RA angiogram helps delineate valve structure
- PA pressure
- *Mean* diastolic transvalve gradient >2 mmHg confirms diagnosis.

Management
Antibiotic prophylaxis against endocarditis indicated.

As with TI the initial management is as for right heart failure. Tricuspid valvuloplasty, commisurotomy or valve replacement are surgical treatment options.

PULMONARY STENOSIS (PS)

Pulmonary stenosis can be subvalvar, valvular or supravalvar. The most common form is congenital, which is often associated with other cardiac defects. The ECG usually shows sinus rhythm with P-pulmonale, RVH and RBBB. CXR shows poststenotic PA dilatation, oligaemic lung fields and, in severe cases, massive cardiomegaly.

TABLE 12.1 Causes and associations of pulmonary stenosis

Defect	Association
Supravalvar pulmonary artery stenosis	Supravalvar aortic stenosis
Rheumatic pulmonary valve stenosis	Other rheumatic lesions (especially mitral)
Non-rheumatic pulmonary valve stenosis	Often isolated Noonan's syndrome Fallot's tetralogy Congenital rubella Carcinoid plaque disease
Infundibular pulmonary stenosis	Fallot's tetralogy (component) VSD Pulmonary valve stenosis

Symptoms
- Depends on the severity of stenosis and associatied lesions. Isolated PS can cause right heart failure symptoms and childhood growth retardation.
- Occasionally 'right heart' angina occurs with severe PS.

Signs
- May be dysmorphic: Noonan syndrome: hypertelorism, short stature, web neck, lymphoedema.
- Right heart failure, as with TI.
- JVP – often 'v'-wave of associated TI, prominent a-wave.
- Palpation – parasternal lift due to RV hypertrophy/dilatation.
- Ejection click (valvular PS only), ESM in pulmonary area and posteriorly, wide split S_2.
- In severe PS S_4 appears (due to RVH) and murmur is more prolonged.
- Murmur is louder on inspiration and after exertion.

Echo (see Chapter 19)
- **High short-axis view**: leaflets thickened, poststenotic dilatation
- **CW Doppler**: pre-:post-valve velocity ratio >1.5:1
- **PW Doppler**: helps assess level of stenosis
- **General**: associated VSD, pulmonary incompetence, mitral lesions.

Cardiac catheterization
- Confirm severity and level of stenosis.
- Saturation 'run' to exclude intracardiac shunt.
- RV angiogram helps document RV systolic function.
- Left-sided catheterization may be needed to study concomitant aortic stenosis.

Management
Antibiotic prophylaxis against endocarditis indicated.

Pulmonary valvuloplasty is an effective treatment for valvular stenosis with resting gradient >60 mmHg. Surgical infundibular resection is indicated for severe infundibular stenosis.

PULMONARY INCOMPETENCE (PI)

Pulmonary incompetence is usually due to pulmonary hypertension and annular dilatation. It can worsen RV failure because of volume overload. PI without pulmonary hypertension is usually well tolerated. Symptoms and physical findings are largely dictated by the presence or absence of pulmonary hypertension. The ECG is similar to that of pulmonary stenosis. CXR may show enlarged pulmonary arteries and cardiomegaly due to right-sided chamber enlargement.

Other causes of pulmonary incompetence

Pulmonary artery dilatation: (idiopathic, Marfan syndrome)
Congenital defect: (absent or malformed leaflets)
Infective endocarditis: iatrogenic (e.g. Fallot's correction)
Rheumatic (rare): carcinoid syndrome (rare)

Symptoms
- Usually relate to primary cause (e.g. mitral stenosis, chronic lung disease)
- Exertional dyspnoea, fatigue
- Often asymptomatic.

Signs
- JVP (severe PI) – 'v'-wave of associated TI, prominent a-wave
- Visible and palpable RV heave, PA pulsation upper left chest
- Right heart failure (severe PI only)
- Non-valvular ejection click (PA expands), loud P_2
- Wide split S_2 (prolonged ejection time), sometimes S_3, S_4
- **With pulmonary hypertension: high-pitched**, decrescendo EDM at upper LSE (Graham–Steell murmur); may be tricuspid PSM
- **Without pulmonary hypertension: low-pitched**, rising and falling EDM at upper LSE
- Murmurs louder on inspiration.

Echo (see Chapter 19)
- **High short-axis view**: colour Doppler shows 'candle flame' jet.
- **CW/PW Doppler**: regurgitant flow in RVOT (velocity declines slowly in pulmonary hypertension, rapidly if PA pressure normal).
- **General**: RV dilatation, TI velocity (associated pulmonary hypertension).

Cardiac catheterization

Not usually required unless uncertain about associated pulmonary hypertension.

MANAGEMENT

Antibiotic prophylaxis only needed if structural (e.g. rheumatic) valve disease.

Most cases do not need treatment. Valve replacement is only indicated in intractable right heart failure.

PROSTHETIC VALVES

Patients with prosthetic valves require regular review to monitor symptoms and valve and LV function. Tissue prostheses in particular have a limited lifespan (~10 years) and regular surveillance helps detect signs of deterioration. Most patients are reviewed annually.

BEFORE CONSULTATION

Ensure that you are familiar with:

- Nature of prosthesis – mechanical or tissue, model, size
- Symptoms and signs at last review
- Resting cardiac rhythm
- Previous CXR and echo findings
- Maintenance medication, including anticoagulants.

CONSULTATION

History

The symptoms of prosthetic valve dysfunction are very similar to those of native valve dysfunction (see earlier). In patients attending the clinic for the first time after valve surgery, also check the following:

- **Improvement in symptoms after surgery**? If not, suspect either prosthetic valve dysfunction, persistent pulmonary hypertension or LV dysfunction as cause.

TABLE 12.2 Classification and suggested anticoagulation targets for prosthetic valves. Tissue valves only require anticoagulation for 3 months after surgery (target INR 2.0–3.0), provided sinus rhythm is maintained

Type	Subtype	Model	Description	Target INR*
Mechanical	First generation	Starr–Edwards	Ball and cage	3.0–4.5
		Bjork–Shiley	Tilting disc	2.5–3.5
	Second generation	Omniscience	Tilting disc	2.5–3.5
		Medtronic–Hall	Tilting disc	2.5–3.5
		St Jude	Bileaflet tilting disc	2.5–3.5
		Carbomedics	Bileaflet tilting disc	2.5–3.5
Tissue	Xenografts	Carpentier–Edwards	Porcine valve	
		Hancock	Porcine valve	
		Wessex	Porcine valve	
		Ionescu–Shiley	Porcine pericardium	
		Hancock	Porcine pericardium	
	Homografts		Cadaveric valve	

* National recommendations vary. The *British National Formulary* recommends INR 3.0–4.5 for mechanical valves. The AHA recommends INR 2.5–3.5 for mechanical valves (2.0–3.0 for patients at increased risk of bleeding). Consult local recommendations before prescribing.

Objectives of review

- Monitoring of valve function
- Educate patient about potential symptoms of valve dysfunction
- Educate patient about dental hygiene and antibiotic prophylaxis
- Prescribe medication (e.g. digoxin, warfarin) if appropriate
- Assess need for redo valve repair/replacement

- **Returned to normal physical activity?** If not, why not? Possibilities are symptom limitation, fear of harming self, overprotective spouse/carer, depression.
- **Returned to work?** Patients in non-physical jobs can return to work after around 2 months; in physical jobs after about 4 months (key limiting factor is allowing sternotomy to heal).
- **Returned to driving?** Normally allowed after around 10 weeks, once sternotomy fused.

Tip: Patients with a poor symptomatic or objective result from surgery should be reinvestigated and a specific explanation determined.

Examination

This should focus on identifying pulmonary congestion, atrial fibrillation, altered or new murmurs (e.g. aortic stenosis), signs of pulmonary hypertension and right-sided cardiac failure. Also check that both an opening and a closing sound are audible with mechanical valves, otherwise valve restriction may be present.

Investigations

These are as for monitoring of native valve disease. Doppler assessment of prosthetic valves is discussed in Chapter 19. It is useful to identify any paraprosthetic regurgitation and to document LV function at the first clinic review after surgery.

MANAGEMENT

First postoperative review

In addition to the factors described above, the first clinic review after valve surgery should be used to check the following:

- Wound healing
- Anticoagulant control: patients with tissue prostheses who maintain sinus rhythm need anticoagulation only for 3 months
- Postoperative pleural or pericardial effusions
- Rhythm: consider cardioversion for patients who develop or remain in atrial fibrillation
- Prosthetic valve function: paraprosthetic regurgitation
- LV function: may become impaired as a result of surgery, or may improve if the left ventricle is offloaded.

Subsequent review

Most patients should be reviewed annually to monitor valve function. Patients with mechanical prostheses can be reviewed every 2 years if stable. The valve type (xenograft, mechanical, allograft), model (Carpentier–Edwards, Starr–Edwards, St Jude etc.) and position (aortic, mitral, tricuspid) should be recorded unambiguously in the patient's records and in all correspondence.

Anaemia

Anaemia can occur in patients with valve prostheses, especially mechanical valves with a paraprosthetic leak. This is relatively uncommon, but occurs because of mechanical haemolysis. Investigations are as follows:

- **FBC**
  macrocytic anaemia (reticulocytes, may be folate deficient)
  red cell fragmentation on blood film
- **Markers of haemolysis**

↑ serum LDH
↓ serum haptoglobins
Coomb's test negative.

Other important causes of anaemia in patients with prosthetic valves are endocarditis and occult blood loss due to anticoagulation.

Embolic complications

Systemic embolism can occur with any prosthesis, particularly in the first month after surgery. The annual risk with anticoagulation is around 1%, although some valves have a higher than average incidence of systemic embolism. For example, the Starr–Edwards prosthesis has an annual event rate of 2.5%, the St Jude valve 1.5% and tissue valves 1%. The embolic risk without anticoagulation is double that with anticoagulation, i.e. 2–5% per year. If embolism occurs despite adequate anticoagulation, consider endocarditis or an extracardiac source. Patients with recurrent embolic events despite anticoagulation can be maintained with a higher INR range, or with the addition of low-dose **aspirin** 75 mg d^{-1}.

Acute prosthetic valve failure or thrombosis usually presents as an emergency (see Chapter 4). Gradual deterioration in function may occur because of obstructive pannus formation or progressive paravalvular regurgitation. If there is clinical or objective evidence of deterioration, further investigation (e.g. with TOE or cardiac catheterization) is necessary to determine whether redo surgery is needed. Redo valve replacement is associated with a greater mortality than first-time valve replacement (5–10% vs 3–5%) and greater morbidity.

Specific advice during surgery and pregnancy

Antibiotic prophylaxis

Antibiotic prophylaxis for dental and upper respiratory tract procedures is as shown in Table 12.3.

Anticoagulation

Patients undergoing minor outpatient procedures, such as day-case operations, cardiac catheterization or dental work, should stop warfarin for two to three doses beforehand. The INR should be less than 2.0 before proceeding to surgery.

For major surgery, or where bleeding incurs a significant risk, warfarin should be discontinued for 4 days and IV heparin commenced when the INR falls below 2.0. The target APTT should be 2.0–3.0. The heparin infusion should be stopped 3–4 hours before surgery and restarted as soon as is considered safe by the surgeon.

Anticoagulation, valve replacement and pregnancy are discussed further in Chapter 2.

TABLE 12.3 Antibiotic prophylaxis against endocarditis. Genitourinary procedures should be treated as special risk under general anaesthesia, except that clindamycin should not be given. Obstetric, gynaecological and gastrointestinal procedures require the same antibiotic cover as genitourinary procedures, but only in patients who have had previous endocarditis or who have a prosthetic valve

	Local anaesthesia	General anaesthesia
No special risk	**Amoxycillin** 3 g orally 1 h before the procedure	**Amoxycillin** 1 g IV at induction, then 0.5 g orally 6 h later *or* **amoxycillin** 3 g orally 4 h before and 3 g orally as soon as possible after the procedure
Special risk*	**Amoxycillin** 1 g IV and **gentamicin** 120 mg IV, then **amoxycillin** 0.5 g orally 6 h later	**Amoxycillin** 1 g IV and **gentamicin** 120 mg IV at induction, then 0.5 g orally 6 h later
Penicillin allergy or received more than a single dose of penicillin in the last month	**Clindamycin** 600 mg orally 1 h before the procedure	**Clindamycin** 300 mg IV over 10 min at induction, then 150 mg orally or IV 6 h later *or* **teicoplanin** 400 mg IV and **gentamicin** 120 mg IV at induction *or* **vancomycin** 1 g IV over 100 min and **gentamicin** 120 mg IV at induction

* Special risk = patients with previous endocarditis or a prosthetic valve. However, patients with prosthetic valves undergoing dental procedures under local anaesthetic can be considered to have no special risk.

SUPRAVENTRICULAR ARRHYTHMIAS

Supraventricular arrhythmias are the most common type of arrhythmia seen in cardiology clinics. This section describes management from the point where the arrhythmia has been diagnosed (from ECG or ambulatory monitoring). This consultation may follow a new patient consultation (e.g. palpitation, Chapter 11; dizziness or syncope, Chapter 11), or inpatient diagnosis (Chapter 7, acute arrhythmias). No assumption is made about underlying electrophysiological mechanisms and arrhythmias are categorized according to the surface ECG appearance, since this is the starting point in the clinic!

Key ECG categories of supraventricular arrhythmia

- Atrial flutter or fibrillation – continuous
- Atrial flutter or fibrillation – intermittent
- SVTs without evidence of pre-excitation
- SVTs with evidence of pre-excitation

Objectives of review
- Assess how symptoms affect patient (e.g. work, physical activity, psychologically)
- Clarify nature of arrhythmia
- Identify underlying cause (e.g. structural disease), precipitants (e.g. alcohol)
- Assess need and suitability for treatments
    medication (e.g. antiarrhythmics, warfarin)
    electrophysiological intervention
- Educate patient about (usually) benign nature of condition

BEFORE CONSULTATION

Ensure that you are familiar with:

- Nature of the arrhythmia
- Symptoms and signs at last consultation
- Resting cardiac rhythm at last consultation
- Previous CXR and echo findings
- Maintenance medications.

CONSULTATION

Go back to the history!

- How long have symptoms been present?
- How frequent and how long are the episodes?
- Are the symptoms interfering with patient's life?
- Are there associated high-risk symptoms (e.g. syncope (could denote SVT associated with severe LV impairment or significant valve stenosis, pre-excited atrial fibrillation, atrial flutter with 1:1 AV conduction, or unsuspected VT), angina or heart failure)?
- Any obvious precipitants (stress, exertion, alcohol, caffeine)?

> **Tip:** Ambulatory recordings often show clinically insignificant asymptomatic atrial arrhythmias. Make sure that symptoms occurred with the arrhythmia before assuming you have identified the cause. Otherwise, keep looking!

Examination

This should focus on the identification of underlying causes of arrhythmia:

- Hypertension
- Cardiac enlargement/signs of cardiac failure
- Murmurs/signs of valve disease

● Non-cardiac causes (signs of thyroid disease, anaemia, chronic lung disease, venous thromboembolic disease).

Investigations
● **ECG**
 – for continuous atrial flutter/fibrillation ensure rate control is adequate (ideally 50–80 bpm). Sometimes exertional symptoms may be marked despite good resting rate control, ETT may unmask an inappropriately brisk rate response to exercise.
 – for intermittent arrhythmias, look for signs of atrial enlargement (tall or bifid P waves), pre-excitation, atrial or ventricular ectopy (which often triggers the arrhythmia), LVH (may indicate aortic valve disease, hypertension or HCM) and previous MI.
 – for narrow-complex SVTs carotid sinus massage or IV adenosine may unmask an accessory pathway by blocking AV nodal conduction. A delta wave ± short PR interval may appear. See Chapter 7 before attempting either manoeuvre.
● **Ambulatory monitoring**. This helps determine whether atrial flutter/fibrillation is continuous or intermittent, as treatment strategies differ. For intermittent symptoms provide a patient-activated recorder for a few weeks: this is more likely to lead to a correct diagnosis than 24-hour tape monitoring.
● **CXR**
 – signs of lung disease
 – intrathoracic masses
 – cardiac enlargement/chamber enlargement
 – pulmonary congestion.
● **Echo**. Echo is mandatory to identify underlying structural heart disease. Supraventricular arrhythmias can be caused by virtually any structural heart problem. The commonest associates are mitral valve disease and IHD with ventricular impairment. Isolated aortic valve disease rarely causes supraventricular arrhythmias.

> **Tip:** Don't forget to check for atrial septal defect: right heart size, tricuspid and pulmonary flows and contrast injection if suspicious.

● **Laboratory tests**. Check FBC, T_4 and TSH to investigate for underlying cause. Check LFTs and mean red cell volume if suspicious of alcohol abuse as aetiology.

MANAGEMENT OF SPECIFIC ARRHYTHMIAS

Continuous atrial flutter/fibrillation
The main choice lies between rate control and restoration of sinus rhythm. Both have advantages and disadvantages. The decision is governed by the

risk of thromboembolic complications, the severity of symptoms and whether the patient is likely to maintain sinus rhythm. Patients with long-standing atrial fibrillation (especially if due to mitral valve disease, hypertension or advanced LV dysfunction) are least likely to maintain sinus rhythm after cardioversion. They have most to gain if cardioversion is successful, because of the importance of the atrial contribution to cardiac output. Most patients merit at least one attempt at cardioversion.

Sinus rhythm strategy

Anticoagulation Four weeks of prior anticoagulation (target INR 2.0–3.5) is mandatory, whether chemical or DC cardioversion is used. (Restoration of atrial mechanical function, not DC shock, causes ejection of clot from the LA appendage.) Digoxin, if prescribed, should be stopped for 48 hours before cardioversion as it reduces the chance of success.

Warfarin should be continued for 4 weeks after cardioversion, then stopped if sinus rhythm is still maintained. Digoxin can be restarted to limit heart rate in the event of recurrence, if the patient tolerates arrhythmia poorly.

Advantages
- Restoration of atrial transport — ↑ cardiac output with exercise
  - appropriate rate response to exercise
- Reduction of atrial stasis — low risk of embolism from atria
  - not exposed to risk of bleeding from anticoagulants

Disadvantages
- General anaesthetic risk (not a major concern for most patients)
- Drugs used to maintain sinus rhythm generally have more proarrhythmic potential than do the AV node-blocking drugs used for rate control.

Antiarrhythmic drugs? Unless the patient has a history of intermittent atrial fibrillation progressing to chronic atrial fibrillation, or has had a previous cardioversion with recurrence, antiarrhythmic drugs are not normally given either before or afterwards. Antiarrhythmic prophylaxis of atrial fibrillation is discussed below under *Intermittent atrial flutter/fibrillation*.

DC cardioversion protocol
- Ensure the patient has had at least 3 weeks of **effective** (INR >2) anticoagulation.

Warning: Cardioversion should not be carried out if the INR is subtherapeutic because of the risk of stroke.

- Some centres stop digoxin for at least 24 hours beforehand. The evidence that this affects outcome is weak.
- Check serum K^+ (success greater if >4.0 mmol l^{-1}).
- Patient fasting >6 h.
- IV access.
- General anaesthetic with short-acting induction agent.
- Cardiovert using following protocol (start at 200 J for atrial fibrillation):
  100 J synchronized shock if fails →
  200 J   "   if fails →
  360 J   "   if fails →
  360 J anteroposterior shock.
- Continue warfarin for at least 1 month if cardioversion successful.
- If cardioversion unsuccessful, consider repeating at later date after pretreatment with antiarrhythmic agent (e.g. amiodarone, sotalol).

Chemical cardioversion protocol The risk of systemic embolism is also significant with chemical cardioversion, as clot ejection is due to the restoration of atrial mechanical function (peak incidence is after 2 days), not the DC shock. Meticulous prior anticoagulation is essential if atrial fibrillation has been present >48 hours. Chemical cardioversion is also appropriate in cases where there is a *clear* history of arrhythmia onset within the previous 48 hours (anticoagulation not required).

- Check U&Es as above
- IV access
- Cardiac monitoring and resuscitation facilities available
- **Flecainide** 2 mg kg^{-1} IV (max. 150 mg) over 20–30 min (stop when cardioversion achieved)
- Same rules as for postcardioversion anticoagulation apply.

Rate control strategy

Anticoagulation Most patients with chronic atrial flutter/fibrillation require long-term anticoagulation with warfarin (target INR 2.0–3.5). Exceptions are patients who, from pooled data from anticoagulation trials, are considered low risk. In these cases low-dose aspirin 300 mg daily is sufficient prophylaxis, but only if all low risk criteria apply.

Advantages
- More appropriate for patients with valve disease or previous failed cardioversions
- Less proarrhythmic potential from rate-controlling drugs

Disadvantages
- Loss of atrial contribution to cardiac output
- Risk of embolic complications

> **Low-risk profile in atrial fibrillation**
>
> Age <65 years
> Structurally normal heart
> Normotensive
> Non-diabetic
> No history of TIA, stroke or systemic embolism.

Drugs for rate control AV node-blocking drugs are used to limit the rate response. A hierarchy of drugs is shown below. Aim for a resting heart rate of 50–80 bpm.

> **Oral drugs for rate control in atrial fibrillation**
>
> **First-line**
> Digoxin 250 µg d^{-1} (after loading ⊗) OR
> β-Blocker (e.g. atenolol 50–100 mg d^{-1})
> Verapamil 240–480 mg d^{-1} OR
> Diltiazem 200–500 mg d^{-1} OR
>
> If digoxin ineffective, ensure blood level therapeutic before adding a second agent.
>
> **Second-line**
> Combination of digoxin AND EITHER verapamil or β-blocker
>
> **Third-line**
> Amiodarone 100–400 mg daily (after loading ⊗).

In atrial flutter rate control is difficult because the AV node-blocking response is not linear and is usually a whole fraction of an atrial rate of around 300 min^{-1}. Thus a therapeutic dose of digoxin may not reduce heart rate from 150 bpm (2:1 AV block), but an additional agent may cause it to fall abruptly to 75 bpm (4:1 block) or lower.

Intermittent atrial flutter/fibrillation
Intermittent atrial flutter/fibrillation is often a precursor to chronic atrial fibrillation, but can exist as a separate entity. The need for antiarrhythmic and anticoagulant treatment is dictated by the severity of symptoms and the frequency and duration of episodes. Ambulatory monitoring is a helpful guide to treatment. Potential precipitants (e.g. hypertension, alcohol, valve disease) should be identified and treated before committing to long-term antiarrhythmic treatment.

Anticoagulation The criteria for warfarin treatment are the same as for chronic atrial fibrillation. Aspirin 300 mg d^{-1} is sufficient for low-risk patients (see earlier) and for those with a clear history of very infrequent, brief episodes.

Antiarrhythmic drugs The choice of oral antiarrhythmic drugs is governed by the patient and their underlying heart disease:

- β-**Blockers** have little proarrhythmic effect and are a sensible first-line agent, especially when ischaemia is implicated as a cause.
- **Sotalol 60–120 mg bd**, which has combined β-blocking and class III activity, is effective but proarrhythmia is more common in women and in patients with LVH.
- Flecainide 50–100 mg d^{-1} is effective but should be avoided in patients after MI (CAST study) with a history of heart failure or ventricularectopy.
- **Propafenone 150 mg bd to 300 mg tid** is as effective as sotalol but shares its proarrhythmic potential.
- **Amiodarone 100–400 mg d^{-1} (usual dose 200 mg d^{-1})** is the safest agent in patients with significant LV compromise. It has many side effects and should be avoided in young patients unless no effective alternative is found. Quinidine can cause hypersensitivity and GI upset. It has been shown to increase mortality in this group of patients and should be avoided.

For all of the above agents, except β-blockers, ambulatory monitoring within the first 5 days of treatment is sensible to identify proarrhythmia.

Other regular SVTs

Diagnosis and management of SVTs is helped by recording a rhythm strip and 12 lead ECG during tachycardia, and a 12 lead ECG during sinus rhythm. This is not always possible if the arrhythmia is occasional, and a rhythm strip is often all that is available to help with the diagnosis. Regular, narrow complex tachycardias have several possible causes in patients who do not have overt pre-excitation (P-R interval <0.12 s ± delta waves) on the 12 lead ECG in sinus rhythm:

- AV node re-entry
- Atrioventricular re-entry (through accessory pathway. Pre-excitation need not be present in sinus rhythm, since many pathways are occult and only conduct retrogradely, from ventricles to atria)
- ectopic atrial tachycardia (EAT)
- inappropriate (pathological) sinus tachycardia
- His bundle tachycardia
- atrial flutter with 2:1 AV block.

> **Tip:** A narrow complex tachycardia with rate 150 bpm is most likely to be atrial flutter with 2:1 AV block.

The key to understanding the underlying mechanism is a systematic examination of the ECG in sinus rhythm and during tachycardia:

- **Pre-excitation in sinus rhythm**? Is P-R interval short (<120 ms) Is there a delta wave? IV adenosine given during sinus rhythm can unmask 'suspected' accessory pathways by slowing AV node conduction and revealing delta wave (see Chapter 7 – How to do an IV adenosine challenge – before attempting this).
- **Arrhythmia initiation** (An atrial premature beat which initiates the tachycardia, and shares the same morphology as tachycardia P-wave, suggests ectopic atrial tachycardia. Gradual onset suggests sinus tachycardia.)
- **P-waves easily visible**? (If not, or buried in the QRS complex, the likely diagnosis is typical AV node-re-entry tachycardia – 'classic SVT'.)
- **P-wave morphology**. If similar to sinus P-waves, suspect pathological sinus tachycardia. If superiorly directed P-wave axis (i.e. negative P in inferior leads) atrial activation is from below, i.e. A-V node re-entry, accessory pathway, or low focus EAT.
- **Is the arrhythmia of 'long R-P' type**? (i.e. the R-P interval > P-R interval).

Causes of long R-P tachycardia

- Sinus tachycardia (physiological or pathological)
- Ectopic atrial tachycardia
- Atypical AV node re-entry (see Chapter 16)
- Permanent junctional reciprocating tachycardia (slowly conducting posteroseptal accessory pathway; tachycardia usually presents in infancy.)
- Accessory pathway remote from AV node (e.g. left lateral bypass tract)

- **How does tachycardia terminate**? Termination with non-conducted P-wave (i.e. AV node blocks tachycardia) virtually excludes atrial tachycardia, which is propagated by an intra-atrial re-entry circuit or automatic focus.

Management is determined by the frequency and severity of symptomatic episodes. An electrophysiological study can be performed if symptoms are troublesome, to determine the mechanism of the tachycardia (Chapter 16). Drug prophylaxis consists of agents that slow AV node conduction (see atrial fibrillation, earlier), or antiarrhythmic drugs (see intermittent atrial fibrillation, earlier).

> Warning: Digoxin and verapamil should be avoided in patients with SVT and Wolff–Parkinson–White syndrome, as they can promote antegrade accessory pathway conduction.

Sotalol, flecainide and amiodarone not only suppress the atrial ectopic activity that often initiates the SVT, but also slow or block conduction in accessory pathways. Radiofrequency ablation now offers a cure for many SVTs, and is an accepted first line treatment for Wolff–Parkinson–White syndrome. There is a small but definite risk attached to ablation procedures which should be explained to patients (Chapter 16).

VENTRICULAR ARRHYTHMIAS

Systematic investigation and follow-up of patients with confirmed ventricular arrhythmias is essential because some are at high risk of sudden death. Treatments are dictated by the type of arrhythmia and the underlying cause. Although essential I_X and R_X will have been done before discharge in patients admitted with symptoms, outpatient clinic follow-up is essential to complete investigation and monitor the effectiveness of therapy.

Key types of ventricular arrhythmia

- Ventricular ectopic beats
- Asymptomatic VT
- Symptomatic VT
- Resuscitated VF or VT cardiac arrest

Objectives of review

- Assess how symptoms affect patient (e.g. work, physical activity, psychologically)
- Clarify nature of arrhythmia
- Identify underlying cause (e.g. structural disease), precipitants (e.g. IHD)
- Risk assessment (is patient at risk of sudden death?)
- Assess need and suitability for treatments
  - medication (e.g. antiarrhythmics)
  - electrophysiological intervention
- Educate patient about condition

BEFORE CONSULTATION

Ensure that you are familiar with:

- Nature of the arrhythmia
- Symptoms and signs at last consultation
- Results of stress testing and angiography, if done
- Previous CXR, ECG and echo findings
- Maintenance medications.

CONSULTATION

History

The same questions apply as for supraventricular arrhythmias (see earlier). In addition, check the following specific factors:

- Family history of sudden death or arrhythmia (familial HCM, long QT syndrome)?

- Coronary risk factors (IHD is the commonest cause of VT).
- Proarrhythmic medication (class I or III antiarrhythmics, tricyclics, theophylline etc.) or diuretic which may lower K^+/Mg^{2+}?
- Does patient take illicit drugs? (e.g. cocaine, 'Ecstasy', amphetamines)?
- Are symptoms associated with exertion or angina episodes (ischaemic trigger)?
- Is patient syncopal? (Poor prognostic indicator, suggests rapid VT, or VT associated with poor cardiac function.)
- Any symptoms to suggest underlying systemic cause (e.g. phaeochromocytoma, systemic infiltrative disorder, e.g. sarcoidosis, carcinomatosis)?

Tip: Asymptomatic ventricular extrasystoles do not require treatment.

Examination
As with SVTs this should focus on identifying an underlying cause for the arrhythmia:

- Cardiac enlargement/signs of cardiac failure/dyskinetic apex (LV aneurysm)
- Hypertension
- Murmurs/signs of valve disease.

Investigations
- **ECG**
  - evidence of IHD: Q waves, persistent ST elevation (LV aneurysm), T-wave inversion, conduction defects
  - LVH voltage criteria (hypertension, ventricular dilatation or HCM)
  - pre-excitation (consider IV adenosine test in sinus rhythm, see Chapter 7)
  - corrected QT interval (long QT syndrome)
  - RBBB may suggest IHD, arrhythmogenic RV cardiomyopathy or Brugada syndrome, but can be normal variant.
- **Exercise testing**. Useful to identify underlying IHD. Even in patients with LBBB or RBBB an ETT may show exercise-induced ectopy or arrhythmia. Patients with symptomatic VT and a positive stress test should have coronary angiography.
- **Ambulatory monitoring**. Establishes relationship between symptoms and arrhythmia and is useful for assessing therapy by giving an index of frequency, duration and heart rate during episodes and for checking for proarrhythmic effects of antiarrhythmic drugs.
- **CXR**. May show cardiac enlargement, signs of cardiac failure, intrathoracic masses.

- **Echo**. Used to identify underlying structural heart disease. Common associates with VT are:
  - LV dilatation
  - regional wall motion defects (especially LV aneurysm)
  - LVH (check for other signs of HCM (see Chapter 13))
  - also look for aortic stenosis, mitral valve prolapse, RV dysplasia (dilated, hypokinetic RV).
- **Laboratory tests**
  serum K^+, Mg^{2+} if patient on diuretics and recurrent arrhythmia
  T_4 and TSH
  24-hour urine collection for metadrenalines if phaeochromocytoma suspected.

MANAGEMENT

Treat precipitants
- Anxiety can heighten awareness of ventricular premature beats (VPBs). In many cases no cause is found. Try and reassure patient they are benign.
- I_x/R_x for ischaemia if VPBs/VT on exercise.
- Treat low K^+/stop proarrhythmic medication.
- Hypertension and poorly controlled cardiac failure are potent precipitants of ventricular arrhythmias in susceptible patients.

Specific antiarrhythmic treatment
This varies according to the specific arrhythmia.

Ventricular premature beats
Patients with symptomatic VPBs are usually seen for follow-up after an initial assessment for palpitation.

VPBs are common in the healthy population. They are not usually associated with IHD or structural heart disease and carry a benign prognosis. The incidence increases with age and VPBs occur more commonly in men. When frequent they are a marker of increased risk in post-MI patients, but treatment of VPBs themselves does not lower the risk (see below). VPBs cause symptoms for several reasons:

- Compensatory pause after VPB gives a sensation of the heart stopping. Post-VPB beat is forceful due to ↑ stroke volume, especially with aortic incompetence.
- Frequent VPBs with retrograde V-A activation cause dizziness, neck pulsation (due to cannon waves) and hypotension.
- Frequent interpolated VPBs (interspersed in normal rhythm without pauses) can dramatically increase heart rate.

Treat precipitants (see above)

Drug treatment Specific treatment of VPBs is indicated only if symptoms significantly affect the patient despite reassurance and R$_X$ of any underlying cause.

● **β-Blockers** (e.g. oral **metoprolol** 25–100 mg bd) are relatively safe and effective and are first-line treatment.
● **Diltiazem** reduces VPBs effectively in hypertensive patients.
● **Amiodarone** is effective at reducing VPBs but in most cases cannot be justified for a benign arrhythmia.

EP interventions (see Chapter 16 for details of procedures)
Occasionally VPBs originating from the right ventricular outflow tract can be treated with RF ablation of the ectopic focus.

Asymptomatic VT
Asymptomatic VT is sometimes identified coincidentally on ambulatory recordings, prompting referral to the cardiology clinic.

It is mandatory to assess for the underlying cause (see above). The prognosis is good in the absence of underlying structural or ischaemic disease, but the treatment of asymptomatic VT (rather than its cause) does not improve prognosis. Check the following:

● Is VT really asymptomatic? An H$_x$ of unexplained presyncope or syncope suggests VT with compromise (see below).
● Is VT monomorphic or polymorphic? Polymorphic VT has a stronger association with sudden death and usually merits admission to hospital for assessment and management (see Chapter 7).
● Does the patient carry a vocational licence (e.g. HGV or pilot licence)? They may have a duty to inform the licensing authority of arrhythmia.

Symptomatic VT
Patients with symptomatic VT attend the follow-up clinic either after initial outpatient assessment for palpitation/dizziness/syncope, or after admission to hospital because of an arrhythmic episode.

Monomorphic VT is characterized by a regular broad-complex tachycardia with complexes of near-identical morphology. There may be similar-shaped VPBs interspersed in sinus rhythm. VT may cause palpitation, flushing,

Warning: Although the frequency of VPBs predicts risk of sudden death after MI, suppression with class Ic (e.g. flecainide, moricizine) or certain pure class III (e.g. D-sotalol) antiarrhythmic drugs increases the risk of death.

dizziness, presyncope or syncope. VT can provoke heart failure or angina in susceptible patients. This section deals with VT not associated with syncope or cardiac arrest.

Careful examination of the ambulatory recording can give useful clues:

- ST depression in the lead-in period suggests an ischaemic aetiology.
- Is VT an escape rhythm from bradycardia? (Pacing may prevent episodes.)
- LBBB morphology suggests RV focus; IHD is still most likely, but consider RVOT tachycardia, RV cardiomyopathy, Brugada syndrome.
- Is VT rate fast (>180 bpm)? (More likely to cause symptoms/compromise.)
- Is VT rate slow? (If VT rate overlaps with patient's normal heart rate range, overdrive pacing using AICD is difficult. Most AICDs use rate criteria for VT detection; inappropriate pacing/shock could result.)

Treat precipitants (see above)

Drug treatment Underlying heart disease will guide the choice of drug. Several different drug strategies have been shown to reduce symptoms and the frequency of episodes:

- **Sotalol** 60–120 mg bd. Contraindicated in long QT syndrome and in patients with *torsades de pointes* VT.
- **Flecainide** 50–150 mg bd. Use with caution after MI ($\uparrow$ mortality in post-MI patients in the CAST trial, although CAST examined a lower-risk group with frequent VPBs, where risk–benefit equation favours risk (of drug)). Flecainide may $\uparrow$ pacemaker/AICD threshold.
- **Amiodarone** 100–400 mg d^{-1} (after loading, 200–400 mg tid for 7 days). Effective but long-term side effects limit use in young patients. Safest agent when LV function poor.
- **Propafenone** 150 mg bd to 300 mg tid. Mild β-blocking effect (caution in asthma/COPD).
- **Disopyramide** 250–375 mg tid is effective for post-MI VT but prolongs the QT interval and can cause anticholinergic side effects.
- **Moracizine** 200–300 mg tid. Relatively new agent; can be proarrhythmic (CAST II trial) and worsen heart failure.
- **Mexiletine** 200–250 mg qid. Effective in post-MI VT but frequent dosing and narrow therapeutic window make it unattractive.
- **Procainamide** up to 50 mg kg^{-1} d^{-1} (in 4–6 daily doses). Long-term side effects (lupus-like syndrome, agranulocytosis) and dosing frequency a problem. Plasma levels should be monitored (target 3–10 µg ml^{-1}; toxic >12 µg ml^{-1}).

(**Verapamil** is occasionally used for a specific VT originating from the interventricular septum, of RBBB morphology. Generally, verapamil should be avoided in patients with VT.)

EP interventions (see Chapter 16 for details of procedures) Right ventricular outflow tract VT can be treated with RF ablation of the VT focus. This tachycardia is characterized by LBBB morphology with an inferior axis.

Resuscitated VF or VT cardiac arrest
Full investigation and planning of treatment in these patients will have been started in hospital during their index admission with cardiac arrest.

Management strategies are discussed in Chapters 4 and 7. The follow-up visit is directed at assessing symptoms and the effectiveness of treatment and follows the general principles outlined earlier in this section.

● **Palpitation or presyncope** should prompt non-invasive reassessment with ETT or Holter monitoring.
● **Syncope** usually necessitates readmission for further assessment and revision of treatment, unless a clear non-arrhythmic cause is known.
● **Ischaemic symptoms** are especially important if ischaemia is implicated in the original event. In patients treated with revascularization as an arrhythmic strategy, ischaemic symptoms may prompt repeat angiography; stress testing may still be helpful in delineating the ischaemic territory.
● **Assess psychological state**. Anxiety and depression are common sequelae of cardiac arrest. Patients may avoid physical or sexual activity because of the fear of sudden death. Cognitive impairment can result from cerebral hypoxia. Formal assessment by a clinical psychologist or psychiatrist may help.
The follow-up of patients treated with AICDs is described in Chapter 17.

CARDIAC FAILURE

Patients with stable cardiac failure and mild symptoms, and who take adequate preventive therapy, do not require regular review unless further intervention is planned. Remember to treat reversible causes and exacerbating conditions, such as hypertension and thyroid dysfunction.

Objectives of review
● Treat symptoms
● Prevent progression of cardiac failure and improve prognosis
● Investigate and manage underlying cause
● Educate patient about condition

BEFORE CONSULTATION

Ensure that you are familiar with:

- Cause of cardiac failure (if not clear, consider further investigation (see Chapter 6))
- Symptoms and signs at last consultation
- Cardiac rhythm at last consultation
- Previous CXR and echo findings
- Maintenance medication
- Results of pending investigations.

CONSULTATION

History
- Ask about dyspnoea (exertional and nocturnal), orthopnoea, fatigue, oedema.
- Note exercise tolerance, NYHA functional class (see Chapter 1).
- High-risk symptoms? (Presyncope, syncope, palpitation.)
- If aetiology not known, ask about symptoms that suggest an underlying cause (e.g. angina, alcohol history).

Examination
This should focus on identifying signs of left- and right-sided cardiac decompensation (see Chapter 1) and any underlying cause (e.g. hypertension, valve disease) and aggravating factors (e.g. anaemia, thyrotoxicosis, arteriovenous shunt).

Investigations
- **ECG**. Check for new atrial fibrillation, sinus tachycardia (both signs of decompensation), inappropriate bradycardia (may aggravate cardiac failure). Voltage criteria for LVH and infarct patterns may give clue to aetiology, if unknown.
- **CXR**. Only necessary if a new presentation, or a change in symptoms/signs since previous visit, or limiting symptoms
    - check heart size and shape, compare with previous films
    - look for signs of decompensation: interstitial oedema, upper lobe venous diversion, Kerley B lines, fluid in horizontal fissure, pleural effusions.
- **Echo** is not needed at every clinic visit, but can be useful:
    - to establish the cause of cardiac failure
    - to monitor LV/RV function
    - to assess the relative contributions of systolic and diastolic dysfunction.
- **Laboratory tests**
    - U&Es – if new or changed dose of diuretic, ACE inhibitor, angiotensin receptor antagonist
    - Hb, TFTs – if not already done, to check for aggravating cause cardiomyopathy screen (see Chapter 6) if cause not known.

The following should also be considered:

- **Ambulatory monitoring**, if suspicion of associated malignant arrhythmia.
- **Stress testing**, if ischaemic aetiology suspected (see Chapter 6).
- **Cardiac catheterization**:
  - identify cause (coronary angiography, identify intracardiac shunts, restrictive or constrictive physiology, valve defects)
  - identify complications (pulmonary hypertension)
  - assessment for cardiac transplantation.

MANAGEMENT

Current treatment for patients with cardiac failure due to systolic LV dysfunction includes:

- **ACE inhibitor**. If not tolerated, consider AT_1 receptor antagonist (e.g. losartan). If renal dysfunction with ACE inhibitor, consider hydralazine/nitrate combination.
- **β-Blockade** – associated with improved symptoms and prognosis in those who tolerate therapy. The evidence base is strongest for oral **bisoprolol** (starting dose 2.5 mg d^{-1}, target dose 10 mg d^{-1}), metoprolol and carvedilol. Careful dose titration is mandatory.
- **Diuretics** are only necessary if there is evidence of pulmonary congestion, peripheral oedema or ascites. Loop diuretics (e.g. oral **frusemide** 20 mg d^{-1}, titrated to response) are the usual first-line therapy. Oral **bumetanide** 1 mg d^{-1}, titrated to response, is reportedly better absorbed in patients with right-sided cardiac failure. Potassium supplements or potassium-sparing diuretics (e.g. oral **amiloride** 2.5–5 mg d^{-1}) may be needed to avoid hypokalaemia. Oral **spironolactone** 50–200 mg d^{-1} is especially useful in treating fluid retention in right-sided cardiac failure and improves the prognosis in patients with severe left-sided cardiac failure.
- Nitrates, e.g. oral **isosorbide mononitrate LA** 30–120 mg d^{-1}, may help relieve dyspnoea and can be prescribed at bedtime to prevent nocturnal symptoms.

Consider the following additional treatments in patients with severe or resistant cardiac failure:

- **Digoxin**: role in sinus rhythm remains controversial but may improve symptoms in some patients and avoid repeated hospitalization.
- **Anticoagulation**: patients in sinus rhythm with LVEF <28% should be

Warning: The combination of an ACE inhibitor or AT_1 receptor antagonist AND potassium supplement/potassium-sparing diuretic can cause dangerous hyperkalaemia, especially if the patient becomes dehydrated. Careful monitoring of U&Es/creatinine is mandatory.

considered for anticoagulation because of the increased risk of embolic complications, especially if an akinetic LV segment or aneurysm is present. Patients with atrial fibrillation and cardiac failure should receive warfarin unless there is a contraindication. The target INR is 2.0–3.0.

Decompensation of cardiac failure

If there is clinical or radiological evidence of decompensation consider increasing the dose of diuretic and/or ACE inhibitor. Resistant fluid retention can be treated with an increased dose of loop diuretic, sometimes in combination with a thiazide (e.g. oral **metolazone** 2.5–5 mg on alternate days) or aldosterone antagonist (oral **spironolactone** 50 mg bd) (see Chapter 6). Inpatient treatment may be necessary to stabilize patients with severe or resistant cardiac failure.

Renal failure

Renal failure is commonly associated with end-stage cardiac failure, due to low cardiac output, renovascular disease, ACE inhibitor and diuretic therapy. A compromise needs to be made between renal function and symptom control: often a significant degree of renal compromise has to be accepted to control symptoms. The oral combination of **hydralazine** (25–50 mg bd) and nitrate (e.g. **isosorbide mononitrate** LA 40–60 mg d^{-1}) is useful where renal failure prohibits the continuation of an ACE inhibitor or AT$_1$ receptor antagonist. Beware of digoxin toxicity in patients with renal failure.

Arrhythmias

Arrhythmias are common in patients with cardiac failure. Atrial fibrillation is a common cause and consequence of decompensation. Anticoagulation and a rate-control or sinus rhythm strategy need to be considered (see earlier). Cardioversion should be considered, as the restoration of sinus rhythm significantly augments cardiac output. The likelihood of immediate and long-term success may be increased by amiodarone therapy.

Asymptomatic non-sustained ventricular tachycardia is a very common incidental finding on ambulatory monitoring. There is little evidence that antiarrhythmic drugs improve outcome. See earlier for the management of symptomatic VT.

Bradycardia occasionally aggravates cardiac failure (e.g. sinus node disease and chronotropic incompetence) and may necessitate permanent pacing.

HYPERTENSION

Hypertension is an important determinant of cardiovascular mortality. Mortality increases with both systolic and diastolic blood pressure. In thin individuals (BMI <23.5) there is a J-shaped relationship between systolic BP and risk of death. Definitions of hypertension are rather arbitrary, but are based on the distribution of BP within a (usually caucasian) population. Although cut-off points are arbitrary they have a large effect on the 'prevalence' of hypertension in the population. Cut-offs for diastolic BP of 90 and 95 mmHg give prevalences of 14.5% and 8.4% respectively for the over-40s. The importance of repeated measurement before committing a patient to a diagnosis of hypertension cannot be overemphasized. Diurnal and environmental factors (especially the 'white coat' effect) substantially affect BP readings.

Effective treatment of hypertension significantly reduces cardiovascular mortality and morbidity. The relative risk of stroke is reduced by up to 40% and of MI by 20%. As the incidence of MI exceeds that of stroke, the absolute risk reductions are similar. Risk prediction graphs are given in Figure 12.1.

DEFINITION

A clinically useful definition of hypertension is a level of BP above which the benefits of treatment significantly outweigh its risks. Definitions are quite variable:

- The **WHO** defines hypertension requiring treatment as BP exceeding 160/95 mmHg.
- Joint recommendations from the **British Hypertension Society, British Cardiac Society and British Hyperlipidaemia Association** indicate that specific antihypertensive treatment is indicated in the following situations:
  sBP ≥ 160 mmHg OR dBP ≥ 100 mmHg on three separate occasions over 1–2 weeks.
  sBP 140–159 mmHg or dBP 90–99 mmHg (sustained) and >15% ten year risk of IHD/end-organ damage (see risk prediction charts, Figure 12.1)

If sBP 140–159 mmHg OR dBP 90–99 mmHg, and ten year risk <15%, annual assessment and review of lifestyle factors is recommended. In normotensive subjects, five yearly BP checks are recommended.

AETIOLOGY

In 95% of cases the precise aetiology is unknown — i.e. 'essential' hypertension. However, (treatable) secondary causes of hypertension will only be found if you look for them and these are relatively more common in younger patients.

Isolated systolic hypertension is sometimes seen in the elderly and in association with a hyperdynamic circulation (e.g. anxiety, thyrotoxicosis, anaemia). Hypertension is more prevalent among black Americans and Japanese, due partly to genetic factors.

BEFORE CONSULTATION

Prior to the consultation, check:

Causes of secondary hypertension

Renovascular disease
    renal artery stenosis
    small/segmental vessel atherosclerosis
    diabetic nephropathy
Renal parenchymal disease
    glomerulonephritis
    polycystic disease
Aortic disease
    aortic coarctation
Pregnancy
    pre-eclampsia
Endocrine disease
    phaeochromocytoma
    Cushing's disease/syndrome
    primary hyperaldosteronism
    hyperparathyroidism
    hyperthyroidism (sBP)
    acromegaly
    congenital adrenal hyperplasia
Drugs
    alcohol
    oral contraceptive
    steroids
    NSAIDs
    sympathomimetics

Objectives of review

- Identify secondary causes
- Identify end-organ damage
- Monitor BP control
- Assess cardiovascular risk factors
- Lifestyle and medical management
- Treat complications

- Appropriate tests for secondary causes done
- Appropriate tests for end-organ damage documented (U&Es, urinalysis, creatinine, ECG, fundoscopy)
- Drug therapy
- Previous BP control.

CONSULTATION

History

Hypertension is usually asymptomatic unless associated with a hypertensive crisis (see Chapter 10) and is often detected at screening examinations.

Headaches and epistaxis occur with equal frequency in hypertensive and normotensive people and are not useful guides. Ask about salt, calorie and alcohol intake and any previously diagnosed cardiovascular risk factors and possible complications (e.g. MI, stroke, renal failure, eye disease).

Examination

Isolated BP measurements may be misleading because of environmental factors. 'White coat' hypertension can give rise to repeated high readings, highlighting the advantage of ambulatory BP monitoring before committing patients to long-term drug treatment. Initial examination should focus on identifying secondary causes (e.g. renal bruit, clinical anaemia and hyperthyroidism, radiofemoral delay). Follow-up examination should include fundoscopy (with grading of retinopathy, see Chapter 1).

Investigations

Assessment of end-organ damage

- Eyes – see Chapter 1 for retinopathic changes.
- Heart – screen for LVH with ECG or, if readily available, echo.
  - assess LV function with echo if ECG abnormal or if symptoms or signs of cardiac failure.
- Kidneys – check U&Es, creatinine. Measure creatinine clearance at least once per year, or more often if U&Es/creatinine deteriorate.
- Arterial tree – check peripheral and carotid pulses, bruits, peripheral perfusion.

Screening for secondary hypertension

- **Renal U&Es, creatinine, urinalysis.** Consider renal ultrasound scan: small or asymmetric kidneys may signify renal artery stenosis. An isotope renogram or renal angiogram should be considered if unilateral small kidney or if ACE inhibition or AT_1 receptor antagonism causes deterioration in renal function.
- **Structural CXR**: look for rib notching, abnormal aortic contour. MRI scanning or aortography are indicated if upper limb BP exceeds lower limb BP by >20 mmHg, unexplained murmur (especially at back), or CXR suggestive.
- **Endocrine/metabolic U&Es** (low K^+ accompanies hyperaldosteronism and phaeochromocytoma, but also diuretic R_x), **calcium, phosphate, glucose, TFTs**. Consider 24-hour urine collection for metadrenalines and cortisol.

Risk factor assessment

Other cardiovascular risk factors should be checked; these are discussed elsewhere in this chapter.

MANAGEMENT

Non-pharmacological

- Weight reduction if overweight (each kg loss yields 3/2 mmHg BP reduction)

- Moderate salt restriction (70–80 mmol d^{-1}) can reduce BP by up to 8/5 mmHg in some individuals
- Minimize alcohol consumption
- Aerobic exercise
- Smoking cessation (does not directly affect BP, but effects of BP and smoking on cardiovascular risk are multiplicative).

Pharmacological

There is a bewildering range of oral antihypertensive drugs to choose from: diuretics, β-blockers, α-blockers, sympatholytic agents, ACE inhibitors, AT$_1$ receptor antagonists, calcium channel antagonists and other vasodilators. A logical approach is to start with agents for which the evidence of benefit (in terms of reduction in end-organ damage and mortality) is strongest.

First-line therapy

- Thiazide diuretics (e.g. **bendrofluazide** 2.5 mg d^{-1}) are effective at reducing BP and preventing complications. The diuretic effect may be poorly tolerated in patients with prostate disease or incontinence problems. Hyperuricaemia and glucose intolerance are reversible side effects.
- β-Blockers (e.g. **atenolol** 50–100 mg d^{-1}, **metoprolol** 50–100 mg bd) are also effective and reduce mortality and morbidity.

Although an unfavourable side-effect profile is often attributed to these agents, the evidence from hypertension trials indicates that β-blockers and diuretics are at least as well tolerated as ACE inhibitors and calcium channel antagonists.

An additional second (and sometimes third) agent may be needed to effectively control BP. Combination therapy using synergistic agents can produce substantial reduction in BP. Ideally, diuretics should be used along with an ACE inhibitor or AT$_1$ receptor antagonist and vasodilators such as nifedipine in combination with a β-blocker.

Comorbid conditions should also influence the choice of agent:

- **Diabetes mellitus**: ACE inhibitors protect renal function in diabetics, and in patients with albuminuria the volume of urinary albumin loss is reduced. Patients with brittle diabetes or hypoglycaemic unawareness may not be suitable for a β-blocker. Thiazides can exacerbate hyperglycaemia, but this does not preclude their use.
- **IHD**: β-Blockers and rate-limiting calcium channel antagonists reduce the frequency of angina symptoms. β-Blockers improve prognosis in patients with previous MI.
- **Cardiac failure**: ACE inhibitors, diuretics and β-blockers (see Chapter 6).
- **Aortic regurgitation**: ACE inhibitors and nifedipine reduce afterload and regurgitant volume.
- **Peripheral vascular disease**: β-Blockers *do not* significantly reduce claudication distance. Moreover, as these patients are at increased risk of

cardiovascular events they have most to gain from β-blocker therapy. However, β-blockers should be avoided in *critical* limb ischaemia.
● **Depression**: β-Blockers and centrally acting sympatholytics (e.g. methyldopa) should be avoided.

Initiation of drug therapy should be considered in patients who are hypertensive despite at least 3 months of lifestyle modification, particularly if there is coexisting cardiovascular disease or risk factors, or evidence of end-organ damage. Monotherapy should be used if possible and the dose optimized before a second agent is prescribed. If monotherapy is ineffective at first it is sensible to change the class of drug used (e.g. from β-blocker to calcium channel antagonist) rather than adding a second agent or trying another drug of the same class. If hypertension is resistant, also check the patient's compliance and secondary causes of hypertension, e.g. 'white coat' effect. Ambulatory BP monitoring helps exclude the latter.

HYPERLIPIDAEMIA

SECONDARY PREVENTION

All patients with IHD should have their lipid profile checked. A random (non-fasting) total serum cholesterol concentration is helpful to screen for hypercholesterolaemia, but many laboratories use a back calculation from HDL and triglyceride concentrations to determine LDL-cholesterol concentration. A fasting sample is needed to determine a full lipid profile. Remember that **following acute illness the serum cholesterol concentration falls**. A sample obtained >24 hours after acute MI may give false reassurance.

In all patients lifestyle modification (e.g. weight reduction, dietary advice and regular aerobic exercise) should be considered. Other coronary risk factors should be identified (see elsewhere in chapter). In patients with premature coronary artery disease (men <55 years, women <65 years) first-degree relatives should be offered screening for hypercholesterolaemia.

As the main treatments that have been shown to alter the risk of death, coronary events and disease progression are based on intervention for hypercholesterolaemia, this section focuses on these.

Total cholesterol ≥5.0 mmol l^{-1}

The baseline fasting lipid profile (total cholesterol, HDL-cholesterol, LDL-cholesterol, VLDL-cholesterol and triglycerides) should be determined. Secondary causes of hyperlipidaemia (below) should be excluded. Patients should receive dietary and lifestyle advice and be started on a statin (e.g. **simvastatin** 10–20 mg d^{-1} or **pravastatin** 20–40 mg d^{-1}). The dose should be titrated until the total cholesterol concentration falls below 5.0 mmol l^{-1} and the LDL-cholesterol below 3.0 mmol l^{-1}. It is of note that the doses shown to be effective at event rate reduction in recent trials (4S, CARE, LIPID) have been simvastatin 20 mg d^{-1} and pravastatin 40 mg d^{-1}). Statins are contraindicated in patients with active liver disease and during pregnancy and breastfeeding.

Secondary causes of hyperlipidaemia
- Hypothyroidism
- Liver disease
- Renal disease, especially nephrotic syndrome
- Diabetes mellitus
- Alcohol excess
- Gout

Choice of statin

At present simvastatin and pravastatin, have the largest evidence base for clinical efficacy. Atorvastatin potently reduces cholesterol concentration and is appropriate in individuals with higher cholesterol concentrations (e.g. >7 mmol l^{-1}).

Total cholesterol <5.0 mmol l^{-1}

All patients should receive dietary and lifestyle advice and have their serum cholesterol concentration rechecked 3–6 months later. Despite evidence of significant event rate reduction in patients with confirmed IHD treated with pravastatin 40 mg d^{-1} (LIPID trial), it is debatable whether patients with cholesterol 4.2–5.0 mmol l^{-1} should receive lipid-lowering therapy. The main determinant of this is likely to be the resources available in a given health-care setting.

PRIMARY PREVENTION

A balance needs to be created between the risk of a major cardiovascular event and the consequences of committing the patient to lifelong lipid-lowering therapy.

Risk assessment
- Age
- Sex
- Blood pressure
- Diabetes mellitus
- Smoking habit
- Family history
- Total cholesterol:HDL-cholesterol ratio >5 indicates significant risk.

Figure 12.1 illustrates the 10-year risk (in the primary prevention setting). This does not incorporate factors such as family history of premature cardiovascular disease or elevated triglycerides, which add to the risk. These charts help guide the selection of patients for intervention. Patients in the high-risk categories (>30% 10-year risk) should initially receive dietary and lifestyle advice and have their profile reassessed after 3 months. If the repeat lipid profile demonstrates total cholesterol $\geq$ 5 mmol l^{-1} or LDL-cholesterol $\geq$ 3.0 mmol l^{-1}, then statin therapy is indicated. The regimen for which there is an evidence base in primary prevention is **pravastatin** 40 mg d^{-1} (WOSCOPS trial).

MANAGEMENT

Resistant hyperlipidaemia
In patients with persistent hypercholesterolaemia, consider:
- Poor drug compliance – if due to side effects, consider an alternative agent
- Reinforce dietary and lifestyle measures
- Change the type of statin (e.g. to atorvastatin)
- Additional lipid-lowering therapy.

There are two major alternative classes of lipid-lowering drug: fibrates and resins. Fibrates (e.g. **bezafibrate** 200 mg tid) significantly reduce cholesterol and triglyceride concentration. Fibrates are particularly useful in mild mixed hyperlipidaemias. Although fibrates can be used in combination with statins, the risk of liver toxicity and myositis may be increased and close monitoring of LFTs and CK is mandatory. Resins (e.g. **cholestyramine** 12–24 g d^{-1}, after careful introduction) are effective but their use is limited by side effects, notably palatability, dyspepsia and flatulence.

Side effects of lipid-lowering drugs
GI upset is common to all preparations and may limit their use. Myositis can occur with statins and to a lesser extent with fibrates, but its incidence is less than commonly thought. Myositis is more likely if statins and fibrates are coprescribed, or if either agent is used in patients receiving cyclosporin or nicotinic acid. Myalgia is a very common symptom in the general population and discontinuation of therapy should be based on elevation of CK (minor elevations are common; CK **>10** × upper limit of reference range *confirms* myositis). Persistent elevation of liver transaminases **>3** × upper limit of reference range is an indication to stop therapy. LFTs and CK should be checked before initiating treatment, at the time of the next cholesterol check (usually 2–3 months after initiating therapy) and at least once per year afterwards.

THORACIC AORTIC ANEURYSM AND CHRONIC AORTIC DISSECTION

Thoracic aortic aneurysms are less common than abdominal aneurysms but carry the same risk of rupture. Patients with thoracic aneurysms are at increased risk of death from aortic dissection and from coexisting atherosclerotic disease. Chronic aortic dissection may be seen *de novo*, following cardiothoracic (especially aortic valve) surgery involving aortic instrumentation, following aortic repair (coarctation, acute dissection) and in association with aortic aneurysm. Both thoracic aneurysms and chronic dissections require surveillance in case medical or surgical intervention is needed.

Objectives of review
- Identify symptomatic deterioration
- Identify expansion/extension of pathology
- Monitor and treat BP
- Plan medical intervention
- Educate patient about any lifestyle restrictions
- Decide whether risk–benefit ratio favours surgery

BEFORE CONSULTATION

Ensure that you are familiar with:

- Aetiology of the aneurysm or dissection (see Chapter 4)
- Symptoms at last review
- Quantitative measures of aortic dimensions and extent of disease.

CONSULTATION

History
Check for symptoms relating to vascular compromise and compression of adjacent structures; ask about any episodes of acute back/chest/abdominal pain that could signify extension of dissection/subacute rupture.

- Back pain   – (nerve compression)
- Dysphagia   – (oesophagus)
- Dyspnoea   – (bronchus)
- Facial swelling – (SVC obstruction)
- Claudication   – (vascular compromise due to peripheral vascular disease, extension of dissection, embolization from aneurysm)
- CNS symptoms – (carotid dissection, cerebral embolism).

Examination
This should focus on monitoring BP, identifying associated aortic regurgitation and any compromise of peripheral circulation.

Investigations

- **CXR**

    sequential monitoring of size of aorta/aneurysm, if visible

    cardiomegaly/cardiac failure due to aortic regurgitation

- **Echo**

    helps diagnosis of aortic root pathology and aortic regurgitation

    TOE can help define disease in descending thoracic aorta

- **CT or MRI**

    the gold standard for monitoring aortic dimensions and extent of dissection, branch vessel involvement

    at least annual scan required for long-term monitoring.

MANAGEMENT

Most patients need intensive antihypertensive therapy, preferably using a β-blocker. Progression and rate of rupture are significantly reduced by β-blocker therapy, the aim of which is to reduce systolic BP below 120 mmHg.

Patients should be considered for surgical repair if they have:

- Thoracic aortic aneurysm >60 mm
- Thoracic aortic aneurysm >55 mm and Marfan syndrome
- Rapid expansion of aneurysm/dissection-related segment
- Aneurysm or dissection-related symptoms
- Significant aortic regurgitation (see earlier).

The balance of risk for surgery is affected by the patient's age and comorbidity. Many patients with thoracic aneurysms die from other cardiovascular diseases, such as MI or stroke, before they succumb to aortic dissection or rupture itself.

CHAPTER 13

MISCELLANEOUS OUT-PATIENT PROBLEMS

CARDIAC TUMOURS

PRIMARY CARDIAC TUMOURS

Primary cardiac tumours are far less common than secondary tumours, with a prevalence of less than 1 in 1000 in most postmortem studies. They are underdiagnosed, often presenting with systemic symptoms such as pyrexia or embolism. Although rare, these tumours are usually treatable with surgical resection, so it is important to consider them in patients with an unexplained systemic illness.

Symptoms and signs of primary cardiac tumour

Symptoms
- Dyspnoea/paroxysmal nocturnal dyspnoea
- Pyrexia of unknown origin
- Weight loss/cachexia
- Dizziness
- Syncope
- Symptoms of systemic embolization

Signs
- Mitral murmurs (LA myxoma)/tumour 'plop' sound – **may be postural**
- Pulmonary oedema (LA myxoma with mitral obstruction)
- Right-sided cardiac failure (sometimes signifies pulmonary emboli and RA myxoma)
- Atrial fibrillation
- Anaemia (normochromic, normocytic on FBC)
- Digital clubbing (<10% of cases)

Myxomas

Characteristics and physical signs

Myxoma can occur anywhere in the heart but the left atrium is the most common site. Myxomas account for 50% of benign cardiac tumours, are solitary in 90% of cases and familial in 10%. The tumour is usually gelatinous and pedunculated, attached to the interatrial septum and moves forward in diastole to partially obstruct the mitral valve. In three-quarters of cases there is a mitral diastolic murmur, which may be intermittent and postural (affects the degree to which tumour obstructs the valve). An added sound in diastole, resembling an S_3, may be heard as the tumour prolapses forward into the valve orifice. Often described as a 'tumour plop', this is usually a retrospective diagnosis once the echo has been viewed!

Investigations
- **CXR** may show LA enlargement, but rarely shows pulmonary oedema. Tumour calcification is very occasionally seen.
- **ECG** shows sinus rhythm. Atrial fibrillation is uncommon (<20% of cases).

- **Echo** is the most helpful investigation and will usually show a large, mobile mass prolapsing into the mitral or tricuspid orifice. Attenuation of late diastolic flow is sometimes seen with Doppler. Transoesophageal echo may be needed for precise delineation of tumour size, number and attachments.
- **Skin biopsy** may be helpful in defining histology if peripheral tumour emboli have occurred.
- **Laboratory tests** are often cited as helpful, but in reality rarely assist with diagnosis. Although the ESR is elevated in 30–50% of cases and elevated γ-globulins are sometimes seen, these findings are non-specific and can also accompany systemic infection and connective tissue disorders.
- **Cardiac catheterization** is not required unless concomitant coronary artery disease is suspected.

Treatment
Tumour resection usually provides a good long-term result. Patients should be followed up annually after surgery to check for recurrence, which occurs in up to 5% of cases.

Fibroelastomas
Fibroelastomas affect the heart valves and surrounding ventricular endocardial tissue. They account for 16% of benign cardiac tumours. They are sometimes multiple and do not usually produce any symptoms. These tumours are frondlike and very mobile. The commonest manifestation is systemic embolization. They may appear after surgical trauma to the heart. Treatment is with surgical excision. Depending on the tumour site, valve replacement and/or implantation of a permanent pacemaker may also be required.

Other benign tumours
Rhabdomyomas are the most common childhood cardiac tumour, usually presenting in the first year of life with heart failure and murmurs due to valve or outflow obstruction. There is a strong association with the systemic disorder tuberous sclerosis. **Fibromas, lipomas and angiomas** collectively account for most of the remainder of benign cardiac tumours.

Malignant cardiac tumours
Only 25% of cardiac tumours have a malignant histology and most are sarcomas. They usually present between the ages of 20 and 50 and most often occur in the atria. **Angiosarcomas, rhabdomyosarcomas and mesotheliomas** account for 70% of primary cardiac tumours. These tumours are aggressive in terms of both local growth and metastatic potential. They often present with progressive cardiac failure due to chamber obstruction. Cardiac tamponade, ventricular arrhythmias and heart block may also occur. Most patients die within 2 years of diagnosis. Surgery is often required to exclude a benign tumour, but results with surgical resection, radiotherapy and chemotherapy are usually disappointing.

SECONDARY CARDIAC TUMOURS

These are far more common than primary tumours and are seen at postmortem in up to 20% of patients who die from malignant disease. Cardiac metastases are usually multiple and most often affect the pericardium and myocardium; the heart valves and supporting structures are usually spared. The likelihood of cardiac metastasis occurring depends on the primary tumour. Occasionally, focal myocardial infiltrates are not due to tumour but to other forms of infiltrative disease (e.g. sarcoidosis, Wegener's granulomatosis).

Tumours commonly associated with cardiac metastasis

- Lung (small cell and non-small cell) carcinoma
- Breast carcinoma
- Mediastinal lymphoma
- Malignant melanoma
- Mesothelioma
- Pancreatic carcinoma

In addition, some relatively rare tumours have a very high propensity to metastasize to the heart, e.g. thyroid carcinoma.

Clinical manifestations

Most cardiac metastases are discovered at postmortem and were previously unsuspected. Symptoms can be produced by local mass effects, pericardial involvement, vascular compression and amyloid deposition.

- **Pericardial effusion** is the most common clinical manifestation. Clinical signs and diagnosis are discussed in Chapter 4. Pericardial aspiration usually provides cytological confirmation of the diagnosis. Most effusions recur after drainage, and subxiphoid pericardiectomy, in which a window is created between the pleural and pericardial spaces, provides palliation of symptoms.
- **Myocardial metastases** present with a variety of symptoms. Cardiac failure may result from infiltration and restriction, chamber encroachment and ventricular outflow tract obstruction. Arrhythmias may also occur. Lung tumours, malignant melanoma and lymphoma most commonly cause myocardial metastases.
- **Restrictive cardiomyopathy** occurs in most cases of systemic amyloidosis, which is sometimes associated with multiple myeloma. Patients present with atrial fibrillation and heart failure. Diagnosis and treatment are discussed in Chapter 6.
- **Superior vena cava obstruction** may accompany mediastinal tumours such as lymphomas and lung carcinomas. Head and upper limb plethora occurs and the patient may complain of headache and facial and arm swelling,

especially when supine or on bending. Collateral veins are sometimes seen on the chest wall. Radiotherapy may provide palliation.

Investigations

The ECG is rarely helpful. CXR may confirm metastatic disease within the lung parenchyma and mediastinal lymph nodes, pulmonary oedema (NB carcinomatous lymphangitis can give a similar appearance), and a globular heart of pericardial effusion. Echo is the most useful investigation and readily identifies pericardial effusion. Myocardial metastases are most often seen as slightly brighter than the surrounding myocardium, speckled and associated with reduced wall motion. Discrete masses are sometimes seen infiltrating the cardiac chambers or outflow tracts.

Treatment

Other than the specific treatments described, it is beyond the scope of this book to cover the treatment of metastatic malignancies.

CARDIAC TRANSPLANTATION

Human cardiac transplantation was first performed in 1967, but did not become an accepted modality of treatment for end-stage heart disease until the 1980s. Refinement of immunosuppressive therapy, rather than improved surgical technique, has been responsible for this. Two major factors limit the applicability of transplantation: the scarcity of donor organs and the cost. Transplants are therefore performed in patients with heart disease refractory to alternative treatment methods and in whom the prognosis is otherwise poor. The registry of the International Society of Heart Transplantation indicates that 5-year survival is 60–65% with a transplant, so a potential recipient's prognosis must be significantly worse than this. It is rare for transplantation to be performed for symptom control (e.g. in intractable angina) alone.

INDICATIONS

A patient may be suitable for cardiac transplantation if he or she has severely limiting symptoms (usually of cardiac failure) and one or more of the following criteria:

- Objective evidence of severe LV impairment, e.g. LVEF <20%
- Reduced maximum oxygen consumption during exercise (VO_2 max <10 ml kg^{-1} min^{-1} assessed using cardiorespiratory exercise testing). A VO_2 max >14 ml kg^{-1} min^{-1} is associated with a relatively good prognosis
- Refractory, frequent ventricular arrhythmias.

Most patients referred for transplantation either have LV dysfunction secondary to IHD or a dilated cardiomyopathy.

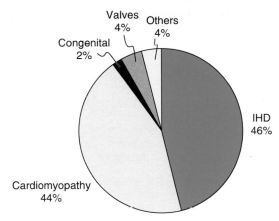

Fig. 13.1 Underlying pathology of patients referred for cardiac transplantation.

CONTRAINDICATIONS

- Irreversible liver, renal or pulmonary disease (heart + lung transplant may be considered in last group)
- Severe peripheral vascular or cerebrovascular disease
- Active infective process
- Insulin-dependent diabetes mellitus with end-organ damage
- Psychiatric illness likely to lead to poor compliance or inability to cope with post-transplant regimen
- Comorbidity which limits prognosis (e.g. untreated malignancy)
- Irreversible pulmonary hypertension (see next section for rationale)
- Advanced age (no absolute cut-off age, but most patients <60).

ASSESSMENT OF SUITABILITY FOR TRANSPLANTATION

In general, patients considered suitable for transplantation have severe functional disability which is refractory to other, conventional modes of treatment. In patients with IHD heart failure is the usual indication, but those with refractory arrhythmias or disabling refractory angina are sometimes considered. A large battery of screening investigations is required to assess suitability.

Cardiovascular function
- **ECG**
- **Left heart catheterization**: assess LV, determine whether revascularization likely to improve LV function/symptoms. May be supplemented with myocardial viability study, e.g. dobutamine stress echo; see Chapter 19.

- **Right heart catheterization**: measure PA pressure, PVR, transpulmonary pressure gradient (mean PA pressure – mean PCWP) and cardiac output. **Pulmonary hypertension** is an adverse factor, as it reflects increased PVR which can lead to failure of donor RV. If PVR >6 Wood units (400 dynes.s cm^{-5}) at rest, further I_x are needed to determine whether the increased PVR is reversible. Some centres use transpulmonary pressure gradient (mean PA pressure – mean PCWP) as index of PVR; should be <15 mmHg. If PVR or transpulmonary gradient high, reassess after the following treatments, aiming for PVR 3 Wood units (200 dynes.s cm^{-5}):
  - Inhaled O_2.
  - 24–48 hours inotrope R_x (e.g. dobutamine 2.5–10 $\mu g\ kg^{-1}\ min^{-1}$) ±
  - Vasodilator R_x (e.g. prostacyclin (epoprostanol), nifedipine, glyceryl trinitrate).

Renal function
- U&Es, creatinine
- Creatinine clearance (24-h urine)
- Isotope renogram if parenchymal renal disease suspected rather than side effect of diuretic/ACE inhibitors.

Ventilatory function
- CXR
- FEV_1, FVC, ratio
- Lung volumes
- ABGs on air in patients with documented lung disease.

Infection screen
IgG titres for:

- Hepatitis A, B and C
- HIV
- CMV
- Toxoplasmosis.

General
- Full blood count + differential
- Fasting blood glucose
- Serum cholesterol and triglycerides.

Tissue typing
This is normally performed by the transplant centre and will provide an index of the likelihood of a suitable donor organ being found. The patient's antibody titres are also a factor, as high levels increase the chances of the donor heart being rejected.

> **Tip:** Blood transfusion should be avoided if possible in patients being considered for transplantation, as antibody titres may increase as a result.

Psychological assessment

This is integral to pre-transplant assessment, in order to detect psychiatric illness associated with chronic heart disease (anxiety, depression), to assess the patient's attitude towards the transplantation of foreign tissue into their body and to assess whether they are likely to comply during the perioperative period, with the drug regimen and with rigorous follow-up.

IMMUNIZATION

Before the patient is placed on the active transplantation waiting list, immunization using the following can be considered by the transplant centre:

- Pneumococcal vaccine
- DTP booster
- Hepatitis B vaccine
- Measles/mumps/rubella (MMR) combination vaccine
- Polio vaccine.

BRIDGING PATIENTS TO TRANSPLANTATION

'Bridging' means any treatment designed to support the patient in the short term while waiting for a donor organ to become available. Bridging treatments include:

- Inotrope support (e.g. intermittent ambulatory dobutamine infusion)
- Intra-aortic balloon counterpulsation (see Chapter 3)
- Left ventricular assist devices (including ambulatory systems, e.g. TCI HeartMate and Novacor devices)
- AICD in patients with recurrent ventricular arrhythmias.

EXAMPLE LONG-TERM POST-TRANSPLANT DRUG REGIMEN

Treatment varies widely between patients and transplant centres. An individual patient's drug regimen is dictated by many factors: renal and hepatic function, immune status, side effects and biopsy histology. **Changes to**

Warning: MMR and oral polio are live attenuated vaccines. Such vaccines are unsuitable for post-transplant patients as they can cause clinically significant infection.

drug regimens should be made only by the transplant centre. The following is an example of a long-term post-transplant maintenance regimen:

- **Prednisolone** 7.5–15 mg d^{-1}.
- **Cyclosporin** 3–6 mg $kg^{-1} d^{-1}$ (newer preparations have greater bioavailability, e.g. Neoral, and doses as low as 2 mg $kg^{-1} d^{-1}$ are now commonly used. Prescription should be brand specific)
- **Azathioprine** 1–2 mg $kg^{-1} d^{-1}$ OR (in azathioprine-intolerant patients)
- **Mycophenolate** 1 g bd–qid.

COMPLICATIONS OF TRANSPLANTATION

Early complications are not seen by most cardiologists as they are dealt with by the transplant centre. These include early acute rejection (treated with high-dose steroids ± antithymocyte globulin) and early infection, commonly with nosocomial organisms (e.g. *Escherichia coli*, *Legionella* spp., *Pseudomonas aeruginosa*, *Staph. epidermidis*). Rejection episodes occur in the first 3 months in 80% of patients. This section covers complications that might be seen at non-transplant centres.

Pyrexial illness

After transplantation, patients check their temperature and weight daily. Pyrexia may simply signify the onset of simple coryzal illness, but could indicate a more serious pathology.

- **Infection with typical organisms**, e.g. *H. influenzae* respiratory tract infection, *E. coli* UTI, is common. Culture blood, urine and sputum.
- **Opportunistic infection** may occur due to immunosuppression:

Candida (oral)	oral **nystatin** 500 000 units qid
(systemic)	oral or IVI **fluconazole** 400 mg stat followed by 200–400 mg d^{-1}
Aspergillus (respiratory)	confirm diagnosis with transbronchial biopsy, R_x usually oral **amphotericin** 100–200 mg qid, but nephrotoxicity renders treatment difficult
Pneumocystis carinii & Nocaridiasis	oral or IVI trimethoprim/sulphamethoxazole (**co-trimoxazole**) 960 mg bd
Toxoplasmosis	graft-acquired, treated with **pyrimethamine** in post-transplant period.

 Warning: Before any new treatments are instituted the transplant centre should be contacted. Diagnosis and treatment of rejection episodes is a specialized area and should not be done by the general cardiologist.

- **Cytomegalovirus infection** presents in many guises and is acquired at some time by the majority of transplant recipients:
    - pneumonitis
    - hepatitis
    - gastroenteritis
    - retinitis.

  Diagnosis is with viral titres or cultures, but these may be negative even with active infection. PCR looks promising for diagnosis. Treatment is initially with IV **ganciclovir** (initially 5 mg kg^{-1} bd), oral preparation sometimes used for prophylaxis (1 g tid, with food).
- **Herpes virus infection** is treated with **acyclovir**. Oral R_x (200–400 mg five times daily for 5 days) is used for herpes simplex infection. IV R_x (5 mg kg^{-1} tid for 5 days) is sometimes needed for herpes zoster infection.

Rejection

Rejection may present with insidious symptoms, e.g. malaise, fatigue, gradual reduction in effort tolerance. New onset of atrial flutter or fibrillation is another clue. The ECG may show reduced QRS voltages and echo may show increased LV wall thickness and reduced isovolumic relaxation time. These are non-diagnostic findings – endomyocardial biopsy (performed by the transplant centre using a bioptome, via the internal jugular approach) is essential for diagnosis and grading (Table 13.1).

TABLE 13.1 Grading of cardiac transplant rejection	
Grade 1a	Focal, mild infiltrate without necrosis
1b	Diffuse, sparse infiltrate without necrosis
Grade 2	Focal, aggressive infiltrate with focal myocyte injury
Grade 3a	Multifocal, aggressive infiltrate with necrosis
3b	Diffuse infiltrate with necrosis
Grade 4	Very severe inflammation ± vasculitis ± haemorrhage and necrosis

Treatment of rejection
- **Mild**

  ↑ oral prednisolone to 30–50 mg d^{-1} for 3 days, then taper over 2 weeks to maintenance dose.
- **Early (<3 months) or moderate/severe**

  methylprednisolone 0.5 g IV bd for 3 days. If biopsy +ve, then: antithymocyte globulin ± anti CD3 lymphocyte globulin ± lymphoid irradiation.

Cyclosporin toxicity

This usually presents with nephrotoxicity, although liver damage can also occur if the cyclosporin level is very high. This should be suspected if there is weight gain and increased serum creatinine; creatinine clearance should then be checked along with trough blood cyclosporin level. Hypertension may result: treat with sustained-release **nifedipine** 20–60 mg d^{-1}. Resistant hypertension can be treated with ACE inhibitors, but renal function should be carefully monitored.

TABLE 13.2 Drugs that interact with cyclosporin	
Increase cyclosporin level	*Decrease cylosporin level*
Amiodarone	Rifampicin
Propafenone	Carbamazepine
Erythromycin/macrolides	Phenytoin
Chloroquine	Barbiturates
Diltiazem	Octreotide
Nicardipine	
Verapamil	
Colchicine	
Methylprednisolone	
Progestagens	
Tacrolimus	

In addition, potentially nephrotoxic drugs (e.g. NSAIDs) may be more hazardous in patients taking cyclosporin. The risk of myopathy with statins is also increased.

Toxicity from other immunosuppressants
- Steroids — Hypoadrenalism, Cushingoid appearance, cataracts, osteoporosis, diabetes mellitus, hyperlipidaemia
- Azathioprine — Bone marrow suppression (especially with concomitant allopurinol), liver toxicity. Alternative agents are cyclophosphamide or mycophenolate
- Mycophenolate — Bone marrow suppression, GI disturbance
- Tacrolimus (FK-506) — A newer immunosuppressant, can reduce requirement for cyclosporin and steroids. Causes QT interval prolongation and hypertrophic cardiomyopathy in young patients. Not often used after cardiac transplantation.

Graft atherosclerosis
Accelerated atherosclerosis is very common in transplanted hearts.

Mechanisms may include immune mediators (antibodies, complement), growth factors (e.g. PDGF), fibrin and thrombin. Elevated serum cholesterol further accelerates the process and CMV infection may also contribute to vascular injury and disease. Annual coronary arteriography is usually performed to monitor for graft vascular disease. Because the donor heart is denervated, ischaemic chest pain does not usually occur. Symptoms are breathlessness (due to ischaemia or silent MI), fatigue and palpitation. Statins (with careful monitoring of liver enzymes and CK) may help prevent graft atherosclerosis.

Other complications
- **Conduction disturbances**: SA node failure common, may necessitate pacemaker insertion. Sinus tachycardia is normal after transplantation due to loss of vagal influence on sinus rate.
- **Malignancy**: affects 10% of patients, usually presents after ~5 years. Squamous cell carcinoma of the skin/lips is commonest, followed by non-Hodgkin's lymphoma and Kaposi's sarcoma.
- Gout.

NEURALLY MEDIATED SYNCOPE

Vasovagal syndrome is characterized by inappropriate vasodilatation and bradycardia in response to a situational trigger, most commonly upright posture. Carotid sinus hypersensitivity and other forms of situational syncope (e.g. cough syncope and micturition syncope) occur because of similar mechanisms. Together, these syndromes form the group of conditions classed as *neurally mediated syncope*. These conditions are underdiagnosed yet can lead to disabling symptoms that put patients at risk of falls and injury and which may preclude them from driving. Chapter 11 describes a systematic approach to assessing patients with recurrent syncope: the most important component is history-taking, aiming to establish any pattern to the symptoms and any potential triggers.

PATHOPHYSIOLOGY OF VASOVAGAL SYNDROME

The normal response to upright posture is initially sympathetic activation, leading to reflex tachycardia, peripheral vasoconstriction and increased force of ventricular contraction. In patients susceptible to vasovagal syncope the Bezold–Jarisch reflex (Fig. 13.2) leads to an inappropriate autonomic response in this situation. When the ventricles contract forcefully in the face of reduced filling (due to venous pooling), mechanoreceptors are stimulated. A brainstem reflex leads to profound vagal stimulation and sympathetic withdrawal, resulting in bradycardia and vasodilatation.

Afferent	Efferent
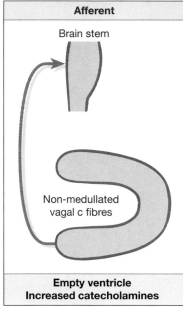	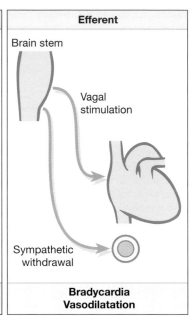
Empty ventricle **Increased catecholamines**	**Bradycardia** **Vasodilatation**

Fig. 13.2 The Bezold–Jarisch reflex.

CLINICAL FEATURES OF VASOVAGAL SYNDROME

Symptoms normally occur during upright posture. This does not include dizziness, that occurs *immediately* on standing – this is postural hypotension, which results from a delayed vasoconstrictor response to the upright position and/or hypovolaemia. In vasovagal syndrome the patient is usually upright for several minutes before symptoms occur. Situational syncope includes syncope in response to noxious triggers, such as pain, micturition, or the sight of blood.

Symptoms
● **Prodromal symptoms** include light-headedness, warmth, sweating, nausea, awareness of heart racing or thumping and loss of colour from the face. A brief period of disorientation/confusion may occur.

● **Syncope** may not always occur, especially if the patient reacts to the prodromal symptoms by sitting or lying. Witnesses may describe loss of colour from the face and a pulse which is slow or difficult to feel.

● **Recovery** is usually quite rapid; there may be a period of flushing/vasodilatation afterwards. Nausea and vomiting may occur after a vasovagal faint and malaise may persist for up to an hour afterwards. Otherwise recovery is quick; in contrast to neurogenic syncope disorientation is usually transient.

TILT TESTING

Vasovagal syndrome is diagnosed with tilt testing. This is essentially a provocation test, during which the patient is maintained in an upright position on a tilt table for a defined period to induce a vasovagal episode. Many tilt testing protocols exist, some of which use adjuvant stimuli to provoke syncope. In general, aggressive tilt protocols have a greater sensitivity for vasovagal syndrome at the expense of specificity, i.e. false positive tests are common. An example tilt protocol is given in the box.

Westminister tilt protocol

- Patient fasted, test performed in morning
- Vasoactive drugs (including diuretics) stopped for approximately 5 half-lives
- Baseline BP and heart rate recorded with patient lying supine for 30 min
- Table tilted to 60° upright angle for up to 45 min; patient is asked to report any symptoms
- Test terminated if bradycardia or hypotension occurs in association with symptoms

---

Steeper tilt angles, which necessitate the use of a saddle support, lack specificity, whereas shallower tilt angles lack sensitivity. The reproducibility of this protocol is 70–90%, with a specificity of 80%. Isoprenaline can be used in cases of a negative passive tilt test, in an attempt to stimulate mechanoreceptors and hence the vagal limb of the Bezold–Jarisch reflex. Sensitivity is improved, but positive tilt tests are seen in up to 16% of healthy asymptomatic individuals. Other adjuvant stimuli, such as the administration of isoprenaline, glyceryl trinitrate or carotid sinus massage, can be used but are less well validated.

Interpretation of tilt test responses

Three key types of tilt response may be seen in vasovagal syndrome:

- **Vasodepressor response**: vasodilatation occurs first and a fall in blood pressure is seen.
- **Cardioinhibitory response**: bradycardia occurs first and slowing of heart rate is seen, often followed by hypotension.
- **Mixed response**: bradycardia and hypotension are seen simultaneously.

Vasovagal syndrome can only be diagnosed if one of these responses occurs *in association with symptoms*.

MANAGEMENT OF NEURALLY MEDIATED SYNCOPE

The most important component is reassuring the patient that their condition is benign and not associated with serious complications such as death or a heart attack. Depending on the frequency of symptoms and whether the patient is able to avoid situations that have provoked attacks, further treatment may or may not be required. Support stockings can help by reducing venous pooling and promoting venous return, but drug treatment may also be necessary.

Drug treatment

This is usually the first-line approach. Drug treatment attenuates both cardioinhibitory and vasodepressor reflexes and, paradoxically, β-blockers help by antagonizing the initial sympathetic response that triggers the vagal reflex. Vagolytics help prevent bradycardia and vasodilatation.

- **β-Blockers**, e.g. atenolol 25–100 mg d^{-1}, or metoprolol 25–100 mg bd.
- **Anticholinergics**, e.g. disopyramide 100 mg bd to 200 mg tid, or scopolamine (hyoscine) 1 mg patch every 3 days.
- **Theophylline** 250–500 mg bd (with monitoring of plasma levels) has been tried, with limited success. Its precise mode of action is unknown, but it modifies adenosine metabolism and may alter vascular tone.
- **Fludrocortisone** 0.1–1 mg d^{-1} has been reported to help by increasing plasma volume, but this agent may cause fluid retention and hypertension and exacerbate cardiac failure.

Many other treatments have been reported to help, but there is little controlled trial evidence to support claims for their efficacy.

Permanent pacing

Pacing may be used as an *adjunct* to drug therapy in patients with a pronounced cardioinhibitory response. AV sequential pacing is required, as AV block may occur during episodes. DDI mode is used (to prevent tracking of sinus rhythm between episodes) with hysteresis (to markedly increase heart rate and augment cardiac output during episodes; see Chapter 17). Pacing alone may only attenuate symptoms because it does not alter the patient's tendency to vasodilatation.

CHAPTER 14

ADULT CONGENITAL HEART DISEASE

GENERAL PRINCIPLES

Advances in paediatric surgery and medicine have led to an increase in the number of adult survivors of congenital heart disease. The main groups are those who have survived with:

- Anomalies normally associated with survival to adulthood life
- Palliative or corrective surgery in infancy or childhood
- Inoperable heart disease.

These patients are increasingly encountered in general cardiological practice, although they are best managed at specialized Grown Up Congenital Heart disease (GUCH) clinics.

PATHOLOGICAL FEATURES OF CONGENITAL HEART DISEASE

The three basic types of anatomical or structural abnormalities are:

- **Obstruction** to blood flow across valves or through the great vessels (the term **atresia** refers to complete obstruction)
- **Communication** between heart chambers or great vessels
- **Transposition** or **anomalous connection** of the great vessels.

Obstruction

Blood flow obstruction produces a pressure gradient across the offending lesion, with abnormally high pressure 'upstream'. This can cause chamber hypertrophy or dilatation and sometimes poststenotic dilatation 'downstream'. Obstructive lesions are usually associated with a murmur.

Communications

Communications are *restrictive* if their small size obstructs blood flow, maintaining a significant pressure gradient between the two chambers. For example, restrictive flow across a VSD produces high-velocity blood flow owing to a large pressure gradient, causing a harsh murmur. Conversely, a large *non-restrictive* VSD allows pressure to equalize between the ventricles, resulting in little or no flow or murmur.

The direction of flow across a defect (*shunt*) is determined partly by the resistance to flow downstream of the communicating chambers. Systemic vascular resistance normally exceeds pulmonary vascular resistance and the direction of flow across a VSD is usually from LV to RV. Flow reversal occurs if pulmonary vascular resistance (and RV pressure) rises, e.g. in Eisenmenger syndrome. Similarly, given that LV compliance is greater than that of the RV, flow across an ASD is usually from LA to RA.

A systolic or continuous murmur in the adult CHD patient is usually a favourable sign as it usually indicates a restrictive lesion which is potentially remediable. This is true even in cyanosed patients, as the murmur may be due to pulmonary stenosis or atresia, which are associated with low PA pressure (this prevents the irreversible pulmonary vascular changes that lead to Eisenmenger syndrome). Conversely, loss of a systolic murmur or the presence of a solitary diastolic murmur suggests an absence of 'protective' pulmonary stenosis, shunt reversal and elevated PA pressure, which may preclude surgery (see later).

Anomalous connections

Survival with transposition of the great arteries (TGA) is not possible unless an associated communication allows mixing of pulmonary and systemic blood, or unless surgically corrected. In *congenitally corrected* TGA, inversion of the ventricular inflows allows saturated blood from the left atrium to enter the morphological right ventricle (which is connected to the aorta) and thus the systemic circulation. Other 'helpful' anomalies include *anomalous pulmonary venous drainage* (pulmonary veins drain into the right atrium) and a VSD with RV outflow tract obstruction (allows blood mixing and prevents pulmonary arterial hypertension). Percutaneous balloon atrial septostomy (Rashkind procedure) or the preservation of ductus arteriosus patency by prostaglandin infusion are palliative manoeuvres that can be used in the postnatal period.

RECOGNITION OF CONGENITAL HEART DISEASE IN ADULTS

Congenital lesions in the adult are indicated by the presence of two or more of the following:

- Precordial murmur (especially continuous)
- Cyanosis
- Digital clubbing
- Abnormal heart shadow or pulmonary vasculature on chest X-ray
- Abnormal ECG (especially RBBB)
- Otherwise unexplained erythrocytosis.

ACYANOTIC CONDITIONS ASSOCIATED WITH SURVIVAL TO ADULTHOOD

BICUSPID AORTIC VALVE

Bicuspid aortic valves usually function normally at birth and can continue to do so throughout adult life. However, fibrosis and calcification often cause progressive stenosis and this lesion accounts for almost half of adult patients who undergo surgery for calcific aortic stenosis.

Specific points
- High risk for endocarditis

- Aortic regurgitation may also develop
- Coexists with other aortic abnormalities (e.g. coarctation)
- See Chapter 12 for follow-up.

ISOLATED PULMONARY VALVE STENOSIS

This accounts for around 10% of cases of congenital heart disease. Familial cases are probably more common than previously thought and pulmonary stenosis can be associated with congenital syndromes (e.g. Noonan syndrome, William syndrome). It usually exists in isolation and with few exceptions is associated with normal adult survival.

Specific points
- The effective orifice area of mild or moderately stenosed valves (Doppler gradients <40 and 60 mmHg, respectively) usually increases as the patient grows in adolescence.
- Hypertrophic subvalvular stenosis or valve calcification can increase RV outflow tract obstruction in severe cases.
- Significant pulmonary stenosis is unlikely in the absence of ECG evidence of right ventricular hypertrophy.
- Low risk for endocarditis.

AORTIC COARCTATION

Adult-type aortic coarctation usually presents in the second and third decades. 50% of patients die before the age of 30 without surgery, although survival is also influenced by coexisting cardiovascular problems, such as hypertension and congenital aneurysms of the Circle of Willis. Aortic coarctation is also associated with VSD, PDA and bicuspid aortic valve.

Surgical correction in childhood usually consists of subclavian flap aortoplasty or resection of the coarctation with end-to-end anastomosis. The role and long-term results of primary balloon angioplasty are not yet clear, although there may be fewer immediate hypertensive complications. This technique is useful for postsurgical recurrence.

Specific points
- Most coarctations are 'juxtaductal', just distal to the left subclavian artery.
- Coarctation can present with aortic dissection (especially in association with bicuspid aortic valve).
- LVF may occur in middle age owing to hypertensive cardiac failure.
- There is a 10% risk of recurrence after surgery (best detected by MRI).
- Resting- and exercise-induced hypertension is common and requires aggressive treatment. Hypertension often does not disappear after surgery, especially if surgery is delayed into adulthood.

CONGENITAL COMPLETE HEART BLOCK

Survival to adulthood is normal, although this condition is not as benign as previously reported. The level of AV block is usually 'high' in AV junction, resulting in a relatively fast, narrow QRS escape rhythm. Despite this, case series report a significant incidence of sudden death in adulthood and permanent pacemaker insertion should now be considered in all patients. Earlier pacemaker insertion should be considered in the following circumstances:

- Syncope or near syncope
- Excessive fatigue
- Widening of QRS complex
- Paroxysmal arrhythmia or slow daytime rate (<50 bpm) on 24 h tape
- Poor chronotropic response to exercise.

LEFT-TO-RIGHT SHUNTS ASSOCIATED WITH SURVIVAL TO ADULTHOOD

OSTIUM SECUNDUM ATRIAL SEPTAL DEFECT

Ostium secundum ASD is often undetected until later life, when 70% of affected individuals aged over 40 will become symptomatic. Secundum ASD and patent foramen ovale account for up to 70% of all atrial septal lesions. Sinus venosus (LA to SVC communication) defects are less common and are associated with partial anomalous pulmonary venous drainage. Ostium primum ASD is discussed in the next section.

Most children undergo secundum ASD closure before adolescence to prevent long-term sequelae. Closure should be considered in young adults with symptoms, a significant shunt (pulmonary to systemic blood flow ratio >2:1; see Chapter 19) and normal PA pressure.

Specific points
- Risk of endocarditis low: isolated secundum ASDs do not merit prophylaxis.
- Symptoms often develop in third and fourth decades.
- May present with palpitation, exertional dyspnoea and fatigue, or paradoxical emboli.
- (Rarely) RV ischaemia can cause angina.
- Mitral valve prolapse occurs in one-third of patients.
- Atrial arrhythmias are common with advancing age, even after surgical correction.
- The role of surgery in the older patient (age >40) is controversial (risk of cerebral embolism, cardiac failure and death significant); newer percutaneous closure techniques may avoid the need for surgery.
- Progressive pulmonary hypertension can lead to right-sided cardiac failure and Eisenmenger syndrome.

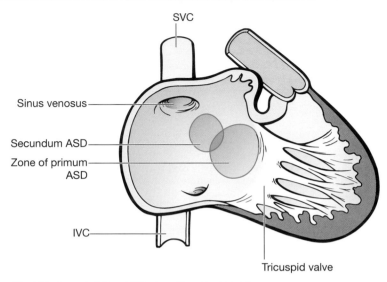

Fig. 14.1 Anatomical sites of ASDs viewed from the right atrium.

PATENT DUCTUS ARTERIOSUS

A large PDA commonly causes cardiac failure within the first year of life, but smaller defects may not cause symptoms until adulthood. The pressure gradient across a restrictive communication between aorta and PA persists throughout the cardiac cycle, resulting in a characteristic continuous murmur. The murmur peaks in late systole and decreases in diastole. It is best heard in the left infraclavicular area.

Specific points
- Significant risk of endocarditis – prophylaxis required.
- PDAs may present with cardiac failure in the adult.
- Survival with large defects is not common unless the LV is protected from volume overload by development of Eisenmenger syndrome (in which case shunt reversal occurs and classic *differential cyanosis* ensues).
- Percutaneous closure devices may in future reduce the need for surgery.

> **Tip:** *Differential cyanosis* is synonymous with PDA and Eisenmenger syndrome. Desaturated blood from the PA streams into the aorta distal to the head and neck vessels, whereas the upper body receives oxygenated blood from the aorta. This results in lower limb cyanosis, with toe clubbing and normal upper body colour and fingers.

VENTRICULAR SEPTAL DEFECT

Two types of defect are commonly seen:

- Those with small restrictive muscular defects (*maladie de Roger*)
- Those with large non-restrictive defects, in whom Eisenmenger physiology has protected the LV from volume overload (Figs 14.2 and 14.3). A left parasternal holosystolic murmur and thrill (without ejection click) is usually heard.

Specific points
- Risk of endocarditis is significant – prophylaxis required.
- The clinical course of small VSDs is benign.
- Large VSDs are rare in adults (pulmonary hypertension develops in childhood)
- Doppler studies help localize the VSD; if flow velocity is high the defect is

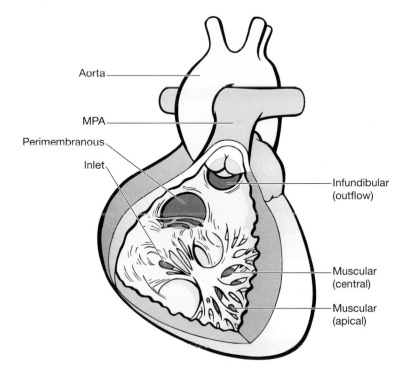

Fig. 14.2 Types and sites of VSDs viewed from the right ventricle.

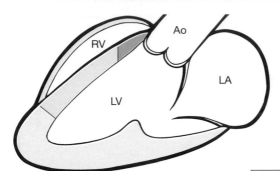

(a) Parasternal long axis view

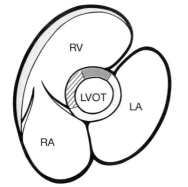

(b) Parasternal short axis at level of LVOT

/////	Perimembranous
	Muscular
	Inlet
	Infundibular

RV	= right ventricle
LV	= left ventricle
Ao	= aorta
LA	= left atrium
RA	= right atrium
LVOT	= LV outflow tract
MV	= mitral valve

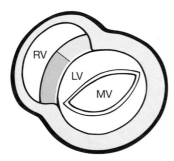

(c) Parasternal short axis at level of MV

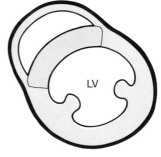

(d) Parasternal short axis at level of papillary muscular

Fig. 14.3 Echo views of VSDs.

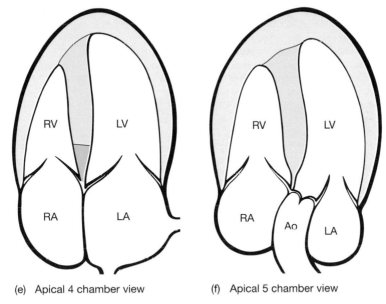

(e) Apical 4 chamber view   (f) Apical 5 chamber view

Fig. 14.3 (cont'd)

likely to be small. Right heart dilatation denotes a large VSD with volume overload ± pulmonary hypertension.

● May be associated with aortic incompetence owing to loss of support of right coronary cusp.

● Consider surgery for large lesions with significant shunts (if PA pressure not significantly elevated).

CORRECTED ANOMALIES AND INOPERABLE LESIONS

PRIMUM ASD AND ATRIOVENTRICULAR SEPTAL DEFECT

Ostium primum ASD is characterized by a defective inferior atrial septum without a ventricular communication. *Atrioventricular septal defect* encompasses defects involving an absent atrioventricular septum. If there is an atrioventricular septal defect the mitral valve is usually abnormal, with a 'cleft' (i.e. tricuspid), and is frequently regurgitant. Complete atrioventricular septal defect comprises a common AV canal, usually with a single common AV valve with two bridging leaflets adjacent to the interventricular septum. AV conduction abnormalities are common. Pulmonary hypertension is common and survival may be limited by shunt reversal.

Specific points

- Risk of endocarditis is significant – antibiotic prophylaxis is required.
- Symptoms similar to secundum ASD (see earlier).
- Coexistent mitral regurgitation increases shunt and symptoms.
- Atrial arrhythmias affect up to 30% preoperatively and 75% postoperatively.
- Median life expectancy with unoperated primum defect is 30 years.
- Surgical treatment is preferable, and consists of patch closure of the defect and repair or replacement of the left AV valve.
- Arrhythmias, conduction defects and progressive valve regurgitation necessitate long-term follow-up.
- Most patients seen in GUCH clinics will have had surgical repair.

TETRALOGY OF FALLOT

Tetralogy of Fallot is the most common form of cyanotic congenital heart disease and consists of:

- Perimembranous VSD
- Infundibular RV outflow obstruction
- RV hypertrophy
- Overriding aorta (aorta overrides the interventricular septum).

The anomaly results from misalignment of the interventricular septum, resulting in a large VSD under the right coronary cusp of the aortic valve. The aortic root usually lies to the right of the PA root, but no actual transposition occurs. Valvular pulmonary stenosis may coexist, but RV outflow tract obstruction is caused mainly by hypertrophy of the infundibular septum. Most patients seen in GUCH clinics will have undergone corrective surgery, although some who have had palliative or no surgery are still seen.

Palliative surgery

Children can undergo corrective surgery at an early age. Previously the practice was for individuals to undergo some form of palliative procedure to allow a period of growth before surgery.

> **Tip:** The most frequently employed operation was the *Blalock–Taussig shunt* (subclavian artery to pulmonary artery graft anastomosis). Other less common systemic–pulmonary connections were the *Waterston* (right PA to ascending aorta) and the *Pott's* anastomoses (left PA to descending aorta).

These procedures increase total pulmonary blood flow, which is otherwise impaired by RV outflow tract obstruction.

Corrective surgery

Complete corrective procedures in tetralogy of Fallot involve VSD closure, incorporating the aorta into the LV and relieving RV outflow tract obstruction. This usually involves resecting the hypertrophied infundibular myocardium, with patch enlargement of the outflow tract. Pulmonary regurgitation can occur and the surgeon may use a homograft valve to reconstruct the ouflow tract.

Long-term complications

Arrhythmia and sudden death
Ventricular arrhythmias are commonly found on ambulatory recording of Fallot patients. However, there is little evidence to support the use of prophylactic antiarrhythmic therapy in asymptomatic patients. Atrial flutter and fibrillation become more common with advancing age.

Right ventricular dysfunction
Patients with corrected tetralogy of Fallot often have impaired exercise capacity, owing to impaired RV function. Residual pulmonary incompetence or stenosis may contribute to this. RV enlargement can be assessed using echo or CXR. Pulmonary valve replacement should be considered if there is significant pulmonary regurgitation.

TRANSPOSITION OF THE GREAT ARTERIES (Fig. 14.4)

Atrial repair
Mustard procedure: The interatrial septum is excised and a 'baffle' or conduit is created using the wall of the common atrium and a pericardial patch to divert the systemic venous return through the mitral valve to the morphological left ventricle. Pulmonary venous return is then committed to flow through the tricuspid valve to the morphological right (systemic) ventricle. The **Senning procedure** creates a similar pathway using atrial rather than patch material (Fig. 14.5).

These intra-atrial repairs have three main long-term complications:

Arrhythmia
Nodal rhythm is common but seldom causes symptoms. Sinus rhythm may return during exercise. Disruption in sinus node function is often due to surgical trauma or alteration in nodal blood flow and pacing is sometimes required.

Late atrial tachyarrhythmias are more sinister. Atrial flutter and atrial fibrillation are poorly tolerated. Sudden death is also a recognized late complication. Ambulatory monitoring can be used to identify at-risk patients.

Right ventricular failure
The RV is surprisingly good at adapting to function as the systemic ventricle, although its ejection fraction often falls during adolescence. Exercise tolerance is usually reduced, but overt right (systemic) ventricular failure is

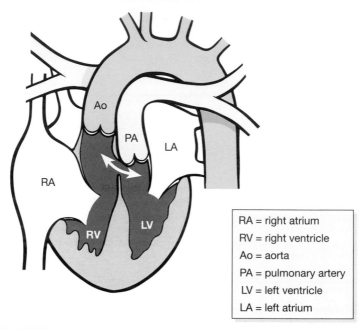

RA = right atrium
RV = right ventricle
Ao = aorta
PA = pulmonary artery
LV = left ventricle
LA = left atrium

Fig. 14.4 Transposition of the great arteries.

surprisingly uncommon. When it does occur it may be exacerbated by tricuspid regurgitation. These patients can be considered for cardiac transplantation, or revision of the Mustard circulation using an arterial switch (see below).

Baffle obstruction

Peripheral oedema, ascites, jugular venous distension and periorbital oedema strongly suggest baffle obstruction. The pulmonary venous circulation can also be compromised, causing symptoms of pulmonary congestion. These symptoms can also be caused by failure of the systemic ventricle.

Interpretation of echo images is not for the novice! Transoesophageal echo is often helpful, as transthoracic echo may not satisfactorily image the atria and baffles. Cardiac catheterization should be considered if there is uncertainty about baffle obstruction, or if transcatheter dilatation of the baffles is being considered.

Arterial repair

The arterial 'switch' operation is a definitive corrective procedure which can

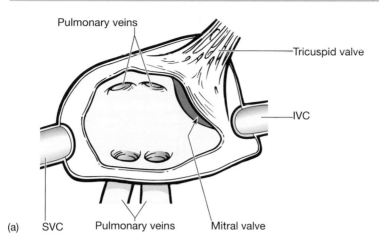

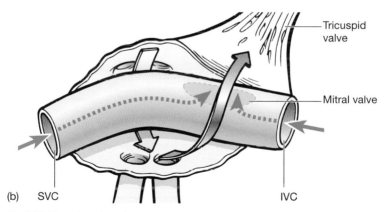

Fig. 14.5 Mustard atrial switch operation – the interatrial septum has been excised.

be carried out in infancy. It is technically demanding and until the 1980s carried a high mortality. The procedure is difficult because the coronary arteries have to be dissected at the ostia and anastomosed to the root of the pulmonary artery. The aorta and pulmonary artery are transected and transposed. The advantage of arterial repair is that the LV functions as the systemic ventricle. Sinus rhythm is usually maintained. Long-term complications include coronary ostial stenosis, supravalvar aortic or pulmonary stenosis, and pulmonary and aortic incompetence.

FONTAN CIRCULATION (Fig. 14.6)

Several congenital defects are associated with an interrupted right heart circulation: tricuspid and pulmonary valve atresia and disorders characterized by a functionally single ventricle, e.g. double-inlet ventricle and hypoplastic right or left ventricles. The *Fontan operation*, its forerunners the *classical Glen* and *bidirectional Glen* shunts, and subsequent modifications including the *total cavopulmonary correction*, were developed to create an atriopulmonary connection. The procedures create a pumpless pulmonary circulation which is driven passively by systemic venous pressure. The role of a left-sided 'drawing' effect is controversial. Maintenance of sinus rhythm and low pulmonary vascular resistance is important in maintaining the Fontan circulation.

> **Tip:** Atriopulmonary corrective procedures
> *Classical Glen shunt*. End-to-end anastomosis of SVC with right PA, with antegrade flow to the left lung from the preserved ventricular connection.
>
> *Bidirectional Glen shunt*. A bidirectional cavopulmonary anastomosis consisting of end-to-side SVC to right PA.
>
> *Fontan-type procedures*. This essentially consists of any procedure that connects the systemic veins (IVC and SVC) to the pulmonary artery, to overcome problems such as tricuspid atresia or a hypoplastic right heart. There are many variations on this theme. Originally an atriopulmonary connection was made between the RA appendage and proximal right PA using an aortic valve homograft; a classical Glen shunt was performed, and a homograft inserted into the IVC. It became apparent that inlet and outlet valves are not essential for acceptable pulmonary circulation.
>
> *Total cavo-pulmonary correction* is one of these variations, in which an intracardiac channel is created within the RA, using a prosthetic patch, directing IVC blood to an anastomosis with the pulmonary artery. The SVC is anastomosed as a bidirectional Glen shunt. This may reduce the frequency of late atrial arrhythmias and AV nodal damage, but long-term outcome is unclear.

Complications of Fontan-type operations

Atrial arrhythmias

The Fontan circulation functions best in sinus rhythm because atrial systole augments pulmonary flow. Atrial brady- and tachyarrhythmias are common. Atrial flutter and, less commonly, atrial fibrillation, are poorly tolerated and **potentially life-threatening**. Early DC cardioversion and discussion with a specialist unit are advised.

Pulmonary blood flow obstruction

The modest pressure gradient between PA and LA is a major component of

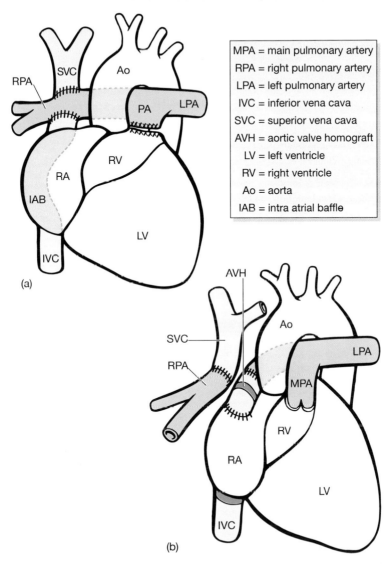

MPA = main pulmonary artery
RPA = right pulmonary artery
LPA = left pulmonary artery
IVC = inferior vena cava
SVC = superior vena cava
AVH = aortic valve homograft
LV = left ventricle
RV = right ventricle
Ao = aorta
IAB = intra atrial baffle

Fig. 14.6 (a) Total cavopulmonary connection; (b) Fontan procedure.

the Fontan circulation. Minor obstructions to pulmonary blood flow have a major haemodynamic effect. This can be caused by atrial thrombosis and 'onion ring' occlusion of Dacron grafts or homograft conduits.

Thromboembolism

Fontan patients are at significant risk of thromboembolism because of venous stasis and clotting factor abnormalities.

Death

The Fontan procedure is associated with a late mortality of around 25% at 15 years. Progressive congestive cardiac failure suggests residual shunting, especially if cyanosis develops. Overzealous diuretic treatment reduces the driving pressure of the Fontan circulation. Expert help should be sought and cardiac transplantation considered.

EISENMENGER COMPLEX AND SYNDROME

The term **Eisenmenger complex** is used to descibe the combination of VSD, severe pulmonary hypertension and consequent right-to-left shunt. The broader term **Eisenmenger syndrome** describes any central communicating defect associated with severe pulmonary hypertension and reversal of a previous left-to-right shunt.

Common causes are:

- ASD
- Non-restrictive VSD
- Large patent ductus arteriosus
- Truncus arteriosus
- Post surgical (Pott's, Waterston's and Blalock–Taussig anastomoses).

Pulmonary hypertension develops because of increased PA blood flow and exposure of the pulmonary circulation to systemic pressure. This causes progressive, eventually irreversible, vascular changes, including intimal hypertrophy, fibrosis and fibrinoid necrosis. Further vascular obstruction is caused by thrombosis and hypoxic vasoconstriction. This in turn increases pulmonary vascular resistance to systemic levels or higher; right-to-left shunting occurs and cyanosis develops. At this stage surgical closure of the communicating defect or *isolated* cardiac transplantation are not feasible, as the RV would fail owing to excessive afterload.

Specific points

- Pulmonary vascular resistance is the factor that determines whether corrective surgery is appropriate.
- Symptoms are exertional dyspnoea, haemoptysis (sometimes fatal), RV angina and exertional syncope (especially if age >20 years).

- Atrial arrhythmias cause significant compromise and are difficult to manage.
- Careful venesection may be necessary.
- Combined heart and lung transplantation is possible in selected patients.

Venesection in Eisenmenger syndrome

- Reserved for patients with severe hyperviscosity symptoms
- Strict aseptic technique is essential
- Two IV cannulae needed for simultaneous venesection and volume replacement
- Colloid or plasma expander used to prevent reduction in circulating volume
- Remove only one unit (approx 500 ml) at a time, over at least 2 h
- Reassess haematocrit after 24 h

The volume of whole blood to be removed can be more accurately estimated as:

$$\text{Volume (L)} = \text{body mass (kg)} \times 0.11 \times \frac{\text{haematocrit}_{initial} - \text{haematocrit}_{final}}{\text{haematocrit}_{initial}}$$

Decompensation in Eisenmenger syndrome

- When well, systemic vascular resistance usually balances with pulmonary vascular resistance and a balanced shunt occurs.
- A reduction in systemic vascular resistance (e.g. due to sepsis, vasodilator medication) increases right-to-left shunting, causing systemic hypoxia and sometimes loss of consciousness.
- Prompt recognition and treatment of arrhythmias is essential.
- Aggressive administration of IV fluids may be useful.
- High-flow O_2 may cause partial pulmonary vasodilatation and reduce shunting.
- Noradrenaline causes predominantly systemic vasoconstriction and may help reduce shunting.
- Do not give agents with systemic vasodilator properties (e.g. dobutamine).

PULMONARY ARTERY BANDING

By artificially creating pulmonary artery stenosis this procedure (employed in infancy) protects the pulmonary circulation from increased flow and pressure, e.g. with non-restrictive VSD. The pulmonary artery can be debanded at the time of definitive surgery.

RASTELLI PROCEDURE

This is an operation that closes a VSD, incorporates the aorta into the LV outflow tract and creates an external RV-to-PA conduit. It is sometimes used to correct a VSD associated with pulmonary atresia.

NON-CARDIAC PROBLEMS

HAEMATOLOGICAL

Regulation of red cell mass

Cyanotic heart disease in the adult is usually associated with secondary polycythaemia. Oxygen delivery can paradoxically be impaired through increased blood viscosity.

Symptoms of hyperviscosity
Headache
Lightheadedness
Paraesthesia
Myalgia
Fatigue
Visual disturbance
Pruritus
Anorexia

Venesection and iron deficiency

Phlebotomy should be reserved for patients with severe symptoms of hyperviscosity. It is rarely needed in iron-replete cyanotic adults with haematocrit ≤ 65%. Venesection is potentially hazardous and the volume of blood removed should be the minimum required for symptom relief. Iron deficiency can cause similar symptoms to hyperviscosity and should be considered as a diagnosis in patients with the above symptoms but a relatively normal haematocrit. Microcytic erythrocytes are less deformable than normal, and so struggle to pass through the microcirculation. Phlebotomy may exacerbate this situation and iron replacement may help. Care is required with iron therapy, as small doses can significantly augment the haematocrit within a week of treatment. **Ferrous sulphate** 325 mg d^{-1} should be given, but discontinued as soon as the haematocrit starts to rise.

Bleeding disorders

Bleeding is common in cyanotic patients, especially those with an elevated haematocrit. It is associated with thrombocytopenia and acquired von Willebrand factor deficiency, and the risk is increased by aspirin, heparin or warfarin treatment of atrial fibrillation. Fatal blood loss can occur after trauma or surgical procedures. Particular care should be taken to ensure that patients do not become iron deficient.

URATE METABOLISM

Hyperuricaemia is common in cyanotic heart disease patients. Acute gout is best treated with IV colchicine, which avoids dehydration through GI upset associated with oral use. Chronic treatment with low-dose colchicine or allopurinol is usually well tolerated.

Considerations for GUCH patients undergoing non-cardiac surgery
- Repeated gradual isovolumic venesection until haematocrit <65%
- Store venesected blood for autologous transfusion
- Meticulous attention to fluid balance: avoid dehydration
- Fresh frozen plasma and platelets may be needed perioperatively
- Fluid filters needed to prevent systemic air and particulate embolism
- Compression stockings and early mobilization to prevent DVT

CHOLELITHIASIS

Cyanotic adults are at risk of calcium bilirubinate gallstones through increased levels of unconjugated bilirubin. Infective endocarditis may result from bacteraemia associated with acute cholecystitis.

PREGNANCY

See Chapter 2.

CENTRAL NERVOUS SYSTEM DISORDERS

Cerebral abscess can occur in adults with congenital heart disease, although the mechanism is not clear. Right-to-left shunts in cyanotic patients allow systemic venous blood to bypass the 'lung filter', thereby allowing bacteria access to the cerebral circulation. Cerebral abscess should be considered in cyanotic patients with headache, fever and/or focal neurological signs. Seizures often occur, and may continue to do so after the infection is eradicated.

Paradoxical embolism is a hazard in patients with a right-to-left shunt, or in whom there is a potential communication from the venous to the systemic circulation. Thrombus from leg or pelvic veins, and air or particulate matter from intravenous lines are all potential risks and should be prevented. Contrast echo helps identify patent foramen ovale or secundum ASD in young patients with stroke due to paradoxical embolism.

The risk of cerebral haemorrhage is increased by oral anticoagulants or antiplatelet drugs: they should only be used if there is a clear indication to do so.

CHAPTER 15

CARDIAC REHABILITATION

PRINCIPLES OF REHABILITATION

Cardiac rehabilitation began as an exercise-based activity to combat the loss of cardiovascular fitness associated with prolonged bedrest after MI. The modern approach recognizes that, in addition to the physical element, there are psychological and social aspects to the rehabilitation process.

World Health Organization definition of cardiac rehabilitation

'... the sum of activities required to influence favourably the underlying cause of the disease, as well as to ensure the patients the best possible physical, mental and social conditions so that they may, by their own efforts, preserve, or resume when lost, as normal a place as possible in the life of the community. Rehabilitation cannot be regarded as an isolated form of therapy, but must be integrated with the whole treatment, of which it forms only one facet.'

Implicit is the central role and responsibility of the patient in rehabilitation and the importance of integrating rehabilitation with other aspects of management. Rehabilitation should involve the patient in 'self-management' of a chronic disease, in the same way as is expected of diabetics. The aims are (i) to modify the disease process (secondary prevention) and (ii) to assist the patient to return to a 'normal' role in society. The process of *behavioural modification* should encourage adaptive behaviours that will achieve those aims.

The following are central to the process of rehabilitation:

- **Pathology**: the disease process affecting the organ, such as coronary atheroma or valve stenosis
- **Impairment**: the negative effect of the pathology on the function of the organ, e.g. ischaemia, LV impairment, low cardiac output
- **Disability**: the functional consequences of impairment for the individual, e.g. reduced exercise tolerance or angina
- **Handicap**: the effects of that disability on the individual's role in society, e.g. unemployment, loss of status, having to give up golf.

Much of contemporary management targets pathology and impairment. Drugs or interventions modify impairments which we think cause the patient's disabilities. Success is often judged by modification of pathology or alleviation of impairment. Given the relationship between pathology, impairment, disability and handicap, we expect that the latter will improve. However, the correlation between pathology or impairment and disability or handicap is relatively poor. There are patients with minimal coronary disease who complain of angina that prevents even light exercise and conversely there are patients with severe three-vessel coronary disease, demonstrable ischaemia and no symptoms. Some of the variance may be explained by physical factors, but often these disparities are due to the psychological state of the patient, their level of fitness, or the demands made of them. This provides a strong argument for an approach which, while recognizing the importance of pathology and impairment, also directly targets disability and handicap. This holistic approach requires consideration of all four elements and therefore integration of rehabilitation with medical and surgical management.

> **Tip:** Ask yourself whether your patient would be symptomatically better if he or she were fitter, whether they would be less distressed if they had a clearer understanding of their condition, whether managing anxiety would improve their quality of life, or whether changing their behaviour might alter the natural history of the underlying disease. If the answer to any of these is 'yes', rehabilitation should play a part in management of their condition.

PHASES OF REHABILITATION

Rehabilitation is not a one-off intervention! It is a process the patient goes through for the duration of their illness. It can be broken down into four phases and is illustrated here for a patient following an acute MI.

PHASE I (IN HOSPITAL)

This is the early (post-diagnosis) phase and is crucial in terms of the potential to do harm. It involves the provision of information, facilitating the understanding of the condition and its implications. The main danger is reinforcement of previously held misconceptions (e.g. the belief that stress at work has caused the MI), or the generation of new ones (e.g. that the patient's heart is irreparably damaged). Such misconceptions can have a major influence on the patient's recovery. This phase involves all health professionals who come into contact with the patient: in the average cardiac unit there are many! There is thus great potential for conflicting information to be given. Good communicators recognize that patients absorb only a small amount of the information given, especially when anxious.

- Information is as powerful a therapeutic tool as any drug and potentially as harmful, so prescribe it accordingly!
- Information should be accurate and **consistent**, with the aim of improving outcome. Provide standardized general information and agree patient-specific information with colleagues.
- As little as 10–20% is retained, so keep it short and **relevant**. The fact that you prevented a massive heart attack by early thrombolysis is not important, but the fact that early thrombolysis has resulted in minimal damage is.
- Uptake is improved by repetition and the provision of written information. Document information given in case notes for the benefit of others who see

the patient after you. Write down anything you particularly want the patient to remember.

● Uptake is reduced by anxiety, which peaks when the patient is transferred out of the coronary care unit and immediately prior to discharge: choose your time to tell the patient things accordingly and use relaxation strategies.

PHASE 2 (RETURN TO OWN ENVIRONMENT)

This encompasses the patient's own efforts to get back to normal and occupies the period from discharge to review in the clinic. Again, information is crucial. This phase will go badly if the patient leaves hospital with a poor understanding of their condition. The primary care practitioner, community nurses or hospital outreach nurse may influence recovery during this period, but can only be effective if they receive prompt, accurate information from the hospital. Information cards, booklets and rehabilitation manuals aid recovery during this phase. Rehabilitation manuals have been shown to reduce anxiety and depression, as well as the need for primary care appointments and unnecessary readmission. Atypical chest pain is the most common reason for rereferral at this stage. From the patient's perspective this phase usually includes decision making about changing behaviours and is important in terms of secondary prevention lifestyle changes.

PHASE 3 ('FORMAL' REHABILITATION)

This phase begins approximately 4–6 weeks after MI and includes several treatment approaches, outlined below. In most rehabilitation units there is a set programme that all patients may be offered, although the concept of a modular approach, geared to the needs of each individual, is gaining favour. Although community-based programmes are increasingly common, this phase is most often delivered in the hospital setting. Uptake in these programmes is approximately 20–30% in the UK, and is influenced by such factors as age, gender, socioeconomic background and the availability of transport.

Phase 3 cardiac rehabilitation programmes usually consist of the following elements, which are described in the next section: exercise, education, relaxation, stress management, goal setting and secondary prevention. Most programmes involve the patients attending a group two to three times per week, for 2–3 hours. Most groups run for 6–12 weeks.

PHASE 4 (MAINTENANCE)

This begins after formal rehabilitation ends and goes on indefinitely. This phase is largely the responsibility of the primary care team. It involves monitoring patients' behaviour and using strategies to maintain good practice. Community-based exercise support groups may be used to reinforce exercise behaviour. Review clinics at primary care level help monitor secondary prevention and the level of disability or handicap.

Cardiologist's role in the phases of rehabilitation
Phase 1   Ensure adequacy, accuracy and consistency of information given
Phase 2   Provide information to patient and primary care team promptly
Phase 3   Assess rehabilitation status and needs at post-MI clinic (see Chapter 12) and refer appropriately
Phase 4   Determine and communicate long-term strategy

COMPONENTS OF REHABILITATION

THE EXERCISE PROGRAMME

There are three main reasons for exercise in patients with cardiovascular disease:

- To improve cardiovascular fitness, so that the patient performs exercise-related tasks more efficiently and with fewer symptoms
- To improve prognosis as part of a lifestyle secondary prevention programme
- To increase confidence and reduce anxiety about exercise.

Improving fitness

Deconditioning is no longer inevitable after MI as prolonged bedrest is no longer advocated and hospitalizations are relatively brief. Appropriate advice during phases 1 and 2 can prevent problems in most cases, but it can take several weeks before patients are able to return to work or to strenuous recreational exercise. Exercise programmes can help prepare them for these activities. Also, patients who are symptomatic during exercise may raise their symptom threshold by improving cardiovascular efficiency. Older patients have less cardiovascular reserve and use it more frequently. They are at least as likely to benefit from exercise training as younger patients, but are less likely to be referred.

The cardiovascular benefits of exercise include reduced sympathetic feedback (and increased vagal tone) from trained muscles. This lowers resting and exercise heart rate and improves the efficiency of O_2 extraction. These effects are mediated peripherally; maximum benefit is derived from exercise which uses a range of large muscle groups, and where a specific training goal is concerned (e.g. fitness to return to a labouring job) exercise should be targeted to that type of activity.

Early studies suggested that to achieve a training effect, exercise had to be undertaken at least twice a week for 20–30 minutes per session. Additional warm-up and cool-down times produce the typical 1-hour exercise sessions seen in most programmes. However, cardiovascular benefits have been recorded with shorter sessions and it is likely that there is a linear relationship between exercise and fitness. Improvements in fitness will equally result from exercise taken outside the class. Teaching the principles of improving and maintaining fitness is an important goal of any exercise programme.

Any increase in risk caused by acute exercise is offset by a reduction in risk at other times. Risk can be minimized by excluding patients with exercise-inducible arrhythmias or hypotension (until treated) and by using moderate rather than high-intensity exercise. Some centres teach patients to monitor their own pulse and maintain exercise to keep the heart rate below 70–80% of the predicted maximum. Other centres use perceived exertion scales, which correlate well with heart rate. Patients exercise so that they feel warm and breathe 'somewhat hard', but not to the point where they cannot speak.

Exercise training can be useful in symptomatic groups, e.g. patients with angina or cardiac failure. The autonomic 'β-blocking' effect is one benefit; some studies also show an *increase* in maximum heart rate and ischaemic threshold which may be due to enhanced collateralization or ischaemic preconditioning. Exercise training improves exercise capacity in moderate heart failure, possibly due to reversal of the myopathy associated with chronic heart failure. This is best achieved if the exercise programme includes strength or resistance training. Benefits are less clear-cut in severe heart failure. Although hospital or community-based exercises are usual, home-based exercise programmes can also be used safely and effectively.

Secondary prevention
See Chapter 12. The main focus should be on identifying an exercise regimen that will improve long-term compliance for the patient (e.g. encouraging activities the patient actually enjoys). Thus the approach for a patient in employment may differ from that for someone who is retired.

Improving confidence
Many patients avoid exercise out of fear. Having exercise recommended by a cardiologist, and receiving instruction from a physiotherapist, is a powerful tool that increases confidence and reduces anxiety.

THE EDUCATION PROGRAMME

Most hospital-based programmes include an education component covering topics such as diet and lifestyle, stress, the benefits of exercise, getting back to normal, and medication. Formal talks may give little opportunity for audience participation and similar information could be given in written format. There is little evidence that lecturing about the dangers of smoking to patients who have already received individual advice alters smoking behaviour. Smaller groups allow more interaction and the session can be used to identify patients' cognitions, beliefs and associated behaviours. Only by addressing these cognitions is it possible to modify behaviour.

RELAXATION AND STRESS MANAGEMENT

Relaxation techniques can be taught individually, in groups or using tapes, and are used by patients to tackle anxiety, panic or associated symptoms. They are often accompanied by breathing retraining, in which diaphragmatic breathing is taught. Shallow breathing, chest breathing and hyperventilation commonly accompany heart disease and are associated with dizziness, fatigue and even chest pain. Anxiety is a normal reaction to cardiac illness and many patients will have symptoms as a result. The tendency to categorize patients' symptoms as 'genuine' and 'non-cardiac' is unhelpful.

When stress is a more fundamental problem, a comprehensive stress management programme helps patients identify stress, stressors and stressful behaviours that can be modified. It is particularly useful in managing angina, where (after exertion) stress is the second most likely precipitant of symptoms.

GOAL SETTING

Rehabilitation programmes employ a goal-setting approach which helps patients return to behaviours that were stopped because of the acute illness. It also helps alter lifestyle behaviours as part of secondary prevention. Although goal setting is most easily applied to exercise, it can also be used for non-exercise activities. It involves teaching the patient the principles of self-pacing and identifying problems such as the 'overactivity/rest cycle' in which the patient overexerts when they feel well and is forced to rest as a result, leading to loss of fitness and confidence.

SECONDARY PREVENTION

Secondary prevention, particularly lifestyle elements, fits well in the practice of rehabilitation. The most commonly used approach is educative, in the expectation that patients will take straightforward advice. Providing the patient with advice *may* initiate a process of contemplating change and in a *minority* of cases a decision to change is followed through. Many patients decide not to change, either because they accept the risk associated with current behaviour (and there is little point in pressing the issue) or because they are not convinced that the advice applies to them. Here, the patient may respond to an approach that challenges their beliefs. Having decided to make a lifestyle change, patients may still fail for a variety of reasons, e.g. nicotine withdrawal symptoms, or peer pressure.

Rehabilitation and the follow-up clinic (see also Chapter 12)
The clinic review should be used to assess whether the patient has decided to

address lifestyle issues and to change behaviour. If not, can they be convinced of the need to change? Fear and badgering *do not work* and may reinforce negative behaviour. A major aim of clinic review and formal rehabilitation programme is to assist the process of change in patients who decide to alter behaviour but who are struggling with the process. This may involve prescribing and monitoring the use of nicotine replacement, identifying behaviours to replace smoking (e.g. exercise and relaxation) and considering alternative approaches such as hypnosis.

At discharge from formal rehabilitation (phase 4) recommendations have to be made to the primary care team for monitoring drug and lifestyle aspects of secondary prevention strategy.

INVESTIGATIVE AND INTERVENTIONAL CARDIOLOGY

ELECTROPHYSIOLOGY

REPORTING ECGs

This section gives an overview of ECG reporting; it does not comprehensively cover ECG interpretation. Separate texts are available that cover this subject in more detail (e.g. Hampton *The ECG made easy* and *The ECG in practice*, Churchill Livingstone). In this section, checklists of important ECG abnormalities and their causes are given and advice about how to report ECGs for wards or for open-access services is included.

Key points in ECG interpretation

- Report the ECG in the light of the available clinical information (e.g. age, symptoms, drug therapy etc.; for example, lateral ST segment depression reflects different processes in settings of hypertension, digoxin therapy and acute chest pain).
- Compare the ECG with previous ones, especially when reviewing patients with acute chest pain.
- Have a systematic approach – rate, rhythm, axis, P waves etc. – then you won't miss anything.

RATE AND RHYTHM

Heart rate is calculated from the RR interval. Count the number of large squares (0.2 s) between successive beats and divide into 300 to obtain heart rate in bpm. In irregular rhythms, average over 5 or 6 beats.

Atrial arrhythmias (see Figs 16.1–16.5)

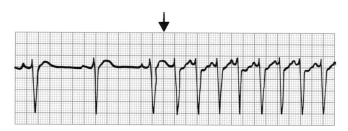

Fig. 16.1 Ectopic atrial tachycardia. Note inverted P waves. (From Hampton J R 1997 The ECG made easy. Churchill Livingstone, Edinburgh, with permission.)

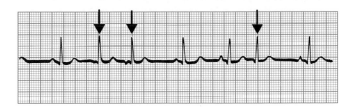

Fig. 16.2 Multifocal atrial ectopic beats – note varying P-wave morphology preceding marked QRS complexes. (From Hampton J R 1997 The ECG in practice. Churchill Livingstone, Edinburgh, with permission.)

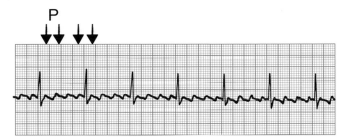

Fig. 16.3 Atrial flutter – note atrial rate of around 300 bpm. (From Hampton J R 1997 The ECG made easy. Churchill Livingstone, Edinburgh, with permission.)

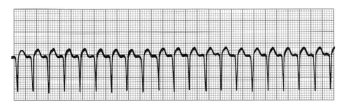

Fig. 16.4 Narrow QRS SVT; could be AV nodal re-entry tachycardia or orthodromic accessory pathway tachycardia. (From Hampton J R 1997 The ECG in practice. Churchill Livingstone, Edinburgh, with permission.)

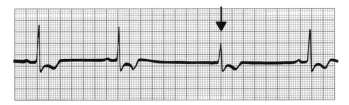

Fig. 16.5 Sinus pause with junctional escape beat. (From Hampton J R 1997 The ECG in practice. Churchill Livingstone, Edinburgh, with permission.)

Junctional arrhythmias (see Fig. 16.6)

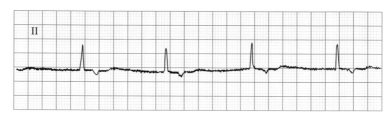

Fig. 16.6 Junctional bradycardia with retrograde P waves.

Ventricular arrhythmias (see Figs 16.7–16.9)

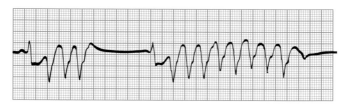

Fig. 16.7 Monomorphic VT. (From Hampton J R 1997 The ECG in practice. Churchill Livingstone, Edinburgh, with permission.)

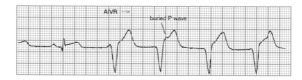

Fig. 16.8 Accelerated idioventricular rhythm, a slow version of VT. (From Jenkins R D, Gerred S J 1997 ECGs by example. Churchill Livingstone, Edinburgh, with permission.)

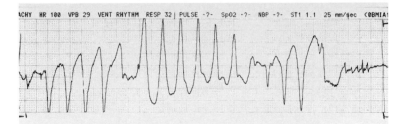

Fig. 16.9 Polymorphic VT – *torsades de pointes* variant: high risk of cardiac arrest.

AV block (see Figs 16.10–16.13)

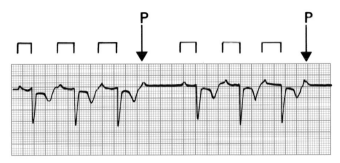

Fig. 16.10 Second-degree AV block – Mobitz type I (Wenckebach). (From Hampton J R 1997 The ECG made easy. Churchill Livingstone, Edinburgh, with permission.)

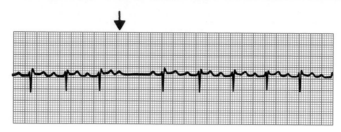

Fig. 16.11 Second-degree AV block – Mobitz type II (infranodal). (From Hampton J R 1997 The ECG made easy. Churchill Livingstone, Edinburgh, with permission.)

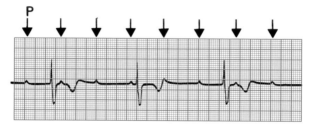

Fig. 16.12 Third-degree AV block with narrow-complex escape rhythm. (From Hampton J R 1997 The ECG made easy. Churchill Livingstone, Edinburgh, with permission.)

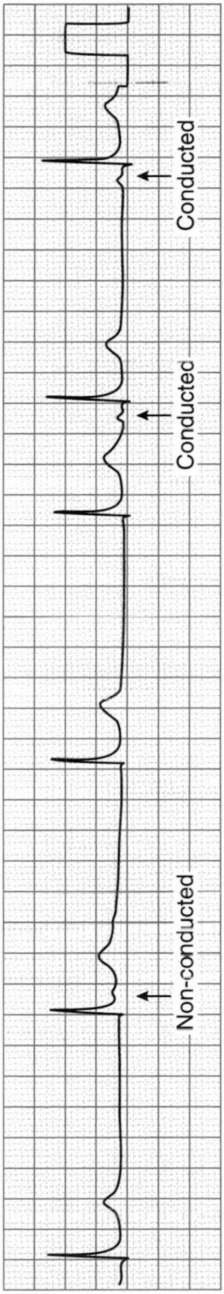

Fig. 16.13 AV dissociation. The intrinsic ventricular rate exceeds the atrial rate. At times P waves are conducted to the ventricles. This is not third-degree AV block and does not require pacing.

Paced rhythms (see Figs 16.14–16.19)

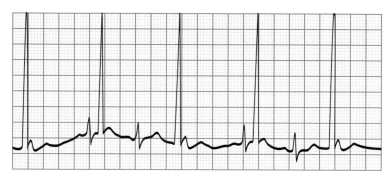

Fig. 16.14 Undersensing in VVI mode. The pacemaker tries to pace because it has not sensed the intrinsic rhythm.

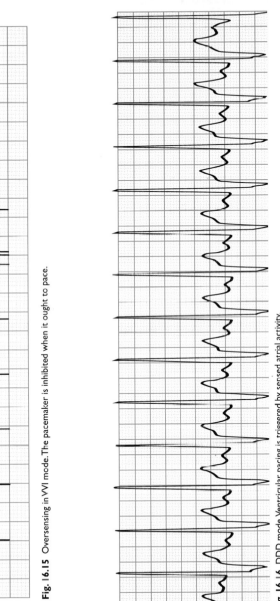

Fig. 16.15 Oversensing in VVI mode. The pacemaker is inhibited when it ought to pace.

Fig. 16.16 DDD mode. Ventricular pacing is triggered by sensed atrial activity.

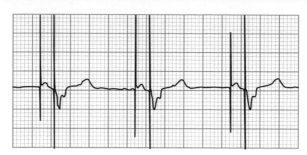

Fig. 16.17 DDD mode. AV sequential pacing.

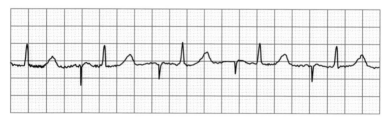

Fig. 16.18 AAI pacing. Note pacing artefact before each P wave.

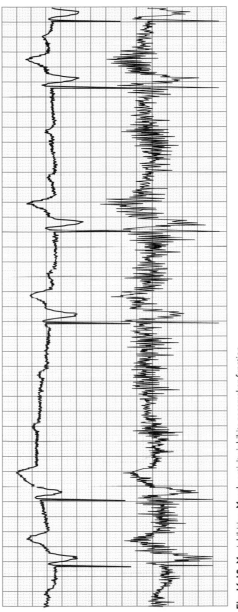

Fig. 16.19 Myoinhibition. Muscle activity inhibits pacemaker function.

FRONTAL AXIS

The mean frontal QRS axis is best estimated using the hexaxial reference system (Fig. 16.20).

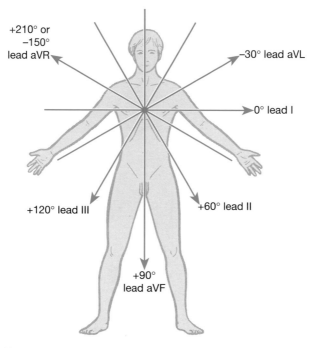

Fig. 16.20 Hexaxial lead system.

Normal axis	−30° to +90°
Left axis deviation	−30° to −90°
Right axis deviation	+90° to +180°
Extreme axis deviation	+180° to −90°

Estimating the frontal axis – quick method (see Fig. 16.21)

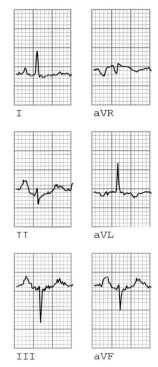

Fig. 16.21 Example ECG for axis calculation.

Example for frontal axis calculation

- Identify a (nearly) isoelectric limb lead. This will lie at right-angles to the mean axis. For example, lead II 'looks' at +60°.

● If this lead is isoelectric, the axis must be about 90° away from it. In this example the axis must be about –30° or +150°.

● To determine which, look at a different lead, at least 45° away from the isoelectric lead. In this example, use lead I (which 'looks' at 0°).

● If this lead is mainly positive, the axis must be near it (–30° in the example). If the lead is mainly negative, the axis must be far from it (+150° in example).

> Very quick method: if leads I and aVF are both mainly positive, the axis is normal.

P WAVES (see Fig. 16.22)

P-wave amplitude is normally <0.2 mV (2.0 mm), duration <0.12 s. The P-wave axis is normally between –50° and +60°. Broad bifid P waves indicate left atrial hypertrophy or dilatation. Tall P waves indicate right atrial hypertrophy or dilatation.

P-R INTERVAL

This is measured from the onset of the P wave to the onset of the QRS complex, normally between 0.12 and 0.2 s. A short P-R interval can occur with pre-excitation and junctional rhythm. A long P-R interval may reflect AV block.

QRS DURATION

Normally <0.12 s. As a quick check, in LBBB the terminal QRS deflection in lead V_1 is usually negative and in V_6 is positive. The opposite is true in RBBB. Right ventricular ectopic beats give LBBB morphology and left ventricular ectopic beats give RBBB morphology.

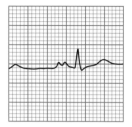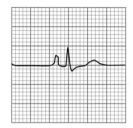

Fig. 16.22 P-mitrale (left) and P-pulmonale.

QRS AMPLITUDE (see Fig. 16.23)

This is affected by ventricular muscle mass, frontal and transverse axis and patient build. Thin patients have larger complexes; obese or barrel-chested patients tend to have smaller complexes. Small complexes also occur with pericardial effusion and hypothermia.

ECG criteria for LVH
- R in I or aVL >12 mm **OR** R in I + S in III >25 mm
- S wave in V_1 + R wave in V_5 **OR** S wave in V_2 + R wave in V_6 >40 mm
- Left axis deviation (axis 'pulled' by ↑ LV muscle mass)
- ST / T-wave abnormalities in I, aVL, V_5, V_6 (abnormal repolarization)
- P-mitrale (left atrium enlarges due to ↑ LV wall stiffness)
- Delayed intrinsicoid deflection V_6 (QRS onset to peak of R wave) >0.05 s

ECG criteria for RVH
- Dominant R wave in V_1
- Dominant S wave in V_6
- R in V_1 + S in V_6 >11 mm
- Right axis deviation (axis 'pulled' by ↑ RV muscle mass)
- P-pulmonale
- Delayed intrinsicoid deflection V_1 >0.04 s

ST SEGMENT

ST segment abnormalities are difficult to interpret in ventricular hypertrophy and RBBB. They cannot be interpreted in LBBB.

- **ST segment elevation** occurs in acute MI, pericarditis, Prinzmetal's angina and with left ventricular aneurysm. Rarer causes are hyperkalaemia, acute pulmonary embolism, stroke and hypothermia. It can be normal (early repolarization) in some individuals, especially Afro-Caribbeans.
- **ST segment depression** occurs in myocardial ischaemia and infarction, digoxin therapy, cardiomyopathies, infiltrative cardiac disease and with many other drugs and metabolic disorders.

> Tip: There are many causes of ST segment and T-wave abnormalities. Clinical information is **essential** for interpretation.

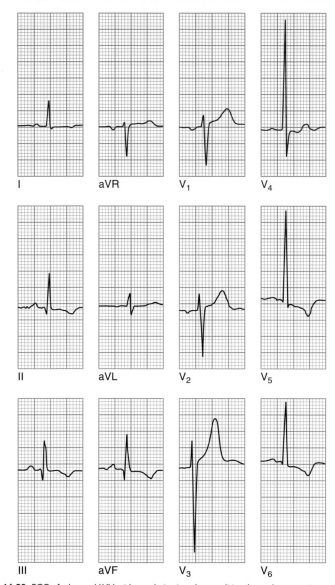

Fig. 16.23 ECG of advanced LVH with repolarization abnormalities due to hypertension.

QT INTERVAL

This varies with heart rate, so a corrected interval (QT_c) is calculated. It is normally between 0.38 and 0.46 s. Long QT interval predisposes to atypical VT (*torsades de pointes*).

$$QT_c = \frac{QT \text{ interval (s)}}{\sqrt{[R\text{-}R \text{ interval (s)}]}}$$

T WAVES AND U WAVES

- **T-wave inversion** is common. It is caused by the pathologies listed under 'ST segment depression' and can occur in many other conditions, e.g. hyperventilation, anxiety, exercise, stroke and allergic reactions. In patients with suspected unstable angina, ST segment changes and T-wave inversion can be used as a component of risk assessment (see Chapter 5).
- **Tall T waves** occur in LVH, hyperkalaemia, acute pericarditis, Prinzmetal's angina and true posterior MI.
- **U waves** occur during bradycardia, with hypokalaemia, digoxin and some antiarrhythmic drugs (especially amiodarone). **Negative U waves** are an early sign of myocardial disease in hypertension.

Causes of QT prolongation

- Electrolyte disturbance ($\downarrow K^+, Ca^{2+}, Mg^{2+}$)
- Antiarrhythmics – amiodarone, sotalol, procainamide, disopyramide, quinidine, bretylium
- Psychotropics – phenothiazines, tricyclics, lithium, haloperidol
- Quinine and related antimalarials
- Other drugs – erythromycin, vasopressin, tacrolimus, terfenadine, cisapride, probucol
- Hypothermia
- Congenital long QT syndromes. May be caused by abnormal left-sided cardiac sympathetic innervation and, in rare cases, sodium channel dysfunction (as in Brugada syndrome). Associated with syncope, high risk of sudden death (>50% die within 10 yrs of diagnosis). Treatments are atrial pacing (shortens QT), β-blockade, AICD and mexiletine (Na^+ channel cases).
  Jervell and Lange-Nielsen syndrome: autosomal recessive, associated with congenital deafness
  Romano–Ward syndrome: autosomal dominant (but more common in females, so may be multiple genes), hearing normal.

SPECIFIC ECG PATTERNS

Acute coronary syndromes
See Chapter 5 for examples.

Acute pericarditis (see Fig. 16.24)

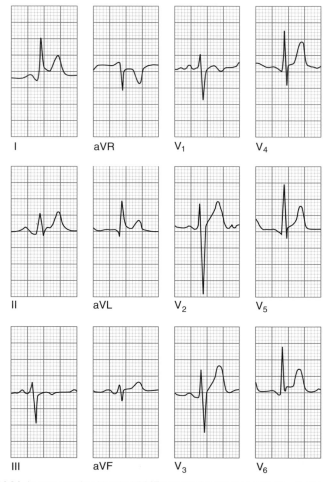

Fig. 16.24 Acute pericarditis. Note 'saddle' ST segment elevation in most lead territories.

Conduction defects (see Fig. 16.25)

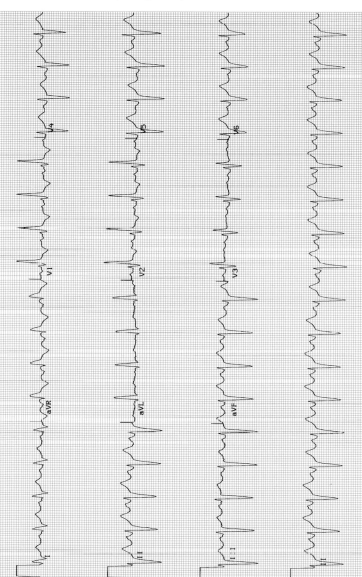

Fig. 16.25 Bifascicular block – RBBB + left axis deviation suggests left anterior hemiblock. If PR interval is prolonged this is termed 'trifascicular block' (see also Chapter 17). (From Jenkins R D, Gerred S J 1997 ECGs by example. Churchil Livingstone, Edinburgh, with permission.)

Pre-excitation (see Fig. 16.26)

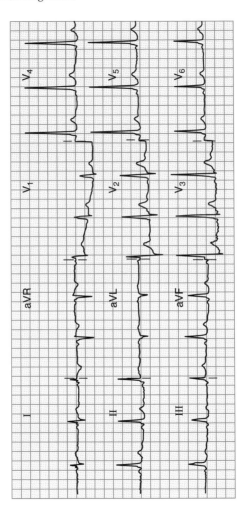

Fig. 16.26 Wolff–Parkinson–White syndrome. The tall R wave in V_1 and positive delta wave suggest a left-sided accessory pathway.

AMBULATORY RECORDING

Ambulatory recordings can be made using continuous recorders (e.g. 24- or 48-hour cassette tape recorders or digital loop recorders), external patient-activated devices (e.g. 'Cardiobeeper' recorder) or, for infrequent sudden episodes, implantable event recorders (e.g. Medtronic Reveal).

● **24-hour 'Holter' recorders** are fine if symptoms occur on an almost daily basis.
● **Patient-activated recorders** are better if symptoms are infrequent (e.g. once a fortnight) but are no use for syncope if there are no warning symptoms.
● **Implantable recorders** are useful for investigating infrequent syncope or presyncope, if non-invasive methods do not produce a diagnosis.

Ambulatory recordings are usually read by an automated computer reader and verified by human eye. The following information is logged:

● **Heart rate histogram**. Look at heart rate variation. A flat trace may indicate inactivity or chronotropic incompetence. A very flat trace may indicate a pacemaker! Sudden jumps in heart rate may signify episodes of arrhythmia.
● **Ectopic beat/episode counter**. This counts narrow- and broad-complex premature beats. Couplets, triplets, VT and SVT episodes and pauses may be counted.
● **Rhythm strips**. A comprehensive log will include the following:
    – main rhythm during recording
    – examples of arrhythmias recorded, including onset and termination
    – rhythm during episodes noted in patient diary
    – rhythm during maximum and minimum heart rate for recorded period.

Checklist for ambulatory recording
● Meticulous electrode site preparation is crucial to obtain clear traces.
● Position leads to obtain clear P waves and as clear a QRS complex as possible.
● Check P waves with patient both erect and supine.
● Explain what symptoms you are interested in to pin down, and show patient how to activate event button. This will mark recording.
● Give an event diary so that patient can log symptoms.
● Encourage patient to lead as normal a day as possible, without immersing device!

Always examine rhythm disturbance in relation to symptoms. Asymptomatic arrhythmias are surprisingly common in healthy people, especially the elderly (see Chapter 11, Palpitation).

Period beginning	QRS	Shape	Prem Norm	SVT	Ab.	Cplt	Trplt	Salvo	VT	Drop. beat	Pause	Brady.	Paced beats	HR min	HR max	Art sec
10:38	1315	0	2	0	0	0	0	0	0	0	0	0	0	55	78	109
11:00	3969	0	5	0	0	0	0	0	0	0	0	0	0	58	83	222
12:00	4026	0	34	0	0	0	0	0	0	0	0	0	0	59	87	66
13:00	4144	0	17	0	0	0	0	0	0	0	0	0	0	63	85	36
14:00	4661	0	25	0	0	0	0	0	0	1	0	0	0	61	119	79
15:00	5959	0	0	0	0	0	0	0	0	12	0	0	0	89	130	349
16:00	5756	0	1	0	0	0	0	0	0	13	0	0	0	90	109	23
17:00	5400	0	1	0	0	0	0	0	0	26	0	0	0	86	114	112
18:00	5542	0	1	0	0	0	0	0	0	27	0	0	0	88	118	133
19:00	5994	0	1	0	0	0	0	0	0	19	0	0	0	90	122	93
20:00	5440	0	3	0	0	0	0	0	0	23	0	0	0	85	111	31
21:00	6111	0	3	0	0	0	0	0	0	19	0	0	0	88	131	161
22:00	5096	0	37	0	0	0	0	0	0	33	0	0	0	74	119	224
23:00	4905	0	26	0	0	0	0	0	0	39	0	0	0	75	95	12
00:00	5079	0	9	0	0	0	0	0	0	41	0	0	0	78	88	0

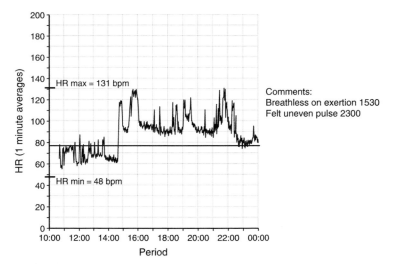

Comments:
Breathless on exertion 1530
Felt uneven pulse 2300

Fig. 16.27 Sample from event log of 24-hour tape recording.

EXERCISE ELECTROCARDIOGRAPHY

Exercise testing is one of the most widely used (and misused!) investigations in cardiological practice. Used correctly, exercise testing helps confirm the diagnosis of coronary disease in symptomatic patients, is useful for assessing functional capacity and provides prognostic information about patients with known coronary disease. Exercise testing is positively **unhelpful** in some groups of patients, particularly when it is applied as a screening test. To understand why, it is important to appreciate that predictive accuracy is affected not only by the test's sensitivity and specificity, but also by the population being studied.

BAYESIAN THEORY

Bayesian theory states that the predictive accuracy of a diagnostic test depends in part on the prevalence of the disease sought in the population which is studied. Overall, the sensitivity and specificity of exercise testing for coronary artery disease are around 68% and 77%, respectively. For diagnosing prognostically important disease (i.e. left main-stem and three-vessel disease) the sensitivity improves to 86%.

● **In a low-risk population**, e.g. asymptomatic middle-aged women, a positive test is more likely to be a *false positive* than a *true positive* (the predictive accuracy is less than 50% – useless!).
● **In an intermediate- to high-risk population**, e.g. elderly men with typical ischaemic symptoms, a positive test is much more likely to be a true positive than a false positive (the predictive accuracy is >90% – useful to *confirm* the diagnosis).

INDICATIONS

Class I (clear-cut indication)
Class IIa (consensus is that testing may be helpful).

Diagnosis of coronary artery disease
● Intermediate probability of CAD (I) (based on age, gender and symptoms)
● Vasospastic angina (IIa).

Risk assessment in symptomatic patients/patients with established CAD
● Initial evaluation of suspected/known CAD (I)
● Suspected/known CAD with significant change in clinical status (I).

After myocardial infarction
- Predischarge (submaximal test, days 4–7) to assess prognosis, determine exercise programme and evaluate treatment (I)
- Early post-discharge (symptom-limited, days 14–21), if predischarge ETT not done (I)
- Late post-discharge (symptom-limited, 3–6 weeks) if symptom-limited test not already done (I)
- After discharge in patients who have undergone revascularization, to plan rehabilitation (IIa).

Exercise testing with ventilatory assessment
- Transplant assessment for patients with heart failure (I)
- Differentiation of cardiac and respiratory limitations in breathless patients where cause is uncertain (I)
- Evaluation of exercise capacity in patients whose own assessment of exercise capacity is not reliable (IIa).

Before and after revascularization
- Demonstration of ischaemia before revascularization (I)
- Evaluation of recurrent ischaemic symptoms after revascularization (I)
- Planning of rehabilitation after revascularization (IIa).

Evaluation of arrhythmias
- Optimizing rate-responsive pacemaker function (I)
- Evaluation of known or suspected exercise-induced arrhythmias (IIa)
- Evaluation of therapy (e.g. ablation) for above (IIa).

 Warning: Exercise testing is only useful when it is applied to an appropriate population. Otherwise it can generate anxiety and lead to unnecessary follow-up tests.

CONTRAINDICATIONS
- Fever/acute viral illness
- Myo/pericarditis
- Severe aortic stenosis
- Aortic dissection
- Uncontrolled hypertension
- Overt cardiac failure
- Unstable angina or acute phase of MI

- Significant resting arrhythmia (e.g. uncontrolled atrial fibrillation, complete heart block)
- Known severe left main-stem or left main equivalent disease
- Physical disability rendering patient unsteady (e.g. osteoarthritis)
- ECG abnormality which renders ST segment assessment difficult (e.g. LBBB, LVH with 'strain', digoxin ECG changes).

EXERCISE PROTOCOLS

The *Bruce* and *modified Bruce* protocols (Table 16.1) are widely used, although there are several other well-validated protocols. The Bruce protocol is used for diagnostic and prognostic evaluation of otherwise fit, stable patients with suspected CAD. In the UK it is also used as a benchmark for vocational licence holders (heavy goods and public service vehicle drivers) with known or suspected CAD. Drivers must complete 9 minutes (stage 3) off anti-ischaemic medication without evidence of significant ischaemia and without symptoms. The modified Bruce protocol is useful for frail and elderly subjects and as a limited protocol for risk assessment in patients stabilized after an episode of suspected unstable angina.

Procedure

Before subjecting your patients to a stress test, try it yourself ! It isn't so easy to balance on the treadmill and although a 14% gradient doesn't look much, Bruce stage 3 is equivalent to walking briskly up a 1 in 7 hill – it's tougher than you think! The following are essential:

- Explain the test. Ask the patient to tell you when symptoms occur.
- Meticulous electrode site preparation, good resting ECG.
- Demonstrate how to use the treadmill. Ensure patient relaxes arms to minimize ECG artefact.

TABLE 16.1 Bruce and modified Bruce exercise protocols

| | Bruce | | Modified Bruce | |
Stage	Gradient (%)	Speed (mph)	Gradient (%)	Speed (mph)
1	10	1.7	0	1.7
2	12	2.5	5	1.7
3	14	3.4	10	1.7
4	16	4.2	12	2.5
5	18	5.0	14	3.4
6	20	5.5	16	4.2
7	22	6.0	18	5.0

- IV access for patients with suspected malignant arrhythmias.
- Check BP during each stage of test.
- Stop test if patient is distressed or very keen to stop, but remember that sensitivity and specificity are improved if patient achieves target heart rate.
- Target heart rate is 85% predicted maximum (220 – age for men; subtract an additional 10 for women).

Indications to terminate test
- Target heart rate achieved
- Worsening angina or excessive breathlessness
- Dizziness
- Fatigue/patient requests test to stop
- Atrial arrhythmia other than ectopic beats
- Frequent ventricular ectopic beats or ventricular tachycardia
- Worsening ST segment shift (elevation or depression)
- Fall or failure to rise in BP
- Exaggerated hypertensive response to exercise (sBP >220 mmHg)
- New high-grade AV block or bundle branch block.

ECG abnormalities often develop during the recovery phase. The patient is monitored until heart rate and BP return close to baseline and any ECG abnormalities have resolved. Delayed resolution of ischaemic ECG abnormalities suggests a critical stenosis of the culprit vessel(s).

Criteria for positive ETT
- Planar ST depression ≥ 1 mm, relative to PQ segment, 80 ms after the J point (junction between QRS complex and ST segment)
- ST elevation
- Increase in QRS voltage (ischaemic LV dilatation)
- Failure of BP to rise during exercise (ischaemic LV dysfunction)
- Ventricular arrhythmias
- (Typical ischaemic symptoms during exercise).

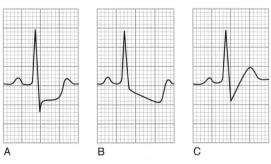

Fig. 16.28 ST segment depression during exercise testing. Planar (A) and downsloping (B) patterns indicate ischaemia, but upsloping (C) ST depression is a poor indicator.

Causes of a false positive ETT

- Cardiomyopathies
- Hypertension (especially with LVH 'strain' pattern)
- LV outflow obstruction (HOCM, aortic stenosis)
- Hyperventilation
- Some resting ECG patterns (LBBB, pre-excitation, digoxin pattern)
- Electrolyte abnormalities
- Tricyclic antidepressants
- 'Syndrome X' – usually middle-aged females with typical ischaemic symptoms but normal epicardial vessels
- Coronary artery spasm
- Sympathetic overdrive (anxiety, adrenergic drugs (e.g. salbutamol))

Features of prognostically important CAD that merit angiography

- ST depression at low workload (<6 min Bruce), in multiple lead groups, persisting into recovery, >2 mm, and downsloping pattern
- Abnormal BP response
- Ventricular arrhythmias

EP TESTING – INTRODUCTION AND INDICATIONS

Cardiac electrophysiology (EP) is a daunting subspecialty – it is very jargonized and intracardiac traces may seem impossible to understand at first. However, as with basic ECG interpretation at medical school a systematic approach renders EP recordings easier to grasp. EP is a very rapidly growing field and indications for EP interventions are expanding rapidly as understanding of arrhythmia mechanisms improves, technology advances and procedures become safer to perform.

MAIN INDICATIONS FOR EP TESTING

These are based on the joint recommendations of the ACC/AHA and NASPE and are summarized in full in *Circulation* 1995;92:673.

Evaluation of bradycardias
- **Sinus node dysfunction**
    - symptomatic patients with suspected sinus node dysfunction, where the link between arrhythmia and symptoms is not established non-invasively
    - known sinus node dysfunction, to evaluate AV node before permanent pacing (usually done in pacing laboratory)
- **AV block**
    - suspected infranodal (His–Purkinje) block as cause of symptoms
    - persistent symptoms despite pacemaker implantation, where another arrhythmia is suspected

- **intraventricular conduction delay**
  - symptomatic patients with intraventricular block, to establish propensity to high-grade block.

Evaluation of tachycardias

- **Tachycardias with narrow QRS complex**
  - frequent symptoms, where EP characterization will determine line of treatment and where drugs ineffective/poorly tolerated/not wanted
- **Tachycardias with broad QRS complex**
  - diagnosis of tachycardia not known from surface ECG, where diagnosis will determine line of treatment
- **Wolff–Parkinson–White syndrome**
  - evaluation for RF ablation
  - patients with unexplained syncope or resuscitated cardiac arrest
  - patients in whom knowledge of accessory pathway properties may determine requirement for treatment (e.g. in high-risk occupations).

Evaluation of unexplained syncope

- Suspected or known structural heart disease, in which non-invasive testing fails to establish diagnosis
- Recurrent, unexplained syncope after negative tilt test (see Chapter 13).

Evaluation of cardiac arrest survivors

- Cardiac arrest in absence of myocardial infarction
- Cardiac arrest >48 h after acute MI, in absence of recurrent myocardial ischaemia
- Cardiac arrest caused by bradycardia.

Evaluation of palpitations

- Palpitations preceding syncopal episode
- Documented inappropriately rapid pulse rate in absence of adequate ECG documentation of arrhythmia.

EP guidance of drug therapy

- VT/VF cardiac arrest, sustained VT
- Rarely used for guiding drug R_x of narrow complex tachycardias, as RF ablation now treatment of choice.

PREPROCEDURE CHECKLIST

- Explain procedure and risks (e.g. of possible need for pacemaker), try to allay anxiety (reduces need for sedation, which compromises induction of arrhythmias)

- Written consent
- Check coexisting conditions (e.g. cardiac failure) well controlled
- Check U&Es, correct electrolyte disturbances
- Stop antiarrhythmics five half-lives before procedure
- Stop warfarin 3 days before procedure: check INR result on the day
- 12-lead ECG of arrhythmia available during procedure (ensures that induced arrhythmia matches clinical arrhythmia)
- Ensure patient is fasting
- IV access
- Blood pressure monitoring
- Set up pressure transducer if transseptal puncture planned
- Check emergency equipment available: defibrillator, resuscitation drugs, intubation kit, pericardiocentesis kit
- Check drugs available (isoprenaline, atropine, adenosine, sedatives and analgesics).

THE EP STUDY AND RF ABLATION

The key to understanding an electrophysiological study (EPS) is to understand the *activation* sequence of the heart. During EPS the activation sequence is examined in several settings:

- **During normal sinus rhythm**
    - allows measurement of normal conduction intervals (see below)
    - identifies possible site of accessory pathway by identifying which part of the ventricles is activated first (pre-excited)
- **During the culprit arrhythmia, induced during the study**
    - identifies activation sequence during SVT, to differentiate accessory pathway from AV nodal re-entry and ectopic atrial tachycardias
    - identifies whether broad-complex tachycardias are ventricular or supraventricular in origin
    - allows localization of VT focus by identifying site of earliest ventricular activation
- **During pacing/paced premature complexes (extrastimuli)**
    - paced atrial extrastimuli allow identification of dual AV nodal conduction by identifying AV nodal pathways with different conduction times and refractory periods (see AVNRT, below)
    - ventricular pacing identifies concealed accessory pathways by identifying which area of the atria are activated first during retrograde VA conduction
    - comparison of complex morphology during ventricular pacing with VT or VPB complexes can be used to locate VT focus ('pace mapping').

CATHETERS AND THE EP TRACE DURING SINUS RHYTHM

Catheter electrodes are placed at strategic positions to help identify the cardiac activation sequence. Signals are displayed at a fast sweep speed (usually 100 mm s^{-1}) to emphasize timing relationships. The ECG thus looks very smeared out. There are many subtleties to EPS recording and this section is designed just to get you started. This is what all those lines are on a standard console (!):

Surface ECG
A signal from at least three leads is usually displayed – usually one inferior, one lateral and one anterior lead.

HRA (high right atrium)
A quadripolar catheter (two pairs of electrodes, one for pacing and one for sensing) is placed in the RA appendage near the sinus node. The sensed atrial signal is usually a sharp spike. Comparison of the atrial signal from here and from lower down (e.g. from the His catheter) identifies whether the atria are being activated retrogradely or antegradely.

RV (right ventricle)
A pacing wire is placed in RV apex, for back-up in case excessive bradycardia or asystole occurs, for pace termination of arrhythmias and for ventricular extrastimulation (see below).

His
A quadripolar catheter is placed across the superior aspect of the tricuspid ring, adjacent to the interventricular septum. Both pairs of electrodes are sensed, giving a 'proximal His' and a 'distal His' recording. A good tracing in sinus rhythm gives three deflections – an atrial deflection (representing low atrial activation), a sharp His spike and a ventricular deflection – known as the A-H-V sequence. This sequence changes during tachycardias (e.g. during VT, retrograde AV conduction may give a V-H-A sequence; during AV nodal re-entry the A and V signal may be superimposed).

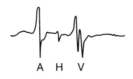

A   H   V

Fig. 16.29 Typical His catheter recording.

CS (coronary sinus)

The coronary sinus os lies posteriorly at the floor of the RA. The sinus runs in the left AV groove and is conveniently placed to measure signals that cross the AV ring (i.e. via accessory pathways). The catheter has four or five pairs of electrodes which measure local potentials, termed CS 1–2, CS 3–4 etc. By convention, CS 1–2 is usually the distal pair (covers left lateral AV ring) and CS 9–10 proximal (at coronary sinus os). The CS signal consists of an atrial (A) and a ventricular (V) deflection. If an electrode pair lies next to an accessory pathway, the A-V interval is shortest at that site, when pre-excitation is present.

Catheters are usually placed via the femoral veins. Once they are in position, baseline measurements are made (see Fig. 16.29), followed by a planned sequence of atrial and ventricular stimulation tests. Drugs are often used to induce AV block (which helps reveal accessory pathway conduction) and to assist arrhythmia induction.

Tip: Anticoagulation

Unfractionated **heparin**, 5000 U IV bolus, followed by an IV infusion, should be given to maintain ACT between 200 and 300. If transseptal puncture is anticipated anticoagulation should be deferred until the procedure is accomplished.

INTRACARDIAC INTERVAL MEASUREMENTS

PA interval

An indirect measure of atrial conduction, measured from onset of the earliest P wave on the surface ECG to the earliest rapid deflection of the atrial electrogram from the His catheter. Normal range 20–40 ms.

AH interval

Represents conduction through the AV node to the His bundle. It is measured from the His catheter, from first rapid atrial deflection to His deflection. It is affected by autonomic tone, pacing and drugs. Normal range 60–120 ms.

HV interval

Represents conduction from proximal His bundle to the ventricular myocardium. Measured from His catheter, from onset of the His deflection to earliest onset of ventricular activation on the surface ECG or ventricular electrogram. It is not significantly affected by autonomic tone. Normal range 30–55 ms.

EVALUATION OF BRADYCARDIA

Evaluation of sinoatrial node function

Sinus node disease causes symptoms because of episodic sinus bradycardia, sinus arrest or sinoatrial exit block. Abnormal sinus node function predicts a favourable response to pacing.

Sinus node recovery time (SNRT)

The HRA catheter is paced faster than sinus rate for >30 s, then abruptly stopped. SNRT is the interval between the last paced beat and the first sinus beat. Normal range <1500 ms. Corrected SNRT (cSNRT) = SNRT – sinus cycle length. cSNRT >600 ms implies mild dysfunction; >3 s implies severe dysfunction.

Sinoatrial conduction time (SACT)

A single paced atrial stimulus is delivered just before the next spontaneous sinus cycle, thereby resetting the sinus node. SACT is calculated from the interval between the paced stimulus to the next sinus beat (return interval).

$$\text{SACT} = \frac{\text{(spontaneous cycle length − return cycle length)}}{2}$$

Normal range 50–125 ms. Prolonged SACT indicates susceptibility to exit block.

Evaluation of AV nodal conduction

EP testing is rarely needed for diagnosis but is useful for identifying the level of block (intra- or infranodal). Infranodal block usually requires pacing as it carries a poor prognosis. Intranodal block is less serious; pacing is only required for symptoms.

EVALUATION AND ABLATION OF SVTs (see also Chapter 7)

EP testing is usually performed in anticipation of subsequent ablation. Although the surface ECG gives clues as to the SVT mechanism, definitive diagnosis usually requires EP testing. EP testing is good at inducing tachycardias due to re-entry or triggered activity, but poor at inducing automatic tachycardias.

Ventricular and atrial extrastimulation

This is used to induce arrhythmia, to test AV node physiology and to unmask accessory pathways which are not obvious in sinus rhythm.

Ventricular extrastimulation

The RV is paced at a fixed rate ('drive cycle') for 6–10 beats, then a paced extra stimulus is added and the subsequent activation sequence recorded. This is repeated, increasing the prematurity of the extra stimulus by 20 ms each time. The following are checked:

- Arrhythmia induction
- Early atrial activation at the CS catheter – accessory pathway conduction
- VA block
- Ventricle is refractory to the paced stimulus (ventricular refractory period).

Atrial extrastimulation

As above, but with atrial pacing. There is a risk of inducing atrial fibrillation with very premature atrial stimuli. Dual AV nodal conduction may be identified (see AVNRT, below). The following are also checked for:

- Arrhythmia induction
- Early ventricular activation at the CS catheter – accessory pathway conduction
- AV block and 'dual' AV nodal conduction (see later)
- Atrium is refractory to the paced stimulus (atrial refractory period).

Example SVT protocol
- SA node function tests (above)
- AV node function tests (e.g. heart rate at which Wenckebach AV block occurs)
- Ventricular pacing (coronary sinus electrogram may identify a short V-A interval, or site of early atrial activation, due to retrograde VA conduction through accessory pathway)
- Ventricular extrastimulation
- Atrial extrastimulation

Once tachycardia is induced, the following observations help establish the mechanism:

- Mode of initiation and termination
- Atrial activation sequence (helps distinguish SA nodal and ectopic atrial from AV nodal and accessory pathway tachycardias)
- Effect of bundle branch block on cycle length (if HR faster during BBB, is *rate-related aberrance*; if HR slower, bundle branch itself must be part of the tachycardia circuit (e.g. slow with LBBB → ipsilateral accessory pathway))
- Effect of atrial and ventricular stimulation during tachycardia
- Effect of AV node blocking drugs on the tachycardia.

Once the mechanism is established, in most cases RF ablation can be performed. This is effective in over 90% of cases of SVT caused by accessory pathways or AV nodal re-entry.

Characteristics of different SVTs

Sinus node tachycardias
Characterized by normal P-wave morphology and narrow QRS. Difficult to
distinguish from physiological sinus tachycardia. These tachycardias may
occur in paroxysms or at a rate inappropriate to the level of activity.

Inappropriate sinus tachycardia
- Automatic tachycardia, cannot be induced at EPS
- Usually idiopathic; can follow accessory pathway or slow pathway ablation
- Sinus node modification or ablation effective in severely symptomatic
  patients; a pacemaker is required after the latter.

Sinus node re-entrant tachycardia
- Sudden onset, paroxysmal tachycardia due to re-entry within the SA node
- Inducible by programmed stimulation
- RF ablation of sinus node and pacemaker implantation is treatment option.

Atrial tachycardias
Ectopic atrial tachycardias (see Fig. 16.1) are characterized by an abnormal
P-wave axis, often a normal PR relationship and narrow QRS. Often
paroxysmal, may be precursor to atrial fibrillation.

Automatic atrial tachycardia
- Uncommon; associated with underlying systemic illness or digoxin toxicity
  and rarely in young adults without structural heart disease
- Usually incessant; may cause ventricular dilatation and cardiac failure
- Exhibits warm-up phenomenon, rate up to 200 bpm, sometimes with AV
  block
- Tachycardia focus is often near the pulmonary veins.

Intra-atrial re-entrant tachycardia
- Paroxysmal and inducible during EPS
- Re-entry usually occurs near the pulmonary veins, interatrial septum, crista
  terminalis and RA appendage
- RF ablation is feasible in some cases.

Atrial flutter (see Fig. 16.3)
- Caused by a large intra-atrial re-entry circuit, usually involving the
  'isthmus' between IVC and tricuspid annulus. Depolarization may occur in
  either direction.
- Atrial flutter is inducible at EPS.
- RF ablation is performed either in sinus rhythm or during flutter. Several
  RF burns are used to create a line of block along the conduction isthmus.
- Recurrence rate is up to 20%.
- Late atrial fibrillation may occur, especially if atria enlarged/diseased.

Atrial fibrillation

● Chaotic atrial rhythm due to multiple interlacing re-entry wavelets, inducible at EPS.

● 'Focal' atrial fibrillation (localized area of tissue considered the site of initiation) can be successfully ablated.

● Other ablation strategies include the performance of conduction corridors around the pulmonary veins, interatrial septum and the right atrium. This procedure is in its infancy.

● His bundle ablation and pacemaker implantation are options in patients whose symptoms are not controlled medically.

AV nodal re-entrant tachycardias (AVNRT)

This is the most common SVT mechanism, caused by the re-entry circuit involving the AV node and atria. Causes regular, usually narrow QRS tachycardia. The 'compact' AV node has two atrial inputs with different conduction properties (Fig. 16.30).

Usually initiated by an atrial premature beat, 'typical' AV nodal re-entry conducts antegradely down the slow pathway and retrogradely up the fast pathway. The P wave is often obliterated because during tachycardia the atria and ventricles are activated almost simultaneously.

Identification of dual AV nodal conduction Done during atrial extrastimulation. The fast pathway cannot conduct when the atrial extrastimulus is very premature. If there is dual AV nodal conduction the A-H

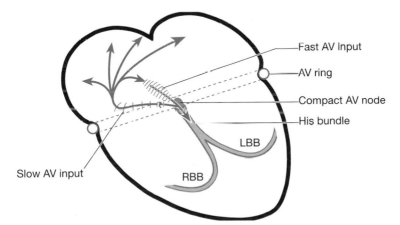

Fig. 16.30 Schematic of AV nodal re-entry circuit. The 'fast' pathway conducts rapidly but has a long refractory period, and the 'slow' pathway conducts slowly but has a short refractory period. This is an example of atypical AV nodal re-entry with antegrade conduction in the fast pathway. An analagous situation occurs in WPW syndrome, in which the accessory pathway acts as the 'fast' AV pathway.

interval 'jumps' by more than 50 ms (compared to that of the previous extrastimulus) when the 'fast' pathway conduction is eliminated (Fig. 16.31).

● Slow pathway ablation is preferred as the risk of AV block is lower.
● Accelerated junctional rhythm occurs during ablation and is usually a marker for success. The endpoint for successful ablation is inability to induce AVNRT.
● The incidence of heart block requiring permanent pacemaker implantation largely depends on operator experience – reported incidence varies from 1 to 20%.

Accessory pathway (atrioventricular re-entrant) tachycardias

These occur in patients with overt pre-excitation (e.g. Wolff–Parkinson–White syndrome) and with 'occult' accessory pathways (not evident on ECG because they either conduct retrogradely, intermittently, or are remote from the AV node). Antegrade conduction is usually down the AV node (orthodromic tachycardia), causing a narrow QRS tachycardia similar to that of typical AVNRT (see Fig. 16.4). Rarer antidromic tachycardias use the accessory pathway for antegrade conduction, giving a broad QRS complex. EPS is helpful as follows:

● **Assess pathway's** *antegrade refractory period*. A short refractory period means the pathway can conduct rapidly and repetitively, suggesting a significant risk of VF and sudden death if atrial fibrillation occurs ('pre-excited atrial fibrillation'). On surface ECG a short R-R interval (<240 ms) during induced or spontaneous AF is associated with a high risk.
● **Localizes the accessory pathway**. Several surface ECG algorithms are available. However, accurate localization (especially with concealed

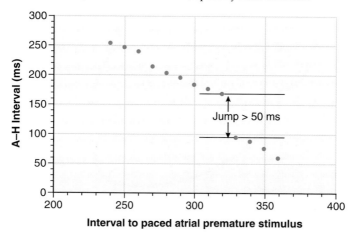

Fig. 16.31 Example of A-H interval jump during atrial extrastimulation.

pathways) requires EPS. Accessory pathways occur anywhere around the AV rings except the isthmus between mitral and aortic valve.

● Ablation is treatment of choice for symptomatic patients and those at high risk.

● Circus tachycardia is usually readily inducible with atrial or ventricular extrastimulation. The pattern of atrial activation during tachycardia is invaluable in accessory pathway localization.

● BBB occurring during tachycardia may influence heart rate. If the accessory pathway is ipsilateral to the bundle branch block, the tachycardia slows.

● Ventricular extrastimulation during tachycardia (when His bundle is refractory) usually advances the atrial electrogram, suggesting that the ventricles are part of the tachycardia circuit. This is not the case in AVNRT.

● >10% of patients have multiple pathways, manifest only after ablation of the most dominant pathway.

With overt pre-excitation ablation is usually performed during sinus rhythm. Rapid atrial pacing, or **verapamil** 5–10 mg IV, can be used to maximize pre-excitation. Left-sided pathways are best ablated using transseptal puncture. Ideally, successful ablation sites are characterized by a ventricular electrogram which commences several milliseconds ahead of the earliest QRS deflection on the pre-excited surface ECG. An accessory pathway potential is sometimes seen. With concealed accessory pathways ablation is performed either during ventricular pacing or during tachycardia. Recurrence rate after successful ablation is low (<5%) and most recurrences are curable at second attempt.

Tip: Ablation of septal accessory pathways carries a greater than average risk of AV block and this should be discussed with the patient.

Rarer forms of accessory pathway tachycardias, such as Mahaim tachycardias and permanent junctional reciprocating tachycardia, are outside the scope of this book.

AV node and His bundle ablation

Indicated in patients with SVTs in whom control of ventricular rate cannot be achieved by other means, or when drug therapy produces intolerable side effects. Ablation is usually done using a right-sided (venous) approach. A permanent pacemaker is required either before or soon after the procedure. There is a significant incidence of lethal arrhythmia after this procedure, which can be avoided by pacing at 90 bpm for at least 3 weeks, gradually reducing to 60–70 bpm. This protects the patient against lethal ventricular arrhythmias.

EVALUATION AND ABLATION OF VENTRICULAR ARRHYTHMIAS

EP testing is used to differentiate broad-complex SVTs from VT, for risk stratification of patients with suspected or confirmed VT and to test the efficacy of antiarrhythmic drug therapy. EP testing for VT utilizes specific extrastimulation protocols. Protocols which are more 'aggressive' (i.e. use multiple extrastimuli, or adjuvant drugs such as isoprenaline) have the greatest sensitivity but relatively low specificity. RF ablation is only appropriate for specific types of VT.

Example 'aggressive' VT protocol

1. Pace from RV apex:
   (a) Drive train of 8 paced beats, cycle length 600 ms (100 bpm), followed by a single extrastimulus, coupling interval 500 ms.
   (b) Repeat, with extrastimulus earlier by 20 ms each time, until ventricle fails to capture (effective refractory period).
   (c) If no VT, repeat steps (a) and (b), with drive train 500 ms (120 bpm).
   (d) If no VT, repeat steps (a) and (b), with drive train 400 ms (150 bpm).
   (e) If no VT, use double extrastimuli.
   (f) If no VT, use triple extrastimuli.
   (With double extrastimuli the first extrastimulus is timed 20 ms longer than the effective ventricular refractory period.)
2. If VT is not induced from RV apex, pace RV outflow tract using above protocol.
3. If VT is not induced from either site, repeat with isoprenaline infusion.

Criteria for positive or negative EPS
- Positive: reproducible >10 beats VT after stimulation
- Negative: no VT induced during study
- Borderline: short episodes VT (<10 beats) induced.

RF ablation for ventricular arrhythmias

Ablation is most successful in patients with a structurally normal heart. The most common variant is RV outflow tract tachycardia, characterized by a non-sustained LBBB-type tachycardia with an inferior axis. It is best induced with isoprenaline or rapid ventricular pacing. It may respond to β-blockers or calcium channel antagonists, but ablation in the RV outflow tract is effective. Other forms of 'ablatable' VT are the fascicular tachycardias (*idiopathic LV tachycardias*) and bundle branch re-entry tachycardia. Ablation of VT caused by cardiomyopathy or post-MI is less successful, but can be used to palliate symptoms in patients with recurrent VT despite drug therapy or AICD.

COMPLICATIONS OF EP TESTING AND RF ABLATION

COMPLICATIONS OF CARDIAC CATHETERIZATION
(see Chapter 18)

COMPLICATIONS OF SUBCLAVIAN/JUGULAR VEIN PUNCTURE
- Pneumothorax/haemothorax
- Subclavian arteriovenous fistula
- Brachial nerve injury.

COMPLICATIONS OF RF ABLATION
- Death (up to 1 in 300 in some series)
- Pericarditis/tamponade
- Transient and permanent AV block
- Radiation burns (with prolonged procedure)
- Stroke (with left-sided procedures and transseptal catheterization)
- MI
- Coronary sinus perforation
- Catheter entrapment within the ventricular trabeculation or valve apparatus
- Aortic or AV valve regurgitation.

PERMANENT PACING

INDICATIONS (see also Chapters 3 (temporary pacing) and 2 (non-cardiac surgery))

Pacing is one of the most rapidly advancing subspecialties in cardiology. Microprocessor, sensor and lead technologies have expanded the indications for pacing, reduced pacemaker-associated symptoms such as pacemaker syndrome, increased device longevity and reduced device size. There has been a marked increase in the number of dual-chamber rate-adaptive and antitachycardia devices implanted in recent years. National guidelines for permanent pacemaker implantation vary from country to country. The ACC/AHA and the British Pacing and Electrophysiology Group (BPEG) have produced recommendations which are broadly similar. This section is based on the AHA/ACC guidelines. After each indication the strength of evidence is indicated, along with the pacing mode usually employed. Pacing modes are described in the next section.

Strength of evidence for treatment

Class I	Consensus is that treatment should be used.
Class II	Treatment is often used, but there is some divergence of opinion about efficacy. Divided into:
Class IIa	Weight of evidence/opinion is in favour of usefulness/efficacy.
Class IIb	Usefulness/efficacy is less well established by evidence/opinion.
Class III	Consensus is that treatment should not be used.

There are six key groups of patient in whom permanent pacing should be considered. The indications given below are not exhaustive; refer to AHA/ACC or BPEG guidelines for details.

AFTER MYOCARDIAL INFARCTION

Inferior MI

Second- and third-degree AV block is relatively common in *inferior MI*. Block usually occurs at AV node level (rather than His–Purkinje level), giving a narrow-complex, relatively fast (>40 bpm) escape rhythm. In most cases AV block resolves within 14 days. Pacing is indicated with:

● *Second- or third-degree AV block persisting beyond 14–21 days.* **CLASS II, DDD.**

Anterior MI

AV block

Third-degree AV block complicating anterior MI is a sinister sign. It often reflects massive infarction involving the His bundle and/or the bundle branches and is often accompanied by haemodynamic decompensation. If the patient survives, dual-chamber pacing is indicated for:

- *Second- or third-degree AV block*, whether persistent or intermittent. **CLASS I, DDD**.

Intraventricular block

In the absence of intermittent second- or third-degree AV block, acquired LBBB or RBBB and bifascicular block are not indications for permanent pacing. Trifascicular block denotes extensive conducting system damage; some centres implant a permanent pacemaker prophylactically. For bi- and trifascicular block complicating anterior MI, extended ambulatory monitoring (up to 48 h) before discharge is warranted to exclude intermittent high-grade AV block.

- *Bifascicular/trifascicular block with intermittent second- /third-degree AV block* on ambulatory monitoring. **CLASS I, DDD**.
- Trifascicular block in absence of intermittent second- or third-degree AV block. **NOT INDICATED, CLASS III**.

Bifascicular and trifascicular block

- **Bifascicular block** occurs when two of the three fascicles do not conduct. Technically this includes LBBB, but bifascicular block usually refers to:
  - RBBB + left anterior hemiblock   OR
  - RBBB + left posterior hemiblock
- **Trifascicular block** implies impaired conduction of all three fascicles without complete AV block. The term usually refers to:
  - RBBB + alternating left anterior and left posterior hemiblock
  - alternating LBBB and RBBB
  - LBBB + long PR interval (denoting either slow conduction in RBB, His bundle or AV node)

(see also Chapter 16, Fig. 16.25)

ACQUIRED AV BLOCK

Third-degree AV block

- *Third-degree AV block* carries a significant risk of death due to asystole and permanent pacing is indicated regardless of symptoms unless a reversible cause can be found. **CLASS I, DDD**.

Second-degree AV block

- *Permanent or intermittent Mobitz type II AV block* requires permanent pacing, as the level of block is infranodal (in the His–Purkinje system) and the risk of asystole relatively high. **CLASS I, DDD**.
- *Mobitz type I (Wenkebach) AV block* is usually benign. Wenckebach conduction is a property of AV nodal tissue and is accentuated by increased vagal tone. It is a common asymptomatic finding in young or athletic individuals. If asymptomatic, pacing is not indicated. Permanent pacing may help if symptoms are *definitely* linked to bradycardia. **CLASS I, DDD**.

> **Tip:** 2:1 second-degree AV block can occur both with Mobitz type I and Mobitz type II conduction; it is not easy to distinguish the two. But complete heart block/asystole is much more likely with type II AV block. An extended period of ambulatory monitoring may help with the diagnosis.

First-degree AV block

Permanent pacing is almost never indicated. An exception is the patient with LV impairment in whom extreme AV conduction delay compromises cardiac output and worsens cardiac failure. In this instance a trial of temporary dual-chamber pacing is indicated first. **CLASS II, DDD.**

AV block associated with atrial flutter/fibrillation

Permanent pacing is indicated if bradycardia is associated with congestive cardiac failure, pauses >3 s, or escape rate <40 bpm. Pacing should also be considered if tachycardia and bradycardia occur and a rate-limiting drug is needed to control tachycardia. **CLASS I, VVI (R).**

CHRONIC INTRAVENTRICULAR BLOCK

Bundle branch block and bifascicular block

- *Intraventricular block with third-degree AV block or Mobitz type II AV block* (permanent or intermittent, both regardless of symptoms). **CLASS I, DDD.**
- *Bifascicular or trifascicular block with symptoms, not documented to be due to AV block*, but where other causes have not been found. **CLASS II, DDD.**
- *Trifascicular block.* Although some centres favour prophylactic dual-chamber pacing, **NOT INDICATED** if symptomatic.

SICK SINUS SYNDROME

This is a conducting tissue disorder (which can affect atrial tissue and the AV node as well as the sinus node) manifest by bradycardias due to sinus node failure and tachycardias, usually initiated in the atria. Pathophysiologically there may be inflammation, fibrosis, degenerative changes and fatty infiltration near the sinus node and in the atria. Sinus node artery disease may mediate the disorder in some cases. It occurs most commonly in elderly individuals without overt structural heart disease. There may be associated AV block. The cardinal symptoms are palpitation (due to tachycardias) and presyncope and syncope (due to bradycardias). Fatigue may occur because of *chronotropic incompetence* (heart rate does not rise with exertion) or *inappropriate sinus tachycardia*. However, sinus node disease is often asymptomatic and ECG features are a common incidental finding on ambulatory recordings.

> **Arrhythmias associated with sinus node disease**
>
> ● **Bradycardias**
> sinus bradycardia
> sinus arrest (junctional or idioventricular escape rhythm)
> sinus arrest with asystolic pauses
> sinoatrial exit block
> bradycardia due to associated second- /third-degree AV block
> ● **Tachycardias**
> ectopic atrial tachycardia
> inappropriate sinus tachycardia
> atrial flutter/fibrillation

Sick sinus syndrome does not cause terminal asystole and studies have failed to show that pacing prolongs life. Common sense tells us that syncope and presyncope are dangerous and indications for pacing are geared to symptom control in:

● *Symptoms associated with documented bradycardia* (remember, dizziness has many causes in the elderly, in whom asymptomatic sick sinus syndrome is common). **CLASS I, AAI or DDD***.
● *Drug-induced symptomatic bradycardia* where drug is considered necessary to limit tachycardias. **CLASS II, AAI or DDD***.

> **Tip:** * DDD implanted if impaired AV node function, e.g. Wenckebach AV block with atrial pacing ≤ 140 bpm, or second- /third-degree AV block on ambulatory recording. Some centres routinely implant DDD devices in case AV block develops after implantation, but the risk of this is only 2% per year.

Pacing is a treatment of last resort for recurrent syncope, where bradycardias are found on ambulatory recording but where a clear relationship between symptoms and bradycardia has not been established. In these cases other causes of syncope (e.g. vasovagal syndrome) should be excluded first. Pacing should **not** be considered if symptoms occur during ambulatory recording in the absence of bradycardia.

HYPERSENSITIVE CAROTID SINUS SYNDROME (HCSS)

HCSS is caused by carotid baroreceptor hypersensitivity, resulting in parasympathetic activation then bradycardia and/or vasodilatation. Symptoms classically occur when pressure is applied to the neck (e.g. wearing a tight collar). Diagnosis is by ECG monitoring and carotid sinus massage (CSM: see Chapter 11 for technique). Pacemaker implantation is indicated for:

- *Recurrent syncope associated with neck pressure.* Asystole >3 s during CSM in the absence of drugs that suppress sinus or AV node function. **CLASS I, DDI + HYSTERESIS.**
- *Recurrent syncope without clear trigger, but with positive CSM test.* **CLASS II, DDI + HYSTERESIS.**

MALIGNANT VASOVAGAL SYNDROME

In this condition a maladaptive reflex results in inappropriate vasodilatation and/or bradycardia in response to venous pooling. This involves (i) initial sympathetic activation, followed by (ii) reflex parasympathetic activation. Reduced venous return initially leads to increased cardiac *sympathetic* activity, in an attempt to augment cardiac output. The ventricles contract vigorously in the face of poor filling and mechanoreceptor stimulation causes profound *parasympathetic* activity leading to a cardioinhibitory (bradycardic) and/or vasodepressor (vasodilatory) response (see Fig. 13.2). The condition is diagnosed with **tilt testing** (see Chapter 13).

First-line treatment is with drugs, either β-blockers to reduce initial sympathetic activation (e.g. **metoprolol** 25–100 mg bd) or vagolytics to reduce subsequent vagal activation (e.g. **disopyramide** modified-release 100–300 mg bd). Other less well validated measures are increased salt intake, compression stockings, fludrocortisone to expand blood volume, and theophylline. Permanent pacing is indicated for:

- *Syncope and positive tilt test with cardioinhibitory response,* where drug therapy has failed and where a trial of temporary pacing during repeat tilt test prevents symptoms. **CLASS II, DDI + HYSTERESIS.**

Miscellaneous

- *Hypertrophic obstructive cardiomyopathy* (see Chapter 6), to induce incoordinate septal and posterior wall function, reducing outflow tract obstruction.
- *Congenital long QT syndrome* (in conjunction with β-blockade) to shorten QT interval.
- *Dilated cardiomyopathy and end-stage cardiac failure.* Short AV delay may improve ventricular filling and cardiac output. The evidence base for this indication is inconclusive.

PACEMAKERS, LEADS AND PACING MODES

Pacemaker technology has generated an entire new vocabulary which can seem daunting at first. This section describes the basic pacemaker device and lead types, along with the basic programmable functions found in standard pacing devices. Antitachycardia devices and AICDs are discussed in the final section.

PACEMAKER LEADS

Lead polarity

● *Bipolar leads* have two terminals at the lead tip; the current path is short and the pacing signal often small or invisible on the surface ECG. Extracardiac potentials (e.g. from chest wall muscle) are less likely to interfere with function.

● *Unipolar leads* have one terminal (–); the device 'can' acts as the positive terminal. These are used less often because pectoral muscle twitching can occur and muscle potentials can interfere with device sensing (*myoinhibition*).

Lead fixation methods

● *Epicardial leads* are attached using a wire suture or screw tip via a thoracotomy or subxiphoid approach. The pacemaker is usually implanted beneath the rectus sheath. Epicardial systems are used in infants, where transvenous leads might be 'outgrown'. Other uses are for AV block occurring during cardiac surgery (especially aortic valve surgery), recurrent infection of the endocardial system and when the patient has a mechanical tricuspid valve replacement.

● *Endocardial leads* are implanted via the cephalic or subclavian veins; tines or fins allow the leads to lodge into trabeculae. Atrial leads are J-shaped, designed to hook into the right atrial appendage. Ventricular leads are longer and straight, designed to lodge in the RV apex.

● *Active fixation leads* use a screw tip to secure the lead into the atrial or ventricular wall. The tip is either retractable or has a rapidly dissolving coating to prevent the lead catching during insertion. During insertion the lead is screwed in over a stiff wire or *stilette*. Indications are: difficulty securing a stable position with passive fixation lead; unexplained lead displacement and massively dilated right heart (RA appendage difficult to locate; RV apex and trabeculae less likely to 'hold' passive RV lead; tricuspid regurgitation displaces lead back into RA). Some centres use these after cardiopulmonary bypass (involving RA appendage cannulation). Although initial pacing thresholds are usually higher than with endocardial leads, long-term performance is good.

● *Steroid eluting leads* are active fixation leads with a steroid eluting tip which reduces inflammation after insertion and improves pacing threshold and sensing.

PACEMAKERS

Pacemakers are usually referred to in terms of the number of chambers paced (single- or dual-chamber), their ability to increase heart rate during exercise (rate-response capability) and their ability to change pacing mode during atrial arrhythmias (mode-switching capability). Other considerations in device implantation are cost, size (e.g. a small device for a very thin patient), event memory (e.g. for patients with intermittent arrhythmias) and longevity (some devices are capable of testing their own pacing threshold, thus minimizing current use).

Dual- and single-chamber devices

● *Single-chamber pacemakers* carry a single lead, either in RA or RV. Single-chamber atrial (e.g. AAI) pacemakers are used in sick sinus syndrome. Single-chamber ventricular (e.g. VVI) pacemakers are used in atrial fibrillation with symptomatic bradycardia.

● *Dual-chamber pacemakers* carry two leads, in RA and RV. This allows sequential pacing of atria and ventricles and also (using DDD mode) ventricular pacing in sequence with the patient's intrinsic atrial rhythm in complete heart block.

Adaptive pacing features (see later for details)

● *Rate-responsive pacemakers* use accelerometer, minute ventilation, temperature or QT interval sensors to trigger an increase in heart rate in response to activity. The degree to which, and rate at which, heart rate increases is programmable.

● *Mode-switching pacemakers* are used for patients with AV block and intermittent atrial tachyarrhythmias. Whereas dual-chamber pacemakers (in DDD mode) attempt to pace the ventricles rapidly in response to the atrial rhythm during tachycardia, mode-switching devices convert to VVI or VVIR mode if the atrial rate exceeds a programmed threshold.

Programmability

● *Telemetry* refers to communication between programming device and pacemaker and vice versa. Modern telemetry links are user-friendly and use a window or menu-driven interface.

● *Multiprogrammability* is the ability to adjust the device's pacing and sensing settings (e.g. rate, output, sensitivity) to suit the individual. All modern devices are multiprogrammable.

PROGRAMMABLE FUNCTIONS

Pacemakers stimulate the heart by generating square-wave electrical impulses which activate conducting tissue. Intrinsic cardiac activity is detected through the pacing lead and the pacemaker can be programmed to inhibit or trigger paced activity in response to this. The amount of energy required to pace the heart varies between patients and may change with time in an individual patient. Also, the sensed electrogram varies between and within patients. Finally, patients' physiological state and requirements may change, and so pacing mode and heart rate may need to be altered to account for this. The aim of pacemaker programming is to optimize pacemaker function in terms of physiological requirements and symptoms, while minimizing energy consumption. The best way to learn about the practicalities of programming is with an experienced technician in a pacemaker clinic. This section should get you started with the commonly programmed functions.

Single-chamber device programming

This section describes the basic programmable functions of single-chamber devices; these are also fundamental to dual-chamber devices. Advanced features such as rate adaptation and mode switching are described later in the chapter. Pacing modes are discussed later in this section.

Paced rate

The interval at which the pacemaker cuts in during VVI or AAI pacing is known as the *lower rate interval*. For most devices this is programmed as a *lower rate* parameter. Patients with intermittent bradycardias need a low programmed rate setting (e.g. 40 bpm). This prevents extreme bradycardia but maintains intrinsic rhythm at other times, and conserves device power. Higher programmed rates can be helpful to increase cardiac output (e.g. in heart failure), but continuous pacing reduces device lifespan and, with VVI devices, may cause pacemaker syndrome (see below). Temporary programming to a low paced rate helps in identification of the underlying cardiac rhythm. Programming to a value higher than the patient's intrinsic rate helps confirm capture, and helps measure pacing threshold.

Pacing threshold and output settings

Energy consumption is dictated by the device **output** (measured in volts) and **pulse duration** (measured in milliseconds). The relationship between these two variables and pacemaker threshold is called the *strength–duration curve*.

Pulse duration/output combinations above the curve achieve capture; those below the curve fail to capture. Pacing *threshold* is determined by fixing the pulse duration and progressively decreasing the voltage from a high value. The threshold is the minimum voltage at which capture is achieved. (Alternatively, voltage can be fixed and pulse duration reduced from a high value; the procedure varies depending on the device model). In Figure 17.1 a threshold of 2.5 V at 0.2 ms (point S) has been determined. To programme an output safety margin there are two options:

1. Increase output to 5.0 V, maintain pulse duration at 0.2 ms (point T), giving safety margin A and threshold A (margin = 5.0/2.5 = 2.0)   OR
2. Increase pulse duration to 0.6 ms, maintain output at 2.5 V (point U), giving safety margin B and threshold B (margin = 2.50/1.2 = 2.1).

The preferred saftey margin is that which consumes the least power. In terms of battery current drain, doubling the output voltage is roughly equivalent to quadrupling the pulse duration. Thus, option (2) is preferable.

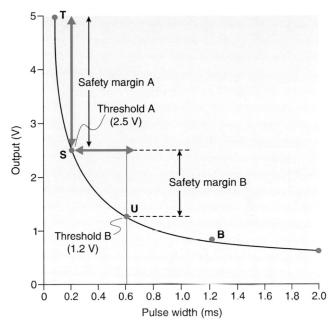

Fig. 17.1 Strength–duration curve (see text).

Sensitivity

Sensitivity is the minimum electrogram amplitude required to register as a sensed event (e.g. sensed P wave in AAI pacing, or QRS complex in VVI pacing). Sensitivity is measured in millivolts. Typical settings are 4 mV for ventricular sensing and 1.5 mV for atrial sensing.

Tip: Numerically low pacemaker sensitivity settings give greatest sensitivity.

If sensitivity is set too low the device may respond to the T wave or an extracardiac potential as a sensed event (*oversensing*). If too high, the device may not respond to a low-amplitude event, e.g. ectopic beat (*undersensing*). In Figure 17.2 a threshold of 6 mV may not detect the QRS complex, whereas a threshold of 3 mV could lead to T-wave oversensing. There is quite a narrow sensitivity window in which sensing occurs appropriately. To avoid this problem, at implantation it is important to obtain a lead position which produces a high-amplitude sensed electrogram (see later).

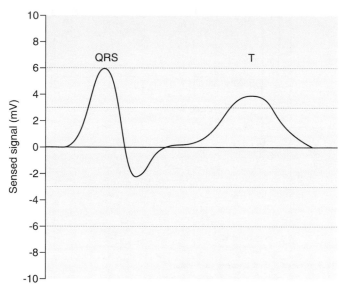

Fig. 17.2 Intracardiac ventricular electrogram, to illustrate sensing (see text).

Refractory period

This is a defined period (in milliseconds) after a paced or sensed event during which the pacemaker 'ignores' the sensed electrogram. A long refractory period minimizes *far field* sensing (e.g. AAI device detecting QRS complex) and T-wave sensing. A short refractory period maximizes sensing of premature complexes. Typical settings are 250–300 ms (ventricular) and 300–400 ms (atrial). Longer refractory periods are needed for AAI pacing to prevent inhibition on the terminal part of the QRS complex.

Polarity

Devices with bipolar electrodes can be programmed to unipolar or bipolar sensing and pacing. The advantages of bipolar pacing and sensing were described earlier. Unipolar pacing is useful during programming of AAI devices as the pacing spike is easily seen on a surface ECG (it can sometimes be difficult to distinguish intrinsic and paced P waves). It is also useful as a holding measure if lead fracture occurs, as only one working lead terminal is needed. Unipolar sensing is sometimes helpful if the sensed electrogram is small in bipolar sensing mode.

Hysteresis

Hysteresis invokes relatively rapid pacing once the heart rate drops below the

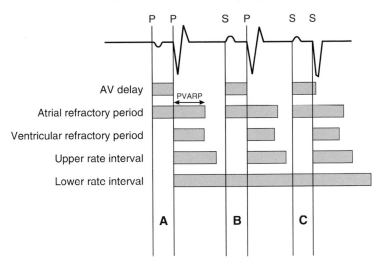

Fig. 17.3 Schematic of DDD pacing (see text).

programmed threshold, e.g. device paces at 70 bpm when heart rate falls below 50 bpm. This function is useful in HCSS and malignant vasovagal syndrome to augment cardiac output during attacks while preserving sinus rhythm at other times.

Dual-chamber device programming

Several additional parameters need to be programmed in dual-chamber devices, to maintain AV synchrony without unnecessary pacing and without inducing a pacemaker-mediated tachycardia. Figure 17.3 illustrates some of these parameters in a device set to DDD mode.

Paced rate

Depending on device model, the lower paced rate is governed by either the atrial or the ventricular channel. If no intrinsic activity is detected during the lower rate interval, either atrial or ventricular pacing occurs. In some devices an *atrial escape interval* can be programmed, which is effectively a lower atrial rate limit.

AV delay

This is a defined interval which starts at a sensed or paced P-wave event. If a QRS event is sensed during the AV delay period, ventricular pacing is inhibited (see Fig. 17.3, complex C). If no QRS event is sensed the device paces the ventricles at the end of the AV delay period (complexes A and B). In intermittent AV block the AV delay is set longer than the patient's intrinsic PR interval, so that ventricular pacing occurs only when AV conduction fails or is significantly delayed. This maintains the normal sequence of ventricular depolarization and conserves device power. Typical programmed AV delay values are 150–250 ms. A longer AV delay can be used if the patient has first-degree AV block, to prevent ventricular pacing during normal rhythm. A short AV delay (50–100 ms) can be used to induce paced bundle branch block for DDD pacing in HOCM and thus reduce left ventricular outflow tract obstruction.

Refractory periods
In DDD pacing the ventricular refractory period is as described for single-chamber pacing. The atrial refractory period encompasses the AV delay interval and extends beyond the start of the QRS complex. This last component is known as the *postventricular atrial refractory period (PVARP)*, and is designed to prevent the atrial channel from sensing and triggering on retrograde P waves occurring after the QRS complex; otherwise an *endless loop tachycardia* could occur. Some devices extend the PVARP automatically in response to ventricular extrasystoles, which commonly trigger these tachycardias (*atrial refractory period extension*).

Ventricular blanking period
The ventricular blanking period is a short period of 10–60 ms initiated by atrial pacing, during which ventricular sensing does not occur. This is designed to prevent the ventricular channel from being inhibited by the atrial stimulus (*crosstalk*).

Upper rate interval/limit
This parameter limits the rate at which the device can track sensed atrial events and so prevents rapid ventricular pacing in response to atrial tachyarrhythmias. When the atrial rate exceeds the upper rate limit, device-mediated Wenckebach-type conduction occurs and limits the ventricular response. Low upper rate limits are helpful in patients who have frequent, symptomatic atrial arrhythmias, but limit the physiological rate response to exercise. Mode-switching devices avoid these problems and are appropriate for patients requiring dual-chamber pacing who are known to have atrial tachyarrhythmias.

PACING MODES
Pacing mode is described using the NASPE/BPEG generic pacemaker code for bradyarrhythmia and antitachyarrhythmia devices. This five-letter code describes several components of pacemaker function (Table 17.1).

TABLE 17.1 NASPE/BPEG generic pacemaker codes

Chamber(s) paced	Chamber(s) sensed	Response to sensing	Rate response	Antitachycardia functions
0 – none	0 – none	0 – none	0 – none	0 – none
A – atrium	A – atrium	T – triggered	R – rate responsive	P – antitachycardia pacing
V – ventricle	V – ventricle	I – inhibited		S – shock
D – both	D – both	D – triggered and inhibited		D – pace and shock

The fourth letter is occasionally used to describe programmability (M = multiprogrammable), but this is usually omitted.

VOO mode

Early pacemakers used this mode, which paces at a fixed rate regardless of the intrinsic rhythm. There is a theoretical risk of inducing ventricular arrhythmias by pacing during the T wave (paced R-on-T phenomenon). VOO mode is no longer used.

VVI mode

Ventricular pacing is inhibited by sensed QRS events and so the inappropriate pacing seen with VOO mode is prevented. VVI devices are cheap. VVIR devices are suitable for those with atrial fibrillation who do not mount a heart rate response to exercise.

Indications

● Atrial fibrillation with complete AV block or symptomatic bradycardia.

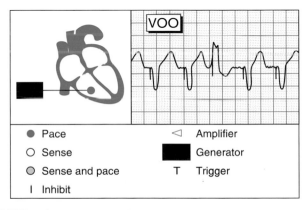

Fig. 17.4 VOO mode.

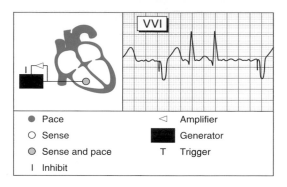

Fig. 17.5 VVI mode.

Disadvantages
● VVI pacing is not appropriate for patients in sinus rhythm with AV block because AV synchrony is lost during pacing. *Pacemaker syndrome* can also occur. VVI pacing in sinus rhythm may also induce atrial fibrillation by retrograde atrial activation.

AAI mode
Atrial pacing is inhibited by sensed P-wave events. AAI devices are also cheap. AAIR devices are suitable for those with chronotropic incompetence.

Indications
● Sick sinus syndrome with intact AV node conduction.

Disadvantages
● Some centres implant dual-chamber devices in these patients because AV block may develop later on, but this occurs in less than 2% of these patients per year. AAI pacing is not appropriate if there is significant conducting system disease (e.g. bifascicular block), Wenckebach AV block with atrial pacing ≤ 140 bpm, or atrial flutter/fibrillation.

DDD mode
In DDD mode the generator can sense and pace both atria and ventricles.

Warning: AAI pacemakers are not appropriate for hypersensitive carotid sinus syndrome or malignant vasovagal syndrome because acute AV block may occur in these conditions.

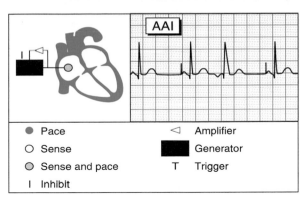

Fig. 17.6 AAI mode.

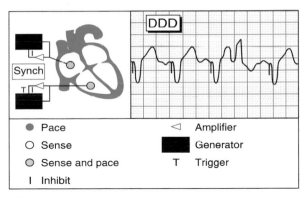

Fig. 17.7 DDD mode.

During sinus bradycardia, atrial (and, if necessary, ventricular) pacing occurs. During AV block ventricular pacing occurs following either a spontaneous or a paced atrial impulse. Thus, ventricular pacing can occur in sequence with sinus activity (*tracking*) and the normal rate response to exercise is maintained despite AV block. DDDR devices are available for patients with chronotropic incompetence.

Indications
● AV block and intact sinus node function.

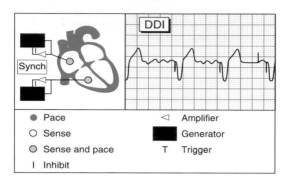

Fig. 17.8 DDI mode.

Disadvantages
● Rapid ventricular pacing may occur during atrial tachyarrhythmias, which may necessitate device reprogramming (see *Upper rate limit*). Mode-switching devices partly circumvent this problem.

DDI mode
Similar to DDD mode, but tracking does not occur in response to spontaneous atrial activity. AV sequential pacing occurs during sinus bradycardia. Ventricular pacing occurs during AV block. During atrial tachyarrhythmias the device effectively operates in VVI mode. DDIR mode can be used in sick sinus syndrome with chronotropic incompetence.

Indications
● Sick sinus syndrome.
● Hypersensitive carotid sinus syndrome (with hysteresis)
● Malignant vasovagal syndrome (with hysteresis).

Disadvantages
● Does not maintain AV synchrony during AV block.

VDD mode
These newer devices have a single ventricular lead but also have sensing electrodes in the right atrium to allow tracking of atrial rhythm. Implantation is simpler than for dual-chamber devices, with less risk of lead displacement and implantation-associated trauma (e.g. pneumothorax).

Indications
● High-grade AV block with intact sinus node function.

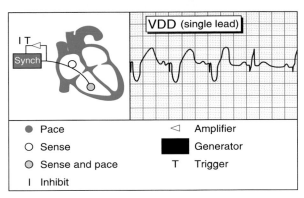

Fig. 17.9 VDD mode.

Disadvantages (see also DDD)
- Atrial undersensing occurs in >5% of cases.
- VVI pacing during sinus bradycardia.

ASSESSING PATIENTS FOR PACING

HISTORY TAKING (AGAIN!)

Although the important elements of history taking from patients with suspected bradyarrhythmias were discussed in a previous chapter, it is always worth re-evaluating the history before committing to pacemaker implantation. A methodical approach may prevent inappropriate device implantation and gives the information required for the procedure to be done as safely as possible. The following checklist outlines the key points.

Check the indication for pacing
- Is there an absolute indication for pacemaker implantation (e.g. third-degree AV block)?
- If not, is there a clear relationship between symptoms and bradycardia?
- If not, have you investigated other potential causes for the patient's symptoms?
- Is there a reversible cause of bradycardia?
    - recent MI
    - ischaemia-induced bradycardia
    - drugs (e.g. digoxin, β-blockers, diltiazem, verapamil, antiarrhythmics)
    - hypothyroidism.

Anatomical considerations

- **Cardiac enlargement** (especially chronic mitral disease, right heart failure and tricuspid incompetence) – active fixation leads may be appropriate.
- **Abnormal anatomy** (especially congenital heart disease – may have left-sided SVC or SVC draining into coronary sinus) – may need to do upper limb venogram/cavogram before implantation.
- **Chronic lung disease** (especially emphysema) – avoid subclavian lead insertion.
- **Recent cardiac surgery** – may use active fixation atrial lead if RA appendage used for cardiopulmonary bypass.
- **Tricuspid valve replacement** – cannot use endocardial RV lead.

Considerations for pacemaker replacement/upgrade

- VVI patients – symptoms of pacemaker syndrome?
- Are old leads working well (high thresholds, abnormal impedence)? Do you expect to replace lead or use old one?
- Are previous leads compatible with new pacemaker (e.g. IS-1 standard)? Will lead adapter be needed? If so, unipolar configuration is required for new pacemaker.

Deciding on device model (see also earlier pacing modes)

- History of atrial tachyarrhythmias? (Mode-switching indicated)
- Is patient very thin? May choose small device at expense of battery size.

Anticoagulation

- Remember to stop warfarin 3–4 days before implantation.
- May need to heparinize after procedure if mechanical prosthetic valve.

Miscellaneous practicalities

- Can patient lie flat for procedure? Oxygen needed?
- Is patient confused/demented? (Sedation? who will provide consent?)
- Allergies? (May need to give opiate analgesia, antibiotic prophylaxis).

EXAMINATION

A full examination will have been done by this stage. Recheck for:

- Thyroid status
- Aortic valve disease (associated with AV block)
- Signs of cardiac failure/enlargement/tricuspid regurgitation – may use active fixation leads, higher paced rate
- Signs of emphysema/chronic lung disease
- Site and orientation of device for replacements/upgrades
    is old lead on top of device? (careful with scalpel!)
    has device migrated? superficial? (may need to create new pocket).

PREPROCEDURE INVESTIGATIONS

ECG/Ambulatory recordings
You will already have looked at the ECG, but don't forget:

- Evidence of recent MI? (AV block may be reversible)
- Chronotropic incompetence? (check ambulatory recording for rate variation and do exercise test if in doubt). Rate responsive device needed?
- Intermittent atrial arrhythmias? Mode switching needed?
- Conduction defects (e.g. bifascicular block) – may influence choice towards dual-chamber pacing
- For device replacement, is there a stable adequate underlying rhythm? You do not want to render the patient asystolic when you unplug the old device.

CXR
- Cardiomegaly (especially right atrial enlargement)
- Chronic lung disease
- Position of existing device and leads.

Echo
There is a good argument to echo all patients before device implantation. Right-sided chamber dilatation and tricuspid incompetence may necessitate active fixation leads. Higher base rates may help optimize cardiac output in patients with ventricular impairment. Significant mitral or tricuspid valve disease may influence choice towards a mode-switching device, as atrial tachyarrhythmias are likely to develop later on.

Laboratory tests
- U&Es to ensure K^+ normal before lead insertion
- INR, if recently warfarinized
- T_4/TSH if sinus bradycardia
- Cardiac enzymes if newly diagnosed AV block.

DECIDING URGENCY

Ideally, once an indication for pacing has been determined a pacemaker should be implanted as soon as possible. Many centres work under the constraints of limited theatre time and patients have to be prioritized. 'Elective' permanent pacing for this section means device implantation within 4–6 weeks.

Symptomatic third-degree AV block
Urgent pacing is required once MI has been excluded as the cause. The risk of asystole/sudden death is significant. Temporary pacing is indicated if a significant delay is anticipated, in the following groups:

- H_x of syncope or presyncope
- Slow escape rhythm (<40 bpm).

All other patients with symptomatic CHB should be kept under observation in hospital prior to device implantation.

Asymptomatic third-degree AV block

If this is identified by chance (e.g. at routine medical examination) it requires prompt permanent pacing. Temporary pacing is not justifiable as the procedure is associated with significant morbidity and the patient has almost certainly had a stable escape rhythm for a significant length of time.

Second-degree AV block

These patients can be paced electively unless there is history of syncope.

Sick sinus syndrome

Although it is widely reported that this condition is not associated with increased mortality, common sense dictates that patients with recurrent syncope should be paced as soon as possible to avoid falls and physical injury. Otherwise, elective pacing is indicated.

HCSS and vasovagal syndrome

Elective pacing is usually indicated, as situations that provoke syncope can be avoided in the interim.

CONSENT AND WHAT TO TELL THE PATIENT

Informed consent is essential prior to pacemaker implantation because complications can and do occur. These are discussed later in the chapter. Patients should be warned of the potential risks in language they can understand. Try not to be alarmist and reassure them that pacemaker implantation is not 'heart surgery' in the same sense as, for example, a bypass operation. Explain that the risk of *major* complications is very low. Patients must also understand the potential risk of leaving their conditions untreated and that device implantation is only contemplated when this outweighs the risk of the procedure itself. Above all, reassure that a normal lifestyle can be resumed soon after the procedure, but do warn about the following:

External interference

It is now rare for external factors to interfere with pacemaker function because of effective shielding of circuitry and the increased use of bipolar sensing. However, the following are potential hazards:

- Unshielded electric motors (device may be triggered to 'magnet rate', or EM pulses from sparks may be sensed by device)
- Large magnets, if adjacent to device (e.g. hi-fi loudspeakers)

- First-generation microwave ovens, if seal broken
- Airport metal detectors (inform security staff, show pacemaker ID card and a manual search will be done instead)
- High-energy transmitters (e.g. radar station) if very close
- Shop-door security systems (do not affect pacemaker, but alarm may be triggered)
- Digital mobile phones (studies show interference to be very uncommon. Advise that phone be held on opposite side to pacemaker)
- TENS machines, interferential physiotherapy devices and neurostimulators may produce impulses that inhibit pacemaker function.

Contact sports
Sports in which the pacemaker site is likely to be hit (e.g. soccer, rugby, martial arts etc.) should be avoided.

Driving
In the UK patients with pacemakers cannot drive heavy goods or public service vehicles. Otherwise, driving is not permitted until one month has elapsed from device implantation (this allows a follow-up check to ensure the pacemaker is functioning and that symptoms have resolved). For patients with AICDs, HCSS and malignant vasovagal syndrome, cases are considered by the driving authority on an individual basis.

PREPROCEDURE CHECKLIST

- Informed consent
- Blood results (e.g. INR)
- Antibiotic prophylaxis*
- Anxiolytic needed? (e.g. **diazepam 10 mg** orally 30–60 min preprocedure, but avoid in confused elderly as it can make confusion worse)
- Sedative needed? (e.g. **haloperidol 2–5 mg** orally or IM, OR **thioridazine 25–100 mg** orally, at least 1 h before procedure). It is impossible to implant the pacemaker if the patient is climbing off the operating table!
- IV access
- Hardware – do you need any of the following :
    - active fixation leads
    - spare dual-chamber pacemaker (for AAI cases, in case AV node function impaired)
    - adapters and lead caps
- Decide lead insertion route
- Isoprenaline needed? – Check underlying rhythm prior to device replacements/upgrades.

(* Used in some units. Suggested protocol is oral **flucloxacillin** 1 g, 1 h before procedure and repeated 1 h and 6 h after procedure. If patient is penicillin allergic, use oral **erythromycin** 1 g, at same time intervals.)

PACEMAKER IMPLANTATION

This can only be learned under the direct guidance of an experienced operator. Exact implantation techniques vary quite widely and this section simply serves as a guide to the main steps involved.

IMPLANTING NEW PACEMAKERS

Local anaesthesia

After cleansing the skin with antiseptic and placing drapes, local anaesthetic (e.g. **1% lignocaine** 10–20 ml) is infiltrated subcutaneously in three sites:

- Along the line of lead insertion (subclavian method) or the deltopectoral groove (cephalic method)
- Along the line of planned incision
- In the area of the pacemaker pocket.

For the latter two sites try to infiltrate just superficial to the pectoral muscle layer.

Lead insertion routes

Cephalic vein access is preferable, since on balance it is a safer technique. However, the risk from subclavian puncture is also low *using proper technique*. There are advantages and disadvantages to both routes (see box).

Subclavian vein access
- To minimize risk of air embolism:
    - ensure adequate hydration
    - use 'head-down' position during puncture (ensure you can see filled neck veins)
    - ask patient not to inhale deeply
    - Valsalva manoeuvre during puncture
    - occlude introducer opening until ready to insert lead.
- Use lateral insertion point to avoid subclavian crush; puncture two-thirds distance from sternoclavicular to acromioclavicular joint and aim for the sternal notch.
- Insert flexible, J-shaped guidewire using Seldinger technique (see Chapter 3). Use fluoroscopy to ensure guidewire does not go headwards.
- Use two separate punctures (unless access is difficult) if dual-chamber device, to avoid tearing the vein when leads are inserted.
- Leave guidewire(s) in place. The main incision and pocket are made (see below) before lead insertion.

Subclavian versus cephalic vein insertion

Subclavian route
- Easier to learn; operator may have used for other procedures (e.g. CVP lines)
- Large-calibre vein, can accommodate multiple leads every time
- Quick, reduces procedure time
- Risks
    - pneumothorax (especially if chest hyperinflated)
    - accidental subclavian artery puncture
    - air embolism (minimized by 'head-down' position during insertion)
    - medial puncture → 'subclavian crush' – lead compressed in angle between clavicle and first rib
    - posterolateral puncture → brachial plexus injury (rare)

Cephalic route
- Safe – risk of trauma much lower as vein cannulated under direct vision
- No risk of subclavian crush
- Takes longer; technically more difficult
- Experienced centres report that vein can accommodate two leads in ~70% of cases, otherwise subclavian approach required.

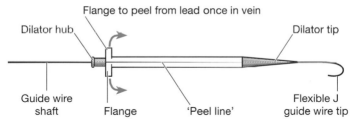

Fig. 17.10 Pacing lead introducer (see text for description of use).

- Most introducers (plastic sheaths used to introduce lead into vein) have a central dilator and can be peeled away from the lead once inserted (Fig. 17.10). Feed the introducer over the guidewire and gently push to its full extent into the vein, dilating it.
- Remove inner dilator, leaving a port of entry into the vein. Cover the orifice with a finger, or blood will leak rapidly.
- **Immediately** feed the lead into SVC using fluoroscopy, then pull the introducer out of the vein and peel away from lead. You can then manipulate the lead into place.

Cephalic vein access
This requires dissection of the (intact!) cephalic vein from the deltopectoral groove.

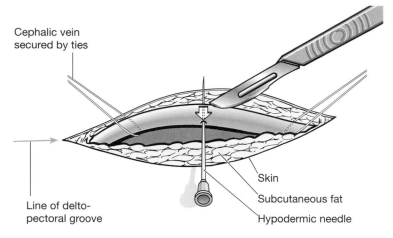

Cephalic vein
secured by ties

Line of delto-
pectoral groove

Skin

Subcutaneous fat

Hypodermic needle

Fig. 17.11 Cephalic vein cut-down (see text for description of technique).

● Make a shallow incision along the deltopectoral groove, from 1 cm below the clavicle. Incision length is determined by device size.
● Dissect carefully to a depth just above the prepectoral fascia. The cephalic vein is usually surrounded by a small amount of fat.
● Free the cephalic vein by blunt dissection and secure loosely with ties.
● Incise the vein transversely across half its circumference. This is best done by placing a needle across the vein and incising on to it (Fig. 17.11).
● Insert flexible J-shaped guidewire into vein; screen until it reaches SVC.
● **Carefully** insert introducer into vein and remove dilator.
● Feed lead into vein until it reaches SVC.

Ventricular lead positioning
Ventricular leads are straight. The target position is the RV apex. Pacemaker leads are supplied with a selection of *stilettes* (thin wires which can be shaped and fed down the centre of lead).

● Make a J curve, about 3 cm across, at the end of a soft stilette.
● Feed stilette into lead and advance into RA. The lead should face the tricuspid valve (Fig. 17.12a).
● Advance lead until it passes through tricuspid and pulmonary valves; that way you know you are pulling back into RV (Fig. 17.12b).
● Take out stilette and place a soft, straight stilette to within 1–2 cm of lead tip.
● Retract lead slowly until it starts to falls towards floor of RV (Fig. 17.12c).
● Advance lead smoothly until it reaches RV apex (Fig. 17.12d).

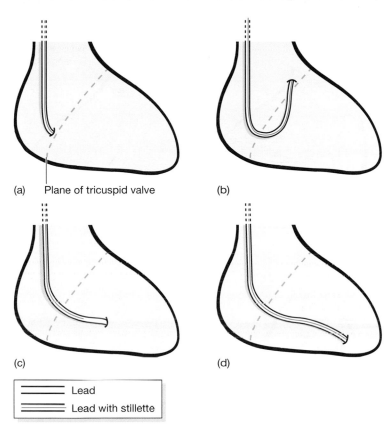

(a) Plane of tricuspid valve   (b)

(c)   (d)

| Lead |
| Lead with stillette |

Fig. 17.12 a–d Ventricular lead positioning as viewed using fluoroscopy.

● Leave enough curve on lead that it does not straighten out with deep breaths.

Atrial lead positioning
Atrial leads are J-shaped. The target position is the RA appendage, which is located anteriorly and superiorly in RA.

● Feed the lead into SVC/RA junction using a straight, soft stilette. Retract stilette and lead should curl up slightly (Fig. 17.13a).
● Advance lead until it slips into RA appendage. It should 'flick' left and right in AP view (if there is spontaneous atrial activity) because of appendage contraction (Fig. 17.13b).

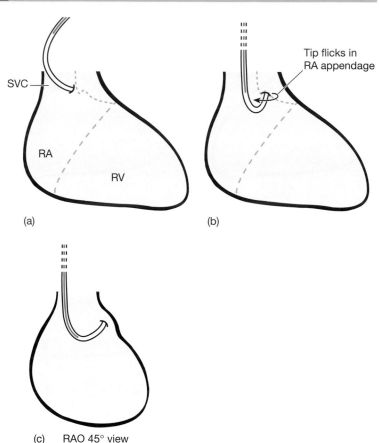

Fig. 17.13 a–c Atrial lead positioning as viewed using fluoroscopy.

- Use RAO 45° view to confirm lead tip is pointing anteriorly (Fig. 17.13c).
- Leave enough 'belly' on J so that lead does not straighten out, but enough tension that it does not fall into body of RA.

Active fixation leads

These are used when it is anticipated that passive lead position will be unstable, when passive leads have displaced, or when apical position gives inadequate electrogram or threshold values. They have either a retractable or a dissolvable tip which exposes a 'corkscrew' after 2–3 minutes in circulation. This gives time to place the lead in position. Target lead position is usually the same as for passive leads, but exact positioning is less critical. Leads are fixed in position by rotating the lead hub, braced over a stilette. Lead thresholds are usually quite high immediately after placement owing to tissue injury, but fall over 5–10 minutes.

Once leads are positioned and satisfactory function is confirmed, secure lead to pectoralis muscle layer using non-dissolvable suture **over lead cuff**.

Testing lead function and stability

Once a satisfactory anatomical position has been obtained, several checks are needed to ensure leads are in a satisfactory *electrical* position. Time spent here can considerably improve device longevity if low voltage thresholds are obtained. Leads vary in their *impedance* characteristics: some are designed to have high impedance (low surface area gives high *current density* and hence lower threshold.) The following tests are recommended.

Electrograms

These are recorded in unipolar or bipolar configuration, depending on planned device programming.

● **Ventricular electrograms** (Fig. 17.14) show 'injury current', with ST elevation, if contact is good. The amplitude should be >6 mV for reliable sensing, otherwise the lead should be resited. A small positional adjustment may give a significant improvement in electrogram amplitude. If satisfactory amplitude cannot be obtained, check *slew rate* (rate of increase in electrogram voltage with time) using pacing system analyser (PSA). A narrow 'surface'-type electrogram is often seen with active fixation leads; if seen with a passive lead, it may have perforated RV wall. The lead can usually be retracted without complication, but echo should be done afterwards to exclude pericardial effusion.
● **Atrial electrograms** are smaller but should be at least 1.5–2 mV for reliable sensing.

Threshold testing

Threshold should be determined using PSA at pulse width 0.5 ms. Implantation thresholds should be <1.0 V for ventricular leads and <1.5 V for atrial leads. If the RV or RA is badly diseased, target thresholds may not be achievable. Active fixation leads should not be repositioned unless threshold remains >2.0 V after a 15-minute wait. Threshold should also be checked during deep inspiration.

 Warning: Do not suture directly over lead insulation as it may become damaged.

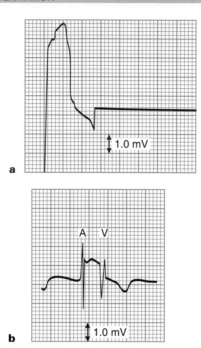

Fig. 17.14 a. Ventricular electrogram showing ST elevation – the 'injury' current. **b.** Typical atrial electrogram.

Lead impedance

This is tested at fixed output (5 V) and pulse width (0.5 ms). Abnormally low impedance (<250 Ω) may indicate damage to insulation; high impedance (>1000 Ω) may indicate lead fracture.

'Ten volt test'

This is pacing at 10 V output to exclude the propensity to diaphragmatic or phrenic nerve pacing from ventricular and atrial leads, respectively. (If this occurs the patient may feel the impulse, an abdominal twitch can be palpated and diaphragm movement is seen with fluoroscopy.)

AV node function

When an AAI system is planned pace atria, increasing the rate until second-degree AV block occurs. If this occurs at rate <140 bpm, then a dual-chamber system is indicated and a ventricular lead should be inserted. Ventricular pacing can be used to check VA conduction time, allowing appropriate programming of PVARP.

> **Tip:** For AAI implants, place an additional guidewire in vein *at the start* in case a ventricular lead is needed. This avoids the risk of damaging the atrial lead with subsequent puncture.

Final checks

If you suspect *at all* that leads may have moved, e.g. during device positioning, recheck threshold. It only takes a few seconds and may prevent a redo procedure. After implantation, check pacing function using a magnet and that atrial sensing is appropriate in DDD mode.

Making the pocket

For cephalic vein access the main incision will already have been made. Blunt dissection (with a finger if possible) is used in the plane of the prepectoral fascia to create a pocket medial to the incision. Do not penetrate the fascia or traumatize the pectoralis muscle, as 'bleeders' are difficult to stop. The pocket should be large enough to accommodate the pacemaker and leads without allowing undue movement. Push leads home and secure appropriate screws on device header. Coil spare lead length under the pacemaker and orientate the device face-up.

The pocket is closed using a layer of dissolvable sutures, between muscle and the opposing subcutaneous layer. This avoids having the device under the incision line (which can be uncomfortable) and minimizes the risk of migration and erosion. One or two further layers of subcutaneous suturing (depending on wound depth) are used to appose the skin edges. Skin closure is ideally done using subcuticular dissolvable sutures, as this gives a good cosmetic result.

PACEMAKER REPLACEMENT/UPGRADE

Depending on the patient device replacement is either very quick and easy, or a long, frustrating procedure. It is vital to be armed with as much information as possible about the existing system before embarking on replacement.

Local anaesthesia

Avoid traumatizing leads while infiltrating local anaesthetic. Infiltrate superficial to the pacemaker, along the planned incision line (see below) and inject ~5 ml **1% lignocaine** into pacemaker pocket. As it can be difficult to anaesthetize the entire pocket, **IV morphine** 5–10 mg should also be given.

Warning: Get assistant to check that correct lead is in correct terminal. Make sure you know which screws to tighten, especially if attaching device to an old unipolar lead.

Check before pacemaker replacement

- Position and orientation of old device (palpation, CXR)
- Is device subpectoral or prepectoral? (general anaesthetic needed to extract subpectoral device)
- Are leads superficial to pacemaker? (palpate over device)
- Is old lead compatible with new pacemaker, or is adapter needed?
- Do you need specific tools (e.g. screwdriver) to disconnect old device?
- Is patient pacemaker dependent?
- For old, unipolar leads, anything to suggest a new, bipolar lead is required?
  - muscle twitching
  - high threshold or impedance
  - under/oversensing
  - myoinhibition
- For single-chamber devices, should patient be upgraded to a dual-chamber device?
  - evidence of AV block/conduction defects (AAI)?
  - pacemaker syndrome (VVI)
  - sinus rhythm and AV block in patient with VVI device.

Pacemaker-dependent patients

For patients who are unable to maintain an adequate spontaneous rhythm, programme paced rate to 50 bpm and set up **IVI isoprenaline** (usual dilution is 2 mg in 500 ml 5% dextrose → 4 mg/ml). Infuse at 1 mg/min, titrate up to maximum of 10 mg/min until spontaneous stable rhythm seen. This allows disconnection of the pacemaker without causing asystole or bradycardia. The infusion rate may need to be reduced if excessive tachycardia or ventricular ectopy occurs.

Opening the pocket

If the existing pacemaker lies in the correct position, incise over its surface medial to the original scar. Make a superficial incision if the lead lies over the device, then dissect down carefully. It is very easy to nick the lead insulation and render it useless. The pacemaker will be surrounded by a dense fibrous capsule, which may be calcified. Blunt dissect down to this layer, which should be obvious by its opalescent appearance. Make a nick in the capsule and open it along the length of the incision. The pacemaker is removed using angled forceps, being careful not to crush the lead.

Checking/replacing leads

Disconnect old device from lead(s). It may be necessary to use careful, blunt dissection to free up lead prior to connection of the new device, or to give enough spare lead if an adapter needs to be fitted. Lead function is checked using a PSA; a new lead will be needed if there is visible damage to the lead; if pacing threshold is excessive (>2.5 V at 0.5 ms for long-term implant); or if impedance is too high or low. If an upgrade is needed or the lead needs to be replaced, the subclavian route is usually preferred (the cephalic vein is either already used or is often difficult to access), avoiding the old lead. The new lead may need to be tunnelled down to the existing pocket after implantation via a small subclavian incision. Redundant leads should be capped and buried deep to the pocket and new device.

Device implantation

If the previous pacemaker has migrated from its original site it may be necessary to create a new pocket deep to the previous site. Otherwise, the new pacemaker is attached and secured to leads and placed in the pocket, which may need to be plicated or reduced to accommodate the smaller size of contemporary devices. Capsule edges are brought together until a firm 'fit' is obtained, so that the pacemaker will not 'flip' or rotate. Closure is otherwise the same as for a new implant.

COMPLICATIONS – PREVENTION AND TREATMENT

Major complications (requiring reoperation or an emergency intervention) affect 1–2% of pacemaker implants. It is important to be aware of potential complications so that they can be recognized promptly and treatment given.

ACUTE COMPLICATIONS

Failed access

- *Failed cephalic vein access* is common because of the variable size and course of the vein and its fragility in some patients.
- *Failed subclavian puncture* may be due to the posterior location of the subclavian vein (where arterial puncture is likely). A lateral puncture may help; failing this, use the contralateral subclavian vein or try the cephalic approach.

Traumatic access

Subclavian artery puncture

This is usually recognized immediately; if not, trauma may be caused by insertion of the dilator. If the artery is punctured, press firmly over puncture site for 5 minutes or until haemostasis is achieved.

Pneumothorax

This more common with lateral puncture sites and in patients with obstructive airways disease. Air may be aspirated during puncture; symptoms of significant pneumothorax are pleuritic pain and dyspnoea. Most are small and resolve spontaneously; a chest drain is only occasionally required.

- *Brachial plexus injury* and *thoracic duct injury* are rare and associated with posterior puncture lines.

Complications of lead insertion

Air embolism
This occurs during introducer/lead insertion when central venous pressure is lower than atmospheric pressure. Symptoms are acute dyspnoea ± haemodynamic collapse immediately following introducer insertion; absent venous backflow through the introducer is a sign of low venous pressure. Measures to minimize the risk of this were discussed in the previous section.

Perforation/cardiac tamponade
Perforation of the right ventricle is relatively common, characterized by a surface-type electrogram, a high threshold, extreme apical position of the lead and often pleuritic pain. A small haemorrhagic pericardial effusion may result. The lead can usually be pulled back without complication. Tamponade is rare (for symptoms and treatment, see Chapters 4 and 3, respectively); echo should be performed if suspected. If tamponade occurs while the lead is still in place, do not remove it or fatal bleeding may occur. Pericardial aspiration is a temporizing measure during acute tamponade and emergency surgery is usually required.

Arrhythmias
Ventricular ectopy/non-sustained VT is common during ventricular lead implantation when the tricuspid valve is crossed. Sustained ventricular arrhythmias are rare. Atrial fibrillation may occur during atrial lead positioning and is a frustration. It is impossible to check atrial lead function with this arrhythmia. Atrial fibrillation may resolve spontaneously within a few minutes; if not, there are several options:

- Aim for optimum anatomical position.
- DC cardioversion under general anaesthetic, then test lead.
- Pharmacological cardioversion using **IV amiodarone** or **IV flecainide** (see Chapter 7 for regimens).

Valve damage
Uncommon; this results from rough handling with lead tines or active fixator caught in tricuspid valve. This is an avoidable complication.

Lead damage
Pacemaker leads are reliable. If lead impedance is abnormally low (<250 Ω) immediately after implantation the chances are you have nicked it with the scalpel! There is no option but to change the lead.

Generator/pocket complications

Failure to pace

If the generator does not function at implantation, double-check that leads have been pushed home and that screws are tightened. Also check programmed parameters. If all of these check out, recheck lead function and position as displacement may have occurred. It is extremely uncommon to have a faulty generator.

Haematoma

This may develop over the first 24 hours after implantation and increases the risk of pocket infection. The pocket becomes swollen, often bruised and painful. The risk of haematoma is minimized by blunt dissection, careful fashioning of the pocket and avoidance of muscle trauma. 'Bleeders' should be cauterized or tied off. Large haematomas require drainage, treatment of the bleeding point and reclosure.

Wound dehiscence

This is rare and is associated with haematoma formation, thin build, inadequate-sized pocket for the device, or poor suture technique.

DELAYED COMPLICATIONS

Lead-related complications

Displacement

- *Macrodisplacement* occurs when a lead displaces visibly from its original position. It is more common with RV dilatation, tricuspid incompetence and suboptimal lead placement (e.g. in mid-RV rather than at apex). If associated with significant rise in threshold or loss of sensing, repositioning or replacement with an active fixation lead is indicated.
- *Microdisplacement* occurs when the lead position is apparently unchanged but sensing ± threshold function alters unfavourably. This can sometimes represent subacute perforation. Management is as for macrodisplacement, although this is a less compelling indication for active fixation lead insertion.

Infection/endocarditis

This is uncommon and the risk is minimized by scrupulous aseptic technique. Symptoms are described in Chapter 8. *Staphylococcus epidermidis/aureus* are the most common culprit organisms. Right-sided endocarditis may result in lung abscess formation. Diagnosis is confirmed by echo/TOE; treatment is pacemaker and lead removal, and antibiotic R_x as described in Chapter 8.

Insulation or conductor failure

- *Insulation failure* occurs with old leads, abrasion (e.g. subclavian crush) and trauma during insertion/device replacement. Impedance falls, typically <250 Ω. Muscle twitching may occur as a result of the current path through pectoral tissue.

- *Conductor failure* is most common with medial insertion and subclavian crush. Acute impedance rise occurs, often accompanied by loss of capture. Temporary reprogramming to unipolar mode may restore function if negative conductor is intact in a fractured bipolar lead. Lead fracture can often be confirmed by penetrated X-ray of the upper thorax. Lead replacement is indicated.

- *Fracture of retention wire*. This complication occurs with some models of atrial J-leads which contain a stilette-type retention wire. These can perforate the lead insulation and RA wall. Patients with these leads require regular fluoroscopic screening of the lead during follow-up.

SVC/subclavian vein thrombosis/occlusion

This is most commonest if multiple leads have been implanted. Symptoms are upper limb ± facial/neck engorgement and headache, especially when bending. Signs are venous distension, bluish discoloration of the affected area and the development of surface collateral veins over the chest. Diagnosis is confirmed by upper limb venography; anticoagulation may help. Chronic SVC occlusion can be treated conservatively or by angioplasty or surgery.

Pacemaker-related complications

Chronic pain

This can result from device erosion or migration, or failure to make an adequate-sized pocket. If severe and persistent, device repositioning may help; otherwise simple analgesia is indicated.

Erosion

Erosion occurs when the pacemaker moves through the skin layers and becomes progressively more superficial. It occurs in thin patients, if the device is not implanted in the correct plane, or if wound closure is inadequate. If the pacemaker is superficial but functions well and does not cause discomfort, it is safe to keep under observation. If complete erosion occurs there is no option but to replace the device in another site.

Migration

This less common now that small lightweight pacemakers are used. Typically a pacemaker may migrate inferolaterally, or behind the breast. No action is required unless there is discomfort, erosion or pacemaker malfunction. Migration can be avoided by securing the device header to the pectoral muscle layer with a permanent suture.

Infection

Usually caused by *Staph. aureus*. Superficial infection (skin redness and heat around the wound) may occur after implantation; take a wound swab and treat with antistaphylococcal antibiotic (e.g. oral **flucloxacillin** 500 mg qid or oral **erythromycin** 500 mg qid). Deep wound infection may initially be silent (especially with *Staph. epidermidis*). Signs are swelling and fluctuance around the pacemaker and tenderness/redness over the incision line. Lack of local signs may denote endocarditis; echo is indicated in all cases. Pacemaker system infection is an indication for device and lead extraction. Extraction is a complicated procedure, beyond the scope of this book.

Miscellaneous complications

● *'Twiddler' syndrome* occurs when the patient 'plays' with the device and flips it repeatedly within the pocket. This results in lead torsion and eventually device malfunction.
● *Device trauma* is rare, but function should be checked if a forceful, direct blow to the pacemaker occurs.

PACEMAKER FOLLOW-UP

Central to learning about pacemaker function and programming is involvement in a pacemaker review clinic. Here, you can learn how to programme commonly used devices and how to deal with problems patients might encounter.

Purpose of pacemaker clinic
● Optimize pacemaker function according to physiological requirements
● Improve device longevity
● Provide patients with information
● Identify malfunctions/complications
● Plan elective replacement

> **Tip:** First, learn the basic functions of pacemaker programmers for commonly used devices – you can then fix simple pacing problems in the middle of the night!

Patients with pacemakers are reviewed at set times in the first few months after implantation. Limited telephone follow-up can be performed for some patients who live a long way from the implanting centre.

TIMING OF PACEMAKER CHECKS

Predischarge check
● Check wound site (haematoma, sutures secure)

- Programme to relatively high output (e.g. usually the preprogrammed nominal device settings) to cope with expected postimplant threshold rise
- Check lead function (see below)
- CXR
    - Macrodisplacement
    - Pneumothorax
    - Device orientation.

1 month
- Check implant site.
- Check lead capture.
- Too early to programme output according to threshold as it may continue to rise at this stage.

3–4 months
By this time lead threshold and sensing should have stabilized and pacemaker parameters can be set accordingly:

- Set output according to threshold (usually reduced from discharge value).
- Adjust sensitivity if needed.
- Perform checks outlined below.

Subsequent follow-up (usually 12-monthly)
Pacemakers typically function for 10–15 years, although this varies according to the model, the number of chambers paced (single-chamber models last longer), output and the frequency of pacing.

Factors determining frequency of follow-up
- Predicted device longevity
- Device output (high output may necessitate more frequent follow-up later on)
- Is patient pacemaker dependent?
- How frequently device is used
- Recent reprogramming: follow-up to assess response
- Patient factors (frailty, geographic factors)
- Device/lead manufacturer recalls

SYSTEM FOR ASSESSING PACEMAKER PATIENT

As with any clinic follow-up the history and relevant examination should be done first. The technical stuff comes later.

History taking
A few well directed questions help you diagnose certain pacemaker problems. Ask about the following:

- *Dizziness* is a non-specific symptom but may indicate pacemaker syndrome

(VVI devices: see end of section), loss of lead capture, under- or oversensing. Exertional dizziness may reflect myoinhibition (especially upper body movement) or chronotropic incompetence.

● *Syncope* should be taken seriously. If the device appears to work well this could reflect intermittent loss of capture (check lead impedance – high if conductor break). Check function with arm raised, behind back; check for myoinhibition. X-ray lead for fracture. Pacemaker patients with HCSS or vasovagal syndrome can remain prone to syncope because of vasodilator response. See also Chapters 11 (dizziness and syncope) and 13 (neurally mediated syncope).

● *Fatigue* is non-specific and common in the elderly. It may indicate that device rate is set too low, especially in patients with cardiac failure, who may benefit from higher paced rates (70–90 bpm). Exertional fatigue may be reduced by adjusting rate response in devices with this function. *Breathlessness* can occur for the same reasons.

● *Palpitation* sometimes indicates atrial arrhythmia (which 'confuses' DDD devices into pacing at the upper rate limit) or pacemaker-mediated tachycardia. Poorly positioned ventricular leads (exerting pressure on tricuspid ring) may trigger VT.

● *Chest discomfort* may arise from the implant site. Ask if positional, related to arm movement. Ask about symptoms of infection (fever, anorexia, malaise). Many patients also have angina, which may be worsened by inappropriately high pacing rates (e.g. with rate-responsive devices).

Examination

Extensive examination is only indicated if the patient reports new symptoms. In all patients check there is no swelling, redness or leak from the implant site. Look at pacemaker orientation and for signs of migration or erosion.

Checking pacemaker function

The following checks should be performed at follow-up visits:

● *Rhythm with patient at rest* – no adjustments made to device.

● *Underlying rhythm* – test intrinsic rhythm either with inhibitor (placed over the pacemaker, this device delivers rapid pulses to inhibit pacing), or temporarily reprogramme lower rate to low value, or temporarily programme output below threshold.

● *Lead thresholds* – devices differ in the precise way in which thresholds are checked. Some automatically check threshold when a magnet is applied to the device (Vario function) by reducing output on successive beats. Others check threshold via programmer telemetry function. It is often necessary to temporarily reprogramme pacemaker function to confirm capture.

● *Atrial leads* – increase paced rate above patient's intrinsic rate. In patients with AV block, where intrinsic ventricular rate does not rise with atrial pacing, it can be difficult to confirm atrial capture if P wave is small; use echo to confirm a-wave on mitral Doppler trace.

- *Ventricular leads* – for VVI, increase paced rate above ventricular rate. For DDD, may need to shorten AV delay to confirm ventricular capture.
- *Lead impedance* – rises with conductor break or faulty connection with pacemaker (usually >1000 Ω); falls with insulator break (usually <250 Ω).
- *Sensing* – it is only possible to check sensing in a given chamber if there is spontaneous activity from that chamber.
    - *Single-chamber atrial and ventricular* – set lower rate below intrinsic rate and ensure device is inhibited.
    - *Dual-chamber* – to check atrial sensing, shorten AV delay (e.g. to 100 ms) and ensure atrial activity triggers ventricular pacing. To check ventricular sensing, lengthen AV delay beyond intrinsic P-R interval to ensure spontaneous QRS complex inhibits ventricular channel OR, in complete heart block, temporarily programme to VVI mode and check as for single-chamber device, above.
- *Myoinhibition* – this is where the pacemaker oversenses skeletal muscle myopotentials and inhibits pacing. It is much more common in pacemakers with unipolar sensing and only needs to be evaluated in these or if myoinhibition is suspected from the history. It is checked using isometric arm exercises or from ambulatory recordings. (In DDD pacemakers myopotentials may be sensed as atrial activity and cause inappropriate acceleration of paced ventricular rate.)
- *Event memory functions* – some devices have built-in memory functions which record the following:
    - frequency of pacing
    - heart rate histograms
    - rate, duration and frequency of arrhythmias
    - mode-switching events.
- *Device longevity* – pacemakers have an internal elective replacement indicator which provides 2–3 months' warning of impending battery depletion. This is checked either by measuring the pacemaker's 'magnet rate', which reduces as the battery depletes, or battery voltage or impedance. Modern programmers provide an estimated device longevity predicted from these data, current output and lead impedance.

SPECIFIC PACEMAKER CLINIC PROBLEMS

Failure to capture

The effect of this depends on the underlying rhythm; it may result in dizziness, syncope or prolonged cardiac arrest. Failure to capture is often intermittent. In dual-chamber devices loss of atrial lead capture is often asymptomatic or may cause reduced effort tolerance owing to loss of atrial systole. The following should be checked:

- Magnet response: does pacemaker capture at all?
- Lead thresholds, impedance

- Sensing (device may be oversensing)
- Programmed settings: has anything changed ('phantom' reprogramming)
- Loss of capture with change in arm position?
- Trauma to pacemaker? external electromagnetic interference?
- Chest X-ray: macrodisplacement?
- Penetrated X-ray of upper thorax: look for conductor break.

An abrupt rise in lead threshold often necessitates lead repositioning or, if chronically implanted lead (>3 months), replacement. If it occurs within 2–3 months of implantation, without macrodisplacement, some centres prescribe steroids (e.g. oral **prednisolone** 40 mg d^{-1} for 1–2 weeks) in case inflammation around the lead has caused *exit block*. Temporary reprogramming to high output may tide the patient through until a definitive procedure can be carried out.

The dizzy patient
Dizziness has many potential causes in pacemaker patients.

Unrelated pathology
Dizziness is common in the elderly and most dizzy pacemaker patients do not have a pacemaker-related problem (see Chapter 11).

Pacemaker syndrome
This occurs in patients with sinus rhythm and a VVI pacemaker. Spontaneous atrial activity and paced ventricular activity occur at different rates. At times atrial and ventricular activity occur in roughly the correct sequence and cardiac output is normal. At other times the atria contract against closed AV valves. This causes jugular and pulmonary venous pressure to elevate and can cause breathlessness, neck pulsation and headache. Also, cardiac output and blood pressure may drop, causing fatigue and dizziness. The best treatment is an upgrade to a dual-chamber device which maintains AV synchrony.

Failure to capture
See Complications.

Arrhythmias
Atrial arrhythmias cause tachycardia in DDD mode owing to the ventricular channel pacing rapidly. In mode-switching devices atrial sensitivity may need to be altered to detect the tachycardia. If mode switching is not available, there are several options:

- Antiarrhythmic drug R$_x$, to prevent atrial arrhythmias.
- Programme upper rate limit to ~100 bpm to limit ventricular response to tachycardia (this also limits response in sinus rhythm during exercise and may cause fatigue and dyspnoea).
- Programme to DDI mode. Unfortunately the device will not track sinus

rhythm, so AV sequential pacing is needed all of the time; this depletes the generator. During atrial tachyarrhythmia the pacemaker effectively switches to VVI mode.

● Replace pacemaker with a mode-switching device.

Pacemaker-mediated tachycardias can also cause dizziness; adjustment of the PVARP and refractory period extension may prevent this. With rate-responsive devices an inappropriately brisk or slow rate response to exercise can cause fatigue or dizziness.

Vasodilatation

In HCSS or malignant vasovagal syndrome permanent pacing alone may not prevent symptoms because inappropriate vasodilatation can still occur.

Suspected system infection

Pacemaker system infection is an uncommon (<1%) but serious complication. *Staph. epidermidis* tends to follow an insidious course, often without external signs of pocket infection. *Staph. aureus* is the usual culprit for florid system infection. Infection is most common in the month following implantation and is more likely to occur during device replacement than during first implant. The presence of a temporary wire during implantation roughly doubles the incidence of subsequent system infection. Symptoms are often non-specific: anorexia, malaise, fever. There may not be obvious signs at the wound site.

Superficial wound infection

For superficial infection (e.g. redness around the suture line without obvious pocket swelling) take a wound swab and treat with antistaphylococcal antibiotics (e.g. oral **flucloxacillin** 500 mg qid for 1 week) and review.

Pocket infection

Boggy swelling, fluid leakage, tenderness and systemic symptoms suggest pocket infection. Echo or TOE is indicated to check for vegetations. Check for clinical stigmata of SBE. Check ESR, CRP, FBC, wound swab and blood cultures. Pacemaker and lead extraction and antibiotic R_x (several weeks if evidence of SBE) are indicated. Open surgical lead extraction is indicated if there are large vegetations adherent to the lead. Temporary pacing may be needed prior to the implantation of a new system on the contralateral side.

Wound swelling without other evidence of infection

In the early phase this may represent haematoma, which may resolve spontaneously. Evacuation is indicated if there is significant discomfort. Assess as above. Wound swelling may also result from trauma or migration of the device. If infection is suspected from clinical assessment and blood tests, system removal is indicated.

Symptoms of systemic infection with normal wound site
This is the most difficult situation; check for other possible sources of infection (e.g. urine, sputum, blood cultures) and assess as for pocket infection. If no other source of infection is found there may be no alternative but to replace the pacemaker system.

RATE-ADAPTIVE AND MODE-SWITCHING PACEMAKERS

RATE-ADAPTIVE PACEMAKERS

Chronotropic incompetence is defined as failure to elevate the heart rate to 70% of the maximum predicted for effort level, or to >100 bpm. Around 40% of patients with sick sinus syndrome have chronotropic incompetence, as do many with AV block. Also, some patients with atrial fibrillation and bradycardias do not elevate heart rate adequately during exercise. These patients may benefit from rate-adaptive pacing, in which the pacemaker rate is increased in response to a sensed physical stimulus. Several different types of sensor are used.

Activity sensors
These use a mechanical or piezoelectric switch and/or an accelerometer to detect physical movement. Although effective, certain activities (e.g. cycling) may not generate much movement and heart rate may not rise. Also, external vibration may cause an inappropriate rise in heart rate.

Minute ventilation sensors
Respiratory activity is detected as a change in transthoracic impedance and minute volume is estimated. Respiratory rate may not rise early in exercise, so these sensors can give a delayed heart rate response. Minute ventilation sensors are not appropriate for patients with chronic lung disease.

QT interval sensors
These work by measuring the paced QT interval, which is shortened by the action of catecholamines. These sensors allow an appropriate elevation of heart rate in response to physical and mental stress, but are dependent on accurate T-wave sensing. Antiarrhythmic drugs and myocardial ischaemia may interfere with sensor function.

Haemodynamic sensors
These devices infer RV stroke volume and RV dP/dt, mainly by measuring changes in transthoracic impedance during the cardiac cycle.

Other sensors
Some pacemaker/lead combinations can detect changes in blood temperature, pH and O_2 saturation.

Sensor combinations

To overcome the problem of inappropriate rate rise, sensor combinations such as activity (brisk early rate response) and minute ventilation (overcomes activity sensor limitations) are used and are effective.

AAIR, VVIR or DDDR pacing modes can be used, according to the underlying pathology. Several parameters are programmed to modify the rate response to the sensed stimulus:

- Maximum heart rate
- Heart rate/activity relationship ('slope')
- Rate acceleration (how rapidly heart rate accelerates to above value)
- Rate deceleration slope.

The effect of programming can be assessed through ambulatory monitoring (ensure that patient is physically active during monitoring period!) and treadmill testing. Aim for approximately 20 bpm rate rise during normal walking, 30–40 bpm rise during brisk walking.

MODE-SWITCHING PACEMAKERS

Atrial tachyarrhythmias affect 20–30% of patients with dual-chamber pacemakers, resulting in inappropriately rapid ventricular pacing in DDD mode. Solutions to this problem are discussed in an earlier section. Mode-switching pacemakers offers a partial solution. These devices can detect atrial tachyarrhythmias and automatically switch to VVI or VVIR mode. Paced rate is then independent of atrial activity. Effective function depends on the detection of atrial activity during tachycardia (adjust atrial sensitivity) and programming of a threshold atrial rate (usually >150 bpm) for mode switching.

AUTOMATIC IMPLANTABLE CARDIOVERTER – DEFIBRILLATORS (AICDs)

AICDs have revolutionized the treatment of ventricular arrhythmias. These devices use advanced pacemaker technology to recognize and treat VT and VF by pacing and defibrillation. Two recent major trials have expanded the indications for AICD implantation to a large subset of patients with ventricular arrhythmias (see box).

Early AICDs were bulky, implanted in an abdominal position and shocked via patch electrodes which were surgically implanted. Most current AICDs resemble a large VVI pacemaker (device volumes are now <100 ml), can be implanted in the pectoral position and apply shock between the lead and the device casing. Dual-chamber AICDs are also available; these improve arrhythmia recognition by sensing atrial as well as ventricular activity and are useful in patients with AV node dysfunction. AICDs are expensive: device/lead combinations typically cost £15,000–£20,000, which limits the scope for implantation in many countries. The indications for implantation need to be interpreted in light of this.

Key AICD trials

MADIT
Criteria: post-MI, LVEF <35%, asymptomatic sustained VT on ambulatory monitor and inducible, non-suppressible VT at EPS
Outcome: relative risk reduction 54% for death over following 5 years

AVID
Criteria: resuscitated VF or VT with syncope or haemodynamic compromise requiring cardioversion
Outcome: trial terminated early; relative risk reduction for death 31% at 3 years

---

Functions of AICD
- Arrhythmia recognition
- Overdrive pacing
- Cardioversion/defibrillation
- Antibradycardia pacing
- Event memory: records arrhythmias, delivered therapy, outcome

---

INDICATIONS

Recent trial results have expanded the indications. The AHA/ACC have published guidelines based on these trials for AICD implantation (see start of chapter for classification of indications); the following indications are based on these.

Class I indications
- Cardiac arrest due to VF or VT, not due to a transient or reversible cause
- Spontaneous, sustained VT
- Syncope of undetermined origin, with haemodynamically significant sustained VT or VF at EPS, where drug therapy is ineffective, not tolerated or not preferred
- Non-sustained VT with prior MI, LV dysfunction and inducible VF or sustained VT at EPS not suppressible by a class I antiarrhythmic drug.

Class IIa indications
- None.

Class IIb indications
(Usually do not apply when cost constraints are restrictive, e.g. UK National Health Service.)

- Cardiac arrest presumed due to VF, where EPS precluded

- Severe symptomatic VT while awaiting cardiac transplantation
- Familial/inherited conditions with high risk of life-threatening ventricular tachyarrhythmias, e.g. long QT syndrome, HOCM
- Non-sustained VT with prior MI, LV dysfunction and inducible VF or sustained VT at EPS *suppressible* by a class I antiarrhythmic drug
- Recurrent syncope of undetermined origin, with haemodynamically significant sustained VT or VF at EPS, when other causes of syncope have been excluded.

CONTRAINDICATIONS

- VT or VF with reversible cause
- VT or VF due to acute MI
- Incessant/very frequent VT (device may deliver frequent shocks and deplete rapidly)
- Prognosis markedly limited by comorbidity, e.g. end-stage cardiac failure
- Psychological instability
- Presence of unipolar pacing system (pacing spike will interfere with AICD function) – may need to be explanted.

IMPLANTATION AND TESTING

AICDs are implanted under general anaesthesia as device testing is unpleasant to the conscious patient and because subpectoral implantation is sometimes preferable to minimize the risk of migration/erosion. Implantation is similar to that of a VVI pacemaker, although a left lateral subclavian approach is often used to accommodate the large-diameter ventricular lead. The mortality from non-thoracotomy AICD implantation is around 1%. The following tests are performed at implantation:

- Standard lead tests (threshold, sensing, impedance)
- Defibrillation electrode impedance test (tested by applying low-energy shock)
- Antitachycardia pacing is tested by inducing VT with timed premature stimuli, then testing the programmed antitachycardia algorithm (see below). Low-energy synchronized cardioversion (between 0.5 and 5 J) may also be tested during VT
- VF is induced by rapid ventricular pacing or a 50 Hz burst to check the defibrillation threshold (energy required for successful defibrillation); this should be below 20 J. An external defibrillator should be charged in case the AICD shock fails.

DEVICE PROGRAMMING FOR ARRHYTHMIA RECOGNITION

Most AICDs use rate criteria to diagnose VT and VF. This is sensitive but not specific and patients can receive inappropriate painful shocks.

> **Causes of inappropriate AICD shock**
> - Supraventricular tachycardias, rate within VT detection zone
> - Sinus tachycardia, rate within VT detection zone
> - Oversensing (e.g. T-wave sensing, myopotential sensing)

To maximize efficacy and minimize the risk of inappropriate shock it is important to know the patient's heart rate range during VT and sinus rate during exercise. If these overlap there is a risk of inappropriate pacing or cardioversion during exertion. β-Blockade can usefully limit sinus rate during exercise. In addition, the following parameters can be programmed to tune therapy.

Rate detection zones
A lower and upper VT rate detection limit can be programmed. Some devices also have a 'fast VT' zone, which is useful in patients with more than one VT rate/morphology. A lower VF detection interval is also programmed.

> **Tip:** The convention is to programme AICD rate detection zone parameters as R-R interval (in milliseconds):
> $$\text{R-R INTERVAL (ms)} = \frac{1000}{(x/60)} \text{ where } x \text{ is heart rate (bpm)}$$

Detection cycles
The number of consecutive cardiac cycles within the detection zone required before antitachycardia pacing or cardioversion is initiated (this ensures that VT is sustained before therapy is delivered). A typical value is 12–16 cycles.

Rate stability
This is the maximum interbeat variation of the R-R interval (in milliseconds) allowed for VT detection. Activation of rate stability detection prevents inappropriate shock for atrial fibrillation, but may prevent the detection of polymorphic VT. Typical settings are 40–50 ms.

'Sudden onset' criterion
This is based on the fact that most VT episodes are characterized by a sudden jump in rate. The use of this function may prevent the detection of VT occurring during stress, when the sinus rate is high preceding VT onset.

QRS morphology
Not available on most devices; QRS morphology criteria are used to identify VT complexes.

DDD devices

Dual-chamber AICDs allow analysis of atrial rhythm during tachycardias to differentiate VT from SVTs.

TIERED VT THERAPY

Tiered therapy is a progressively aggressive strategy for treating VT. Typically, the device is programmed to attempt overdrive pacing, then a low-energy shock, followed by a high-energy shock. Overdrive pacing is appropriate for VT with which the patient is likely to be haemodynamically stable, i.e. cycle length >300 ms (HR <200 bpm). Several parameters can be programmed:

- **Number of attempts** – number of consecutive attempts at a given mode of antitachycardia therapy before device moves to next tier of therapy.
- **Burst pacing** – a constant cycle length burst of paced beats is delivered, usually with an interval 80–90% of the tachycardia cycle length. More rapid bursts are more likely to induce VF.
- **Ramp pacing** – as above, but each successive cycle in the burst is shorter than the previous one.
- **Number of beats** – number of paced beats in each ramp or burst cycle, usually 6–10.

Example of tiered therapy for VT, cycle length 350 ms:

(a)	Burst pacing	8 beats	cycle length 90%	3 attempts
(b)	Ramp pacing	8 beats	10 ms decrement	3 attempts
(c)	Low-energy shock		5 J	1 attempt
(d)	High-energy shock		34 J	1 attempt

CARDIOVERSION/DEFIBRILLATION

Low-energy shocks are less likely to terminate VT than high-energy shocks. For many patients low-energy shocks are just as unpleasant, in which case the low-energy shock tier can be omitted. The sensation associated with DC shock varies between patients, ranging from no symptoms to the sensation of a painful kick to the chest or back. The only appropriate therapy for VF is a high-energy shock (e.g. 34 J). VF therapy is usually set to deliver repeated 34 J shocks until cardioversion is achieved. Shocks significantly deplete the AICD battery, although most devices can deliver more than 100 shocks.

INTERPRETING DEVICE MEMORY FUNCTIONS

AICD interrogation provides information from several sources:

- **Marker channel**: records the timings of sensed and paced events.

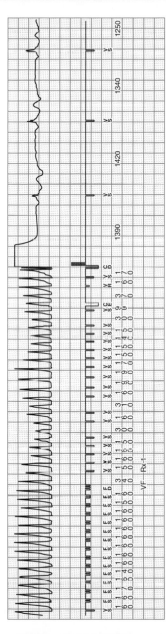

Fig. 17.15 Sample AICD record of VT cardioversion. The two traces are intracardiac ECGs and the marker channel. Tachycardia cycle lengths are within the VF detection zone (FS = VF cycle sensed); after several cycles the device diagnoses this as VF (FD = VF detected). The device charges and cardioversion is delivered (CD) with restoration of sinus rhythm (VS = ventricle sensed).

- **Stored electrogram**: records the intracardiac ECG waveform before, during and after an arrhythmia.
- **Event memory**: records the number of sensed arrhythmias and therapies that have been delivered and whether or not successful.

WHAT TO DO IF AICD DELIVERS A SHOCK

AICD shocks cause considerable anxiety to patients. It is important not to cause panic, but it is best to assess the patient as soon as is reasonable, ideally within 24 hours of the shock. If there are new symptoms (e.g. chest discomfort preceding the shock, dyspnoea etc.) assess the patient immediately.

- **History**: prodromal symptoms, dizziness, syncope, awareness of antitachycardia pacing
- **Examination**: pulse rhythm (?new onset atrial fibrillation), cardiac failure (increases likelihood of VF/VT)
- **AICD check**
    what was rhythm preceding shock? (often difficult to tell from intracardiac ECG)
    if atrial fibrillation, consider adjusting rate stability function
    if sinus tachycardia, consider altering detection zones, or β-blockade to limit sinus rate
    if VT or VF, check for precipitants (e.g. electrolyte disturbance, cardiac failure) and consider either:
      – more aggressive antitachycardia pacing regimen
      – antiarrhythmic drug therapy.

SOCIAL AND PSYCHOLOGICAL ASPECTS

Practical restrictions with AICDs are minimal and similar to those with permanent pacemakers. In the UK the driving authorities will consider individual cases for reissue of a personal driving licence if no symptomatic arrhythmias or DC shocks have occurred within the preceding 6 months.

Anxiety and depression are common among AICD patients, especially in those who have received shocks. Minimizing inappropriate shocks is pivotal to minimizing psychological upset. Psychological support is needed after implantation: some patients benefit from input from a clinical psychologist. AICD support groups exist in some regions and offer practical advice and help from fellow patients.

 Warning: Antiarrhythmic drugs, e.g. amiodarone, flecainide, may increase the defibrillation threshold. This may need to be rechecked if drug therapy is introduced.

CHAPTER 18

CARDIAC CATHETERIZATION AND INTERVENTION

INDICATIONS FOR DIAGNOSTIC CARDIAC CATHETERIZATION

The following list of indications for diagnostic coronary angiography is based on AHA/ACC guidelines and is not exhaustive. See Chapter 17 for classification of indications. Class II indications, for which the strength of evidence is less clear-cut, are often not applied in countries in which angiography is less freely available than in the United States. Angiography is only one aspect of cardiac catheterization. Haemodynamic assessment and right heart catheterization are integral to the assessment of patients with valvular and congenital heart disease and cardiomyopathies.

CORONARY ARTERY DISEASE

Asymptomatic patients
- Inducible ischaemia at low workload during stress testing   (class I)
- Resuscitated cardiac arrest   (class I)
- After MI, with positive (but not high-risk) stress test   (class II)
- Prior to non-cardiac surgery, with positive stress test   (class II)
- After cardiac transplantation   (class II)

Stable angina
- Limiting angina despite optimal medical therapy   (class I)
- Inducible ischaemia at low workload on stress testing   (class I)
- Before major vascular surgery (e.g. AAA repair) if patient has angina or positive stress test   (class I)
- Resuscitated cardiac arrest   (class I)
- Pulmonary oedema suspected to be due to ischaemia   (class I)
- (Occasionally) diagnostic purposes in patients with chest pain and inconclusive or negative stress test   (class II)
- Males <40 with angina, females <40 with angina and positive stress test, patients <40 with previous MI   (class II)
- CCS class III or IV angina which responds to medication   (class II)

Unstable angina
Although unstable angina is listed as a class I indication for angiography in the AHA/ACC guidelines, its role in the acute phase is far from clear. Early conservative and early interventional approaches are both valid and the degree to which angiography is used depends on local resources and policy. Angiography should be performed in the following situations:

- Unstable angina with symptoms refractory to drug therapy
- Unstable angina with persistent high-risk features (see Chapter 12)
- Inducible ischaemia at low workload after episode of unstable angina.

Acute MI

Primary angioplasty is a valid effective approach recommended as an alternative to thrombolysis in the 1996 AHA/ACC *Guidelines for the Management of Patients With Acute MI* (JACC 1996; 28: 1328–1428). Most centres do not do this because it requires 24-hour immediate access to cardiac catheterization facilities. Angiography can be considered for patients with acute MI and:

- Absolute contraindication to thrombolysis (see Chapter 5)
- Failed thrombolysis. The evidence base for this is weak, but 'rescue angioplasty' can be considered in the following situations:
  - haemodynamic instability (e.g. cardiogenic shock)
  - ongoing chest pain
  - within 8 h of onset of symptoms.

In addition, cardiac catheterization is indicated for:

- Suspected acute mitral regurgitation or VSD (class I)
- Suspected subacute free wall rupture (pseudoaneurysm) (class I)
- Recurrent post-infarct angina (class I)

VALVULAR HEART DISEASE

Echo is the main diagnostic modality in these patients. Cardiac catheterization provides supportive information and may be needed for the following:

- Pressure gradient across stenotic aortic or mitral valve
- Assessment of mitral and aortic regurgitation using ventriculogram or aortogram
- PA pressure, cardiac output and other haemodynamic variables
- Identification of coexisting coronary artery disease.

In addition, indications for *coronary angiography* in patients with valve disease are if surgery is being contemplated in:

- Patients with ischaemic symptoms (class I)
- Males ≥ 35 years and postmenopausal females (class I)
- Males <35 years and premenopausal females undergoing left heart catheterization to assess mitral or aortic valve (class II)
- Multiple coronary risk factors (class II)

CONGENITAL HEART DISEASE

Cardiac catheterization is not a prerequisite for all types of corrective surgery, but is required prior to balloon intervention for aortic coarctation, congenital aortic stenosis, restricted Mustard baffle etc. It is also useful to determine the size of intracardiac shunts. *Coronary angiography* is required in patients who develop angina, older patients requiring corrective surgery (rules for valvular disease apply) and in patients with suspected anomalous coronary anatomy.

MISCELLANEOUS

- Aortic dissection
- Unexplained congestive cardiac failure
- Diagnosis and assessment of patients with cardiomyopathies.

CORONARY ARTERY AND BYPASS GRAFT ANATOMY

CORONARY ARTERIES

Figure 18.1 shows the six standard angiographic views of the left coronary artery (LCA) and two standard views of the right coronary artery (RCA). Coronary anatomy is variable; common variations include:

Abbreviations used for coronary anatomy	
LMS	left main stem
LCA	left coronary artery
RCA	right coronary artery
LAD	left anterior descending coronary artery
Cx	circumflex coronary artery
ICA	intermediate coronary artery
OM (e.g. OM_1, OM_2)	first, second obtuse marginal branch (of Cx)
D (e.g. D_1, D_2)	first, second diagonal branch (of LAD)
PD	posterior descending artery

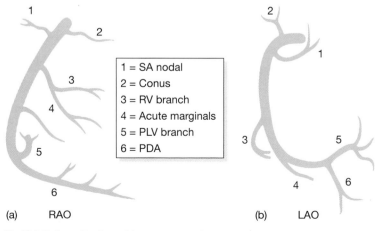

1 = SA nodal
2 = Conus
3 = RV branch
4 = Acute marginals
5 = PLV branch
6 = PDA

(a)   RAO

(b)   LAO

Fig. 18.1 Radiographic views of the coronary arteries.

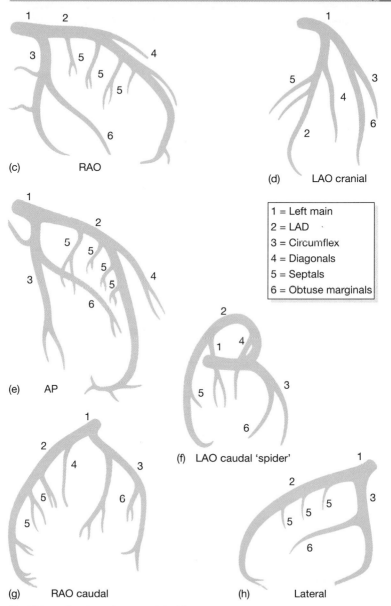

(c) RAO

(d) LAO cranial

(e) AP

1 = Left main
2 = LAD
3 = Circumflex
4 = Diagonals
5 = Septals
6 = Obtuse marginals

(f) LAO caudal 'spider'

(g) RAO caudal

(h) Lateral

Fig. 18.1 c to **h**: radiographic views of the left coronary artery.

- **Intermediate coronary artery (ICA)**. The LCA trifurcates into the LAD, Cx and an intermediate vessel, which is effectively a diagonal branch. It may be large and subtend a significant territory.
- **Left main stem (LMS)**. This may be absent, in which case the LAD and Cx have separate origins from the aorta. Suspect this if LAD or Cx is absent during 'LCA' injection.
- **Tributaries** of the main coronary arteries are very variable in number and size, especially obtuse marginal (OM) branches of the Cx and diagonal branches of the LAD.
- **Posterior descending artery (PDA)** normally arises from the distal RCA ('right dominant' anatomy), but may arise from the Cx ('left dominant').

The following anomalous coronary configurations may also be seen:

- Cx arising from the right sinus of Valsalva, adjacent to RCA. This is the most common anomaly (~1 in 150).
- Single coronary artery, or origin of all three arteries from non-coronary sinus. Sometimes a coronary artery passes between the pulmonary and aortic roots – the vessel may become compressed, with the risk of ischaemia and sudden death during exercise.
- RCA arising from the left sinus of Valsalva adjacent to LCA.
- High anterior origin of RCA.
- LCA arising from the pulmonary artery. Ischaemia occurs in early life and only 25% survive to adolescence or adulthood.
- Coronary artery fistulae may also occur. Most drain into the right heart chambers or pulmonary artery.

CORONARY ARTERY BYPASS GRAFTS

Saphenous vein grafts are anastomosed to the ascending aorta approximately 5–10 cm above the aortic valve, in a (usually!) predictable manner.

- PDA grafts originate from the right anterior aspect of the aorta and run vertically to the inferior surface of the heart.
- OM grafts originate from the left anterior aspect of the aorta and arc towards the posterolateral surface of the heart.
- LAD and diagonal grafts originate from an intermediate position and run laterally towards the anterior interventricular groove.

The left and right internal mammary arteries arise from the proximal subclavian arteries, taking off at approximately 90°. They are most often anastomosed to the LAD and RCA, respectively.

IMAGE ACQUISITION

Catheterization laboratories use either single-plane or biplane imaging. The latter uses two cameras to record simultaneous images from different angles.

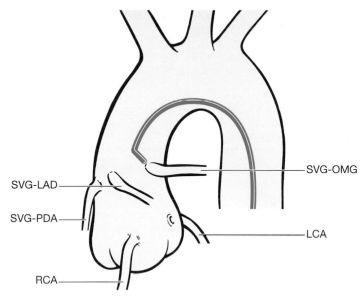

Fig. 18.2 Orthodox position of saphenous vein bypass grafts.

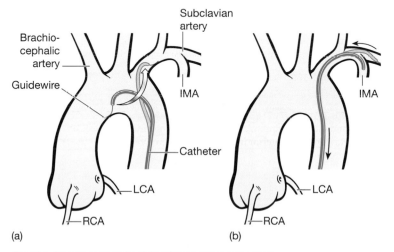

Fig. 18.3 Selective angiography of the left internal mammary artery.

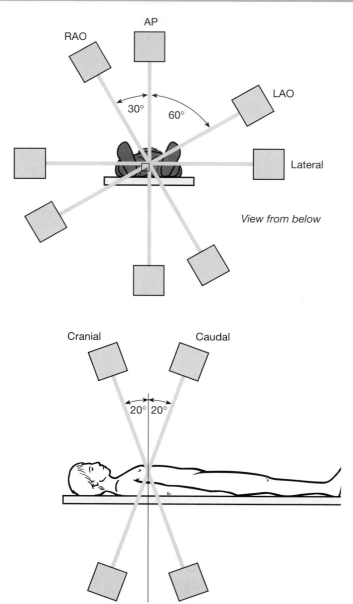

Fig. 18.4 Orientation of imaging cameras during coronary angiography.

With practice, the biplane system allows faster image acquisition and halves the amount of contrast agent needed during the study. Images can be stored in various formats. Ciné film has been largely superseded by digital image acquisition, which gives greater flexibility for manipulation and analysis. Catheter studies can be archived on videotape or optical disc.

RADIATION PROTECTION

It is essential to attend a recognized radiation protection course before carrying out any procedures that use X-ray screening. National requirements vary but focus on the protection of patients and staff. It is sobering that in the UK the incidence of haematological malignancy among cardiologists is well above the national average.

Radiation monitoring badges, which contain a small patch of X-ray film, should be worn at all times in the catheterization laboratory. A badge is worn over the thorax and on the thyroid collar. Badges are normally checked monthly to ensure radiation exposure is within recommended limits.

MINIMIZING PATIENT EXPOSURE

Reducing radiation exposure minimizes risk to patients, operators and other staff. Simple measures can dramatically cut down exposure:

- Minimize screening time – keep your foot off the pedal!
- Minimize distance between intensifier and X-ray tube.
- Use the *cones* to focus on the area of interest. This targets X-rays at a smaller area of the patient.
- Only use high-intensity imaging to record images you *need*.
- Minimize imaging time during each coronary injection (but not at the expense of important data; e.g. long runs may be needed to identify late filling of collateral vessels).

MINIMIZING OPERATOR EXPOSURE

Operators must protect themselves and must not screen if laboratory staff are not wearing protective clothing. Most of the operator's X-ray exposure is due to reflection and scatter from the table and the patient. Exposure is minimized by:

- Wearing a lead apron and thyroid collar
- Leaded spectacles: reduce risk of cataract
- Shielding between patient and operator, e.g. lead apron below the table and leaded glass screen between patient (not X-ray camera) and operator
- Minimizing distance between intensifier and X-ray tube (reduces scatter)
- Using fluoroscopy in views with the least X-ray scatter. AP views expose the operator to less radiation than lateral views

- Maximizing distance between operator and X-ray tube (i.e. standing back)
- Minimizing imaging time, as described above.

PREPROCEDURE CHECKLIST

Cardiac catheterization should only be carried out by (or under the direct supervision of) trained operators, in a properly equipped and staffed catheterization laboratory: most have trained radiographers, cardiac technicians and nurses. Operator experience has an important bearing on the safety of catheterization procedures.

BEFORE ATTENDANCE (e.g. in outpatient clinic)

Explain to the patient:

- Day case or overnight stay?
- What the procedure involves. Reassure that it is minimally uncomfortable.
- Potential risks.
- Potential benefits (e.g. allows planning of future R_x, identifies whether prognosis might be improved by revascularization).
- Where appropriate, to discontinue oral anticoagulants 2–3 days before the procedure. All other medications (except diuretics) should be taken on the day of the procedure.
- Recovery phase: possibility of local haematoma, not able to drive immediately afterwards.

BEFORE PROCEDURE ITSELF

- Double-check history and examination:
  - previous angiograms and findings
  - previous interventions (PTCA, stents, CABG), sites treated, types of bypass graft used
  - changes in clinical status since last reviewed (e.g. has angina got better? Is the procedure still indicated?)
  - check peripheral pulses to confirm access route.
- Obtain written consent for diagnostic procedure *and any anticipated interventions*.
- Laboratory tests:
  - full blood count
  - blood group

 Warning: Patients with suspected or confirmed contrast allergy should receive oral prednisolone 50 mg bd the day before and 50 mg stat 4 h prior to the procedure.

- INR if normally taking oral anticoagulants (INR should be <2.0 before elective cardiac catheterization)
- U&Es, creatinine (contrast agents are nephrotoxic)
- fasting glucose and lipid profile if not already done.
- Ensure up-to-date ECG available for comparison.

PREPROCEDURE TREATMENTS

- Fast for at least 4 hours.
- IV access.
- **Premedication**
  oral **diazepam** 10 mg 1 h before procedure
  IV **diazepam** 5–10 mg in addition if anxious at time of procedure.
- **Renal impairment** (e.g. creatinine >200 μmol l^{-1}) is associated with significant morbidity after cardiac catheterization. Contrast agents are nephrotoxic and renal decompensation may occur after the procedure. The risk of this can be minimized by sensible precautions:
  - IVI 0.9% saline 500 ml over 8–12 h before procedure*
  - use least nephrotoxic contrast agent available
  - use echo if possible to avoid contrast load with LV angiogram/aortogram
  - minimize use of 'test injections' before coronary injection
  - use minimum amount of contrast needed to properly opacify arteries
  - IVI 0.9% saline 500 ml over 12 h after procedure*
  - check U&Es, creatinine the morning after the procedure; monitor daily if renal function deteriorates, encourage good fluid intake.
- **Diabetic patients** should be scheduled so that they do not miss a main meal. If this cannot be arranged (e.g. patient first thing on morning list) and patient is insulin dependent, the following are options:
  glucose–potassium IV infusion, with separate IV insulin infusion adjusted according to capillary glucose level

Example scale for insulin infusion during cardiac catheterization	
BLOOD GLUCOSE LEVEL	INFUSION RATE
<4 mmol l–l	0.5 U/hr
4–8 mmol l–l	1.0 U/hr
8–15 mmol l–l	2.0 U/hr
15–20 mmol l–l	4.0 U/hr
>20 mmol l–l	review

  glucose–potassium–insulin (GKI) IV infusion (e.g. 8 units soluble insulin and 10 mmol KCl in 500 ml 10% glucose, infused at 125 ml h^{-1}). A new infusion bag, with an adjusted quantity of insulin, may be needed depending on capillary glucose level
  give usual SC insulin, and infuse glucose at rate dictated by capillary glucose level.

* Caution in patients with severe LV impairment or history of cardiac failure.

Diabetic patients with renal impairment should not take metformin on the morning of the procedure (increases risk of nephrotoxicity).

ARTERIAL ACCESS

Evaluate the access site carefully *before* bringing the patient in for the procedure! It is no use discovering that your patient has no femoral pulse when he or she is on the table. Double-check the limb pulses before scrubbing.

ACCESS SITE

The right femoral artery is most often used because it is easiest to access, is associated with a low complication rate and (unlike the brachial approach) doesn't get in the way of the X-ray cameras. Despite this, there are situations in which brachial or radial artery access is safer and preferable:

- Aortic coarctation (prevents effective steering of catheters from leg)
- Severe aortoiliac disease or aortoiliac surgery
- Patient taking oral anticoagulants
- Uncontrolled hypertension (haemostasis easier from brachial route).

The femoral and brachial approaches will be described here.

Femoral artery access
The right groin is cleansed and draped after identifying the anatomical landmarks. The femoral artery is palpable just below the inguinal ligament, midway between the anterior superior iliac spine and the pubic symphysis. (Femoral canal anatomy: from medial to lateral: vein, artery, nerve.)

- Palpate femoral artery.
- Infiltrate ~5–10 ml 1% lignocaine into subcutaneous tissues, about 2–4 cm below the inguinal ligament over the femoral pulse. Angle needle 45° to skin, aiming for a point over which the pulse can be felt. Infiltrate carefully over, not into, artery.
- Insert access needle (16–18 gauge Cook's needle) at same site and aim in same direction to puncture artery. A brisk 'spurt' confirms arterial puncture. Sluggish backflow indicates either venous puncture or that the needle is not properly in the artery.
- Use Seldinger technique to introduce guidewire, then haemostatic sheath into artery (see Chapter 2). Choose sheath appropriate to intended catheter gauge (5–8 Fr catheters have outer diameter 1.7–2.7 mm).

Brachial artery access
The brachial artery is smaller than the femoral artery and cannulation is associated with a higher incidence of vascular complications. The brachial artery can be approached using a cutdown method or by simple percutaneous

puncture. The arm is hyperextended, using a pad beneath the elbow and the wrist pronated and secured using a bandage. The artery is palpated medially in the antecubital fossa. After cleansing and draping, a skin incision is made (taking care not to traumatize the artery) before insertion of the access needle. The Seldinger technique is used for sheath insertion; a 6 Fr sheath (or smaller) is normally used.

SHEATH REMOVAL

Sheath removal is one of the most important parts of any catheterization procedure. Done carelessly it can cause serious complications. It should be done as soon as possible after elective catheterization to minimize the risk of complications. If the sheath has to be left in place (e.g. if an intervention is planned later that day), an obturator should be inserted and IV heparin (10 U/kg^{-1} IV bolus, followed by 1000 U h^{-1} IVI, adjusted to APTT) given to prevent arterial thrombosis.

The sheath is removed with a single, smooth movement of one hand, while pressing gently over the femoral pulse 2–3 cm above the puncture site with the other hand. Firm pressure is applied once the sheath is removed, for approximately 10 minutes. Pressure is then gently released and the puncture site examined for bleeding. If bleeding occurs, a further 5 minutes of continuous pressure should be applied. Watch for swelling around where pressure is being applied, as haematoma formation can occur. Distal limb pulses should be checked hourly for 4 hours after sheath removal.

If the sheath has been left in place for more than an hour, analgesia is needed (IV **morphine** 5–10 mg, with an antiemetic). Tissues around the access site should be infiltrated with local anaesthetic (e.g. 5 ml **1% lignocaine**) before sheath removal. IV **atropine** 0.5–1.0 mg may be needed if a vasovagal reaction occurs.

> **Tip:** When a sheath has been inserted through a **peripheral arterial graft**, extra care is needed during removal. There is a significant risk of graft thrombosis, so less pressure should be used to allow some flow in the graft while securing haemostasis.

TROUBLESHOOTING

Unable to cannulate the artery

Cannulation should not be attempted if the artery cannot be palpated. A weak femoral pulse may indicate significant peripheral vascular disease, which increases the risk of limb ischaemia during and after cannulation. An alternative access site should be considered.

If the pulse is adequate, recheck the anatomical landmarks. Ensure that the insertion needle is flushed and free of obstructing thrombus and debris. If venous blood is obtained on needle insertion, the puncture is too medial. Shooting pains affecting the leg indicate femoral nerve irritation, suggesting that the puncture is too lateral.

Poor flashback of arterial blood
This suggests:

- Femoral vein puncture – dark venous blood
- Poor arterial flow – peripheral vascular disease
- Incomplete cannulation of the arterial lumen
- Puncture of small branch artery.

Advancing the needle slightly may bring it fully into the arterial lumen; if so, a brisk flashback occurs. If flow remains poor withdraw the needle very slowly and watch for flashback, as you may have exited the back wall of the artery. Reinsert after compressing the puncture site for 2–3 minutes. If in doubt about which vessel has been punctured, use X-ray contrast to identify the vessel (ensure you can freely aspirate blood first).

Unable to advance the guidewire
The guidewire should pass easily down the introducer Cook's needle. **Never force a guidewire**, as this may dissect the artery, rupture a plaque or cause acute vessel closure.

If the guidewire meets immediate resistance it may be extravascular – this can be confirmed with fluoroscopy. Reposition or reinsert the needle. In obese patients, in whom the angle of access is by necessity steeper, flatten the angle of the needle (relative to the artery) and gently advance the guidewire.

If resistance is met after initially smooth passage of the guidewire the problem is likely to be with vascular anatomy (e.g. iliac artery stenosis or tortuous vessels). After insertion of the arterial sheath a contrast injection will define the vascular anatomy. Tortuous iliac vessels can be negotiated with a straight angulated soft-tipped guidewire. A long sheath may help minimize tortuosity, which makes steering of catheters very difficult.

Pain during sheath insertion
This suggests either inadequate local anaesthesia, or trauma or dissection of the femoral artery. Contrast injection helps identify whether the sheath is extravascular, or if the artery has been dissected. If limb perfusion is compromised seek immediate help from the vascular surgery team.

Difficulty with haemostasis
Despite prolonged pressure persistent bleeding may occur at the sheath site (see later). The risk of this is increased by:

- Obesity

- Aortic regurgitation
- Hypertension
- Coagulopathy: thrombocytopenia, warfarin therapy etc.

Check for and correct any coagulopathy. A mechanical clamp, such as a Femostop, should be used at mean arterial pressure to stop bleeding. After 30 minutes, pressure can be slowly reduced over 30–60 minutes. Alternatively, devices are available (such as VasoSeal) which instil bovine collagen along the tract from the arterial adventitia to the skin surface. This achieves rapid haemostasis and can be used in fully anticoagulated patients. These devices use large sheaths to deliver the collagen and care must be taken not to inject collagen into the artery!

CATHETERIZATION PROCEDURE

Before starting, run through all of the information required from the catheterization procedure. Is a right heart catheterization needed? How many bypass grafts should be sought? Is an aortogram needed? Saturation measurements? Short cuts lead to incomplete assessment, the need for a repeat procedure and perhaps to the patient receiving the wrong treatment.

Vascular access is obtained as described earlier (arterial) and in Chapter 3 (venous). If the procedure lasts more than 20 minutes, **unfractionated heparin** 50 IU kg^{-1} should be given IV to minimize the risk of thromboembolism. After the procedure anticoagulation can be reversed using **IV protamine** (1 mg per 1000 IU of heparin given). Protamine allergy is relatively common and is a special risk in patients who have previously used protamine insulin, in those with fish allergy and in infertile men or men who have had a vasectomy (see Complications).

CARDIAC CATHETERIZATION PROTOCOLS

Most patients undergoing cardiac catheterization need, as a minimum, coronary and LV angiography. The LV angiogram can be omitted if a satisfactory non-invasive assessment can be made (e.g. echo) or to minimize contrast load (e.g. in renal failure or pulmonary oedema).

Right heart catheterization should be considered for:

- Valvular or congenital heart disease
- Cardiac failure of unknown aetiology
- Cor pulmonale or pulmonary disease
- Suspected constrictive pericarditis or restrictive cardiomyopathy
- Assessment for heart transplant.

Aortography is helpful in patients with suspected aortic valve disease, thoracic aortic aneurysm, ruptured sinus of Valsalva or aortic dissection. It may also assist in the location of bypass grafts, or if an anomalous coronary artery origin is suspected.

LEFT HEART CATHETERIZATION

Before inserting catheters into the circulation, ensure the *pressure manifold* is working properly. This consists of a syringe, connector tubing, a series of three-way taps which connect the catheter to a pressure transducer, a saline flush circuit and a contrast agent reservoir. Always connect catheters to manifold tubing while flushing with saline: the 'wet-to-wet' or 'flush-to-blood' connection. Always check that there is no air in the catheter and tubing by aspirating blood back from the catheter before starting any series of contrast injections.

LV angiogram

A pigtail catheter is inserted via the femoral sheath, over a guidewire. The guidewire is advanced to the level of the carina (tracheal bifurcation, easily visible on fluoroscopy). The pigtail catheter is advanced over the wire into position in the descending thoracic aorta. The guidewire is removed and the catheter connected to the manifold and advanced over the aortic arch to the aortic root. Ascending aortic pressure can be recorded from this site.

To cross the aortic valve the catheter is gently advanced. When it reaches the aortic valve it flexes. Applying clockwise torque while gently advancing and retracting the catheter usually causes it to jump through the aortic valve into LV. The catheter should be advanced towards the cardiac apex, to avoid catheter-induced mitral regurgitation and so that complete LV opacification occurs during ventriculography. LV pressure (including end-diastolic pressure) can be recorded from this site. Small adjustments in catheter position may be needed if ventricular ectopy occurs.

The LV angiogram is performed using RAO (right anterior oblique) 30° and LAO (left anterior oblique) 60° views (see Fig. 18.3), during inspiration. The patient should be warned to expect a hot flushing sensation and sometimes transient urinary urgency. A power injector is used to inject approximately 40 ml of contrast over 2–3 s into the LV. The volume of contrast agent used can be modified according to the anticipated size and function of the ventricle, as well as the degree of mitral regurgitation.

After LV angiography, LV pressure should be recorded. The transaortic pressure gradient can be measured by continuous pressure recording during withdrawal of the catheter from the LV. If intracavity or subvalvar obstruction (e.g. HOCM or subaortic membrane) is suspected, the withdrawal gradient should be measured using an end-hole rather than a pigtail catheter.

Aortogram

If needed, an aortogram can be performed after LV angiography. The same camera angles are used. The pigtail catheter is positioned 3–7 cm above the aortic valve to avoid catheter-induced aortic regurgitation. Using the power injector, 40–60 ml of contrast are injected into the aorta over 1–2 s. If aortic regurgitation is suspected the LV should be included in the image field.

For single-plane imaging the ventriculogram and aortogram are usually obtained in one view only: the RAO 30° view for the ventriculogram and the LAO 60° view for the aortogram.

CORONARY ANGIOGRAPHY

Judkins catheters are used as standard for coronary angiography via the femoral approach (Fig. 18.5). The left Judkins catheter has two angled segments near the tip and is designed to engage the left coronary ostium while bracing against the opposite aortic wall. The right Judkins catheter is straight other than at the tip and is designed to be torqued into the right coronary ostium.

In 95% of cases Judkins size 4 catheters are adequate for catheterization of the LCA and RCA. Some operators give sublingual GTN before angiography, to dilate the vessels to maximum diameter. The catheters are advanced, positioned and flushed in the descending aorta, as described for the pigtail catheter above. As the catheter engages the coronary ostium, **watch for damping of the pressure waveform. This may indicate an ostial stenosis or catheter-induced spasm**. The catheter should be quickly and gently removed if this occurs.

Left coronary artery

Using the AP view the left Judkins catheter is advanced over the arch. Care is needed to prevent the catheter from folding over on itself. The catheter usually 'finds' the LCA naturally. Images are obtained during inspiration in the standard six radiographic views: AP, lateral, LAO cranial, RAO, LAO caudal and RAO caudal (see Figs 18.1 and 18.4). Cranial and caudal views use approximately 20° angulation.

- A steep RAO cranial view helps separate the LAD from overlapping diagonal vessels.
- The AP caudal view 'opens out' the left main stem.

Right coronary artery

Using the LAO view the right Judkins catheter is advanced to the level of the aortic valve, then withdrawn gently and torqued clockwise. The catheter tip should rotate from aortic lumen to aortic wall and slip into the right coronary ostium. Images are obtained during inspiration in the standard two radiographic views: LAO and RAO (see Figs 18.1 and 18.5). The distal RCA is opened out using the LAO cranial view during expiration.

Bypass grafts

Using the AP or the LAO view, the right Judkins catheter is advanced into the ascending aorta. Radio-opaque markers or clips may be left by the surgeon, indicating the sites of the graft ostia, but these cannot be relied upon (see

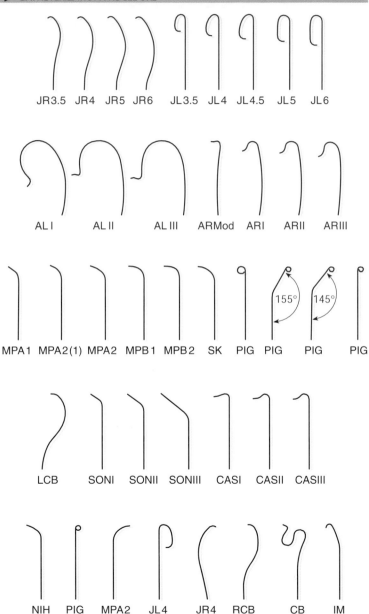

Fig. 18.5 Range and shapes of coronary catheters.

Fig. 18.6). The catheter is gently manipulated around the ascending aortic wall in the LAO and ROA views and torqued as for RCA catheterization. The catheter tip usually 'jumps' forwards when it encounters a graft ostium. LAD and OM grafts are usually easy to cannulate in this way. RCA grafts may require a straighter (e.g. multipurpose) catheter because the graft take-off is at an acute angle to the aorta. Specially designed left and right coronary bypass catheters can also be used. Images are obtained during inspiration in the LAO and RAO views; the LAO cranial view is sometimes needed to delineate the RCA graft insertion point.

Internal mammary grafts

The internal mammary arteries are cannulated with the arm positioned at the patient's side. Warn the patient of a flushing sensation in the arm during contrast injection. A right Judkins or internal mammary artery catheter is positioned in the aortic arch and rotated clockwise to advance it towards the internal mammary artery via the left subclavian (LIMA graft) or the innominate and right subclavian (RIMA graft) artery. Location of the subclavian arteries may be assisted using the guidewire.

- **The LIMA** arises anteroinferiorly from the left subclavian artery, 3–5 cm distal to the origin of the vertebral artery. Because it takes off at approximately 90° angle to the subclavian artery, the more angulated internal mammary catheter is often needed to selectively cannulate it.
- **The RIMA** arises from the equivalent position on the right side. As the innominate artery has to be negotiated, care is needed not to cannulate or traumatize the right internal carotid artery when locating the right subclavian artery. During inspiration, digital images are obtained in the standard two radiographic views: LAO and RAO.

RIGHT HEART CATHETERIZATION

This should be performed as described in Chapter 3. In addition to the haemodynamic measurements described in Chapter 3, the following may be helpful:

- Simultaneous LV and PCWP measurements, to estimate the transmitral pressure gradient in mitral stenosis.
- Simultaneous LV, RV and RA pressure measurements in suspected constrictive pericarditis/restrictive cardiomyopathy.

Depending on the indication for right heart catheterization, O_2 saturation can be measured from blood samples taken at several sites. Where congenital heart defects or intracardiac shunts are suspected, **all** sites should be used:

- PA
- RV – subvalvar, mid-cavity and apex
- RA – high, mid and low
- SVC – high and low

- IVC
- LV
- Aorta.

TROUBLESHOOTING

Unable to advance or manipulate the catheter

If resistance is felt while advancing the catheter or guidewire, don't force it, as vessel trauma, plaque rupture, dissection or embolization might occur. There are several reasons why there may be resistance:

- Vessel tortuosity
- Iliac/femoral artery stenosis
- Guidewire not in vessel lumen
- Guidewire in wrong vessel (e.g. small branch artery).

Use screening to identify the tortuosity of the iliac artery or aorta. If there is brisk backflow of blood through the introducer needle, inject a little contrast to see where you are. A straight, soft-tipped guidewire may help you negotiate a tortuous segment and a long sheath may partly straighten out the artery. Once negotiated, catheters should be exchanged over the guidewire so that the tortuous segment is not damaged.

Tortuosity also makes catheter manipulation difficult because torque is not transmitted to the catheter tip. Excessive torque makes the catheter kink and this damps the pressure trace. Once kinked, a catheter is useless and must be replaced. To avoid this, the guidewire may be kept in the catheter (well away from the tip) to brace it while applying torque, until the coronary artery is engaged. Only do this as a last resort, as the pressure trace cannot be observed until the catheter is reconnected to the transducer. If the catheter cannot be engaged using this method, consider an alternative arterial access route.

Unable to cross the aortic valve

Sometimes the pigtail catheter will not cross the aortic valve. It can be braced with a guidewire but should not be forced: torque rather than brute force is required! If there is significant aortic stenosis the pigtail will not cross the valve. Do an aortogram to identify the aortic valve orifice and any associated aortic regurgitation. Through the pigtail catheter, a straight-tipped floppy guidewire can be used to cross the valve: brisk back-and-forth movement is needed, otherwise the forceful aortic jet deflects the guidewire. Once the valve is crossed the catheter is advanced over the guidewire into the LV. If this method fails, a Judkins right coronary catheter may help the guidewire traverse the

 Warning: Be very careful not to cannulate one of the coronary arteries while trying to cross the aortic valve – power injection into a coronary artery can be fatal.

valve: it is more 'steerable' than the pigtail. Once the right coronary catheter is in LV, record LV pressure and a withdrawal gradient. If LV angiography is required (and it usually isn't, if echo images are good), the right coronary catheter must be exchanged for a pigtail catheter over a long ('exchange') guidewire.

Unable to selectively cannulate the coronary arteries

Consider ostial occlusion or severe ostial stenosis if the ostium is reached but cannot be properly cannulated. Sinus of Valsalva injection may reveal whether the artery is patent. An aortogram helps identify whether coronary arteries or bypass grafts are patent.

- *Left coronary catheter folds up.* The catheter is too small (the aorta may be large, unfolded or aneurysmal). A Judkins left, size 5 or even 6, catheter may be needed.
- *Catheter tip does not reach left main stem at correct angle to engage.* The catheter may be too big; try a Judkins left size 3.5.
- *Right coronary artery take-off goes upwards.* Here the Judkins right catheter will not engage the ostium properly, or slips out during injection. An Amplatz right coronary catheter may be needed; these come in different sizes. With difficult or anomalous coronary arteries trial and error with differing catheter types (e.g. multipurpose) may be necessary.

Damping

If the catheter wedges into and occludes an artery the pressure trace may 'ventricularize' (low diastolic pressure) or flatten. Always watch out for this, as hypotension and arrhythmias may follow; withdraw the catheter gently to restore flow. These indicate one of the following:

- Catheter impacted in stenosed coronary ostium
- Catheter has 'superselected' branch artery, e.g. LAD
- Catheter is directed at aortic wall (damping only) and is not engaged
- Catheter is in LV (ventricularization ± damping).

Contrast injection in the sinus of Valsalva may reveal an ostial stenosis. Cautious movement of the catheter into or just below the ostium should allow a quick angiogram to be taken; do not inject forcefully and disengage the catheter immediately. Unnecessarily forceful hand injections may precipitate VF.

Inadequate opacification

This usually occurs because the catheter is not properly engaged. Further manipulation or a change of catheter may be needed. If the coronary arteries are very large or coronary blood flow brisk (e.g. associated with severe LVH), a more rapid injection is needed to achieve adequate opacification. It may be difficult to obtain good images in obese patients because of tissue attenuation.

Coronary artery spasm

See section on Interpretation.

COMPLICATIONS OF DIAGNOSTIC ANGIOGRAPHY

Life-threatening complications are rare (~1 in 1000), but include MI, stroke, aortic or coronary dissection, cardiac rupture, air embolism, arrhythmia and peripheral vascular damage. Complications are more common in patients with serious disease, e.g. left main stem disease, aortic or peripheral vascular disease. Other complications are quite common and include haematoma at the puncture site, angina, vasovagal reactions and allergies to contrast agents and drugs.

PERIPHERAL VASCULAR COMPLICATIONS

Haematoma

This is a very common complication. The likelihood of haematoma formation is related to:

- Length of time sheath left in place
- Size of sheath
- Anticoagulation
- Technique of sheath removal
- Presence of hypertension or aortic regurgitation
- Obesity.

Most haematomas do not require intervention, although analgesia may be needed. If the 'haematoma' is tense, expansile, associated with a bruit or very tender, consider the alternative diagnosis of femoral artery pseudoaneurysm.

Pseudoaneurysm

Pseudoaneurysms should be suspected in any patient with a tense, tender, expansile groin swelling. A pseudoaneurysm represents a partial rupture of the femoral artery, with formation of a false aneurysm involving the media and adventitia. Ultrasound is used to confirm the diagnosis. Simple pseudoaneurysms (small, with a narrow neck) can be treated using prolonged (20–30 min) compression under direct ultrasound guidance. Large or complex pseudoaneurysms require surgical repair.

Haemorrhage

If, despite prolonged pressure (>30 min), bleeding occurs from the puncture site, use a mechanical clamp or haemostatic device to prevent blood loss (see earlier). Check a coagulation screen and, if necessary, reverse the effects of heparin with protamine, or warfarin with Factor IX concentrate. Remember that excess protamine acts as an anticoagulant; 1 mg protamine neutralizes 100 units of mucous heparin; less protamine is required if heparin is given more than 15 min previously.

Infection

If the puncture site exudes or becomes inflamed, or if pyrexia occurs, consider local infection. Take wound and blood cultures and treat with antistaphylococcal antibiotics (e.g. oral flucloxacillin 500 mg qid) if the site is clearly infected.

Limb ischaemia

This is rare and usually occurs in patients with significant peripheral vascular disease. It is always useful to check the popliteal and pedal pulses *before* cardiac catheterization to give a comparison afterwards. The signs of acute limb ischaemia are paralaysis, paraesthesia, pallor and loss of peripheral pulses. If these occur, ask for an urgent review by the vascular team.

CONTRAST AND PROTAMINE REACTIONS

Mild reactions

Urticaria, mild pyrexia and rigors may settle without intervention, although oral or IV chlorpheniramine 10 mg reduces symptoms. Nausea may necessitate an antiemetic. Protamine can cause loin pain; opiate analgesia is usually required along with IV hydrocortisone 100–200 mg and IV chlorpheniramine 10 mg.

Anaphylaxis

Anaphylaxis is treated with IV hydrocortisone 200 mg, chlorpheniramine 10 mg ± IV plasma expander and IM adrenaline 0.5–1 mg (see Chapter 4).

VASOVAGAL REACTIONS

Patients are often anxious during the procedure and vasovagal reactions are common. If hypotension and bradycardia occur:

- Disengage catheter
- Elevate patient's legs
- Give IV atropine 1 mg
- Give IV plasma expander 200–500 ml rapidly
- Ask patient to cough repeatedly to raise blood pressure.

ARRHYTHMIAS

Supraventricular arrhythmias are often transient and usually do not need treatment. Brief episodes of VT or salvoes of ventricular ectopic beats are common, particularly when instrumenting the tricuspid valve or LV. These usually settle spontaneously. VF may occur during coronary injection, especially when excessive pressure is used in a small artery. Arrhythmias should be managed as described in Chapter 7.

CORONARY ARTERY DISSECTION

See next section.

INTERPRETING THE CORONARY ANGIOGRAM

This requires a careful, methodical approach. Each set of images should be inspected carefully during the procedure, so that any necessary extra views can be taken at the time. It is very easy to miss significant coronary stenoses or to misinterpret angiograms if you rush. Also, review the angiogram again after the procedure and before making a report, so that nothing is missed.

Familiarize yourself with the coronary anatomy (see earlier). The LAD follows the skyline in the AP and RAO views and reaches the apex. The circumflex lies posteriorly and is closest to the spine in the standard views.

The severity and eccentricity of coronary artery stenoses should be assessed from several views. Some quite severe but elliptical stenoses may appear insignificant in some views because of the imaging plane and/or foreshortening. Coronary stenoses usually need to cause >70% diameter reduction before they become haemodynamically significant (see later), but angiography often underestimates the true extent of a stenosis. The severity of coronary stenoses is usually assessed as the estimated amount of luminal loss, and is graded as mild (70–80% reduction in cross-sectional area), moderate (80–90%) or severe (90–99%). Remember that there is a 'squared' relationship between cross-sectional area and vessel diameter. Stenosis severity is graded using either an 'eyeball' estimate or quantitative coronary angiography (QCA), where the lumen margin is traced on a computer screen to compare the diameter of the stenosis with that of a reference segment.

SPECIAL CONSIDERATIONS

Ostial stenoses

Ostial stenoses are easy to miss. They may only be visible in one plane; often the catheter and vessel obscure the 'pinched' segment at the origin of the vessel. The pressure trace often damps when the catheter is engaged and contrast may not reflux into the aorta during injection. If there is doubt about the presence of an ostial stenosis, try extra views (e.g. AP caudal view to outline left main stem) or use intravascular ultrasound (IVUS).

Coronary spasm and myocardial bridging

Apparent coronary stenoses can be caused by coronary spasm. Spasm often occurs at the site of an atheromatous plaque and should be suspected if the stenosis is inconstant, occurs during vessel instrumentation, or is associated with chest pain. If in doubt, give sublingual or intracoronary GTN and repeat the angiogram.

Cyclical focal stenoses are sometimes seen during systole. This occurs because a section of the artery (usually proximal or mid-LAD) has an intramyocardial course. Myocardial contraction constricts or occludes the coronary artery during systole – this is known as *myocardial bridging*. This is a

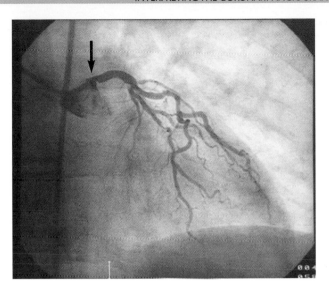

Fig. 18.6 Ostial left main stem stenosis (arrow).

common incidental finding and is of doubtful clinical significance, as coronary blood flow mostly occurs in diastole.

Filling defects

In situ thrombus appears as a filling defect in the vessel lumen. It is usually seen in patients with recent unstable angina or MI. Sometimes a discrete defect is not seen but the lumen appears hazy. Coronary dissection (spontaneous or iatrogenic) may also cause a filling defect, which can be difficult to discriminate from thrombus (Fig. 18.7). A linear 'flap' is usually seen in some views. False filling defects may be seen as a result of 'streaming' of contrast, especially distal to a severe stenosis or around an intracoronary guidewire. Filling defects in saphenous vein grafts may be caused by valves, which are usually distinguishable from thrombus or graft stenosis. If there is doubt about the presence or nature of a filling defect, IVUS is extremely helpful.

Occluded vessels

An occluded branch artery is easy to miss, especially in the left coronary system. An occluded distal LAD (Fig. 18.8) may be missed because a diagonal branch is preserved and asssumed to be the missing vessel. Check systematically for all of the major vessels and ensure that any wall motion abnormality is accounted for by a diseased or absent vessel. Look for late

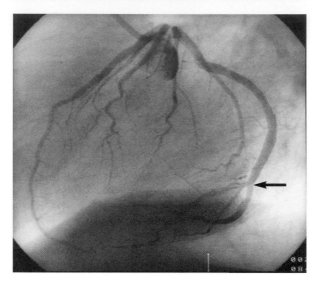

Fig. 18.7 Chronic dissection of posterior descending branch of the circumflex artery (arrow). Patient was a transplant recipient, the donor having died in a traumatic road traffic accident.

collateral filling or 'ghosting' images of the occluded arteries – a prolonged coronary injection may be needed to show this. The stumps of occluded grafts are often found with a 'roving catheter', but an aortogram is sometimes needed to confirm that grafts are not patent.

Collateral circulation

Occluded or tightly stenosed arteries often receive blood via collateral arteries arising from a nearby vessel. For example, the circumflex may feed collateral vessels that perfuse the posterior descending branch of the RCA. Also, antegrade collaterals may arise from the proximal part of an occluded artery and feed the distal vessel ('bridging' collaterals). Competitive flow may be seen in a diseased vessel (dye shunts back and forth) because anterograde flow competes with retrograde collateral flow. This is often seen in bypass grafts, where native coronary flow competes with that from the graft.

Superimposed/foreshortened vessels

The complex arborization of the coronary tree means that in some views vessels will be superimposed on one another. This can obscure some focal stenoses. This is a particular problem with the LAD and its diagonal branches. Depending on individual patients' anatomy, additional views (e.g. AP caudal and steep RAO cranial) may be needed to separate out these vessels (Fig. 18.9).

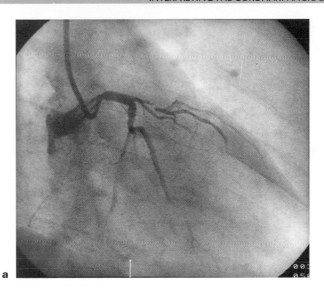

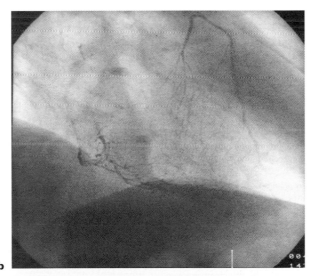

Fig. 18.8 Occluded LAD with retrograde filling from the RCA.

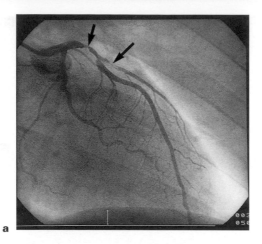

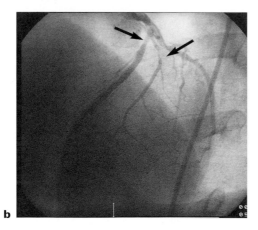

Fig. 18.9 Severe proximal LAD and D$_1$ stenoses (arrows). The LAD stenosis is seen in the RAO view but not the LAO cranial view.

QUANTITATIVE ASSESSMENT OF CARDIAC FUNCTION

The left ventriculogram, aortogram, pressure traces and blood oxygen saturations provide information about:

● Cardiac output and LV function

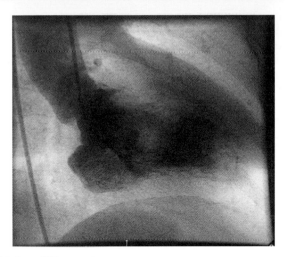

Fig. 18.10 Inferior wall LV aneurysm.

- Severity of aortic valve disease
- Severity of mitral valve disease
- Presence and severity of left-to-right shunts
- Systemic and pulmonary vascular resistance.

CARDIAC OUTPUT AND LV FUNCTION

Volume estimations
LV ejection fraction and (in combination with measurement of LV wall thickness) LV mass can be estimated.

> **Tip:** Left ventricular end-diastolic and end-systolic volumes (LVEDV, LVESV) can be calculated using the Dodge formula. LV length (L [cm], aortic valve to apex) and area (A [cm^2]) are obtained in systole and diastole from the RAO 30° profile of the left ventriculogram.
>
> $$\text{Ventricular volume (ml)} = \frac{0.849 \times A^2 \times f^3}{L}$$
>
> where f is the magnification factor, usually obtained by calibrating the image against a reference such as the catheter diameter.

Cardiac output
Cardiac output is most often measured using the thermodilution method with

a pulmonary flotation catheter (see Chapter 3). Cardiac output can also be estimated using the Fick principle. This uses the difference between the pulmonary arterial and aortic O_2 saturation to estimate cardiac output. For accurate estimation, additional measurement of O_2 consumption is needed (e.g. using a Douglas bag), but in practice an assumption is made. This may introduce errors because patients may be hyper- or hypometabolic, with associated increased or decreased O_2 consumption.

> **Tip:**
>
> $$\text{Cardiac output (l min}^{-1}) = \frac{\text{Oxygen consumption (ml min}^{-1})}{(\text{Ao SaO}_2 - \text{PA SaO}_2) \times \text{Hb} \times 1.34}$$
>
> where Hb = haemoglobin concentration (g l^{-1}). This equation ignores the small amount of O_2 dissolved in plasma, although for every 10 kPa of O_2, 0.34 ml of O_2 is dissolved in 100 ml of plasma.
>
> Mean O_2 consumption can be estimated from the product of the O_2 consumption index (see Fig. 18.6) and the body surface area $\left(\text{BSA} = \sqrt{\dfrac{\text{height (m)} \times \text{weight (kg)}}{36}}\right)$

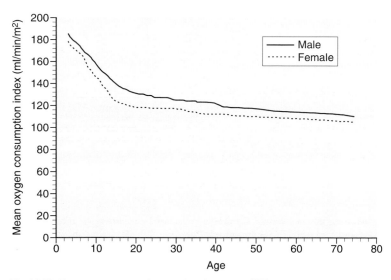

Fig. 18.11 Mean oxygen consumption assuming a heart rate of 70 bpm.

VALVE DISEASE

Valve stenosis

Information can be obtained during diagnostic catheterization about peak-to-peak gradient (e.g. peak aortic and peak LV pressure in aortic stenosis), mean gradient and, in combination with cardiac output measurement, valve orifice area. In patients with atrial fibrillation, filling pressure and stroke volume vary from beat to beat, so that average values derived from 10 cardiac cycles are needed to calculate valve area. Several parameters can be measured:

- **Peak-to-peak gradient**. Aortic and LV pressures are recorded during withdrawal of the pigtail catheter across the aortic valve. The 'withdrawal gradient' is the difference between peak aortic and peak LV pressure. Although this is often used to estimate the severity of aortic stenosis, it can be inaccurate because there is a significant time delay from peak LV to peak aortic pressure in aortic stenosis (see Fig. 18.12a).
- **Peak instantaneous gradient**. More accurate; measured using a double-lumen pigtail catheter which simultaneously records pressure in LV and aorta. The peak instantaneous gradient is the highest pressure gradient at any time during the cardiac cycle and this is what is estimated during Doppler echocardiography.
- **Mean gradient**. This is the mean pressure gradient (during ejection) measured using planimetry of the area bounded by aortic and LV pressure traces (see Fig. 18.12). This value is used to calculate valve area.

Tip: The Gorlin formula

Simultaneous pressure recordings permit the estimation of the valve area according to the Gorlin formula, which states:

$$\text{Aortic valve area (cm}^2) = \frac{\text{Cardiac output (ml min}^{-1})}{44.3 \times \text{SEP} \times \text{HR} \times \sqrt{\text{Mean aortic gradient (mmHg)}}}$$

$$\text{Mitral valve area (cm}^2) = \frac{\text{Cardiac output (ml min}^{-1})}{37.7 \times \text{DFP} \times \text{HR} \times \sqrt{\text{Mean mitral gradient (mmHg)}}}$$

where SEP = systolic ejection period, the length of time (s) blood is ejected from LV every beat (i.e. LV pressure > aortic pressure)

DFP = diastolic filling period, the length of time (s) blood is filling LV every beat (i.e. PCWP > LV pressure).

Pulmonary and tricuspid valve areas can be estimated using similar equations for the aortic and mitral valves, respectively. The Gorlin formula underestimates valve area when cardiac output is low.

Mitral valve area is estimated in a similar manner, mean valve gradient

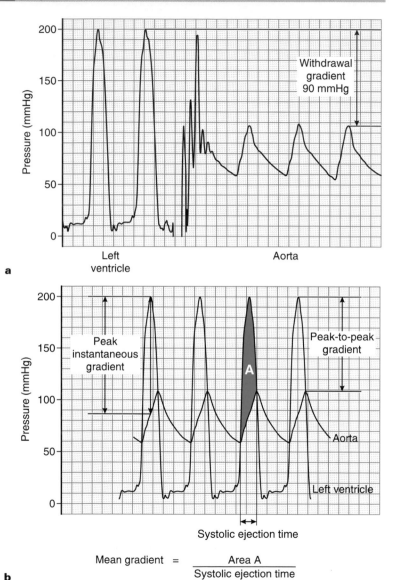

Fig. 18.12 Pressure tracings. (a) Withdrawal pressure trace in aortic stenosis. (b) Simultaneous LV and aortic pressures in aortic stenosis. (c) Simultaneous LV and pulmonary artery wedge pressures in mitral stenosis.

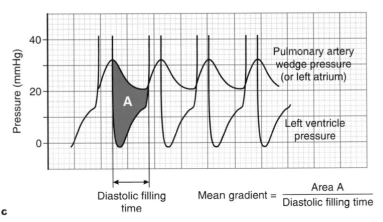

Fig. 18.12 (cont'd)

calculated from simultaneous pulmonary capillary wedge and LV pressure recordings (see Fig. 18.12c).

Valve regurgitation

The severity of aortic and mitral regurgitation can be estimated from the aortogram and left ventriculogram, respectively. Severe aortic regurgitation is associated with opacification of LV within one or two beats of contrast injection, whereas severe mitral regurgitation causes reflux of contrast into LA and the pulmonary veins. Catheter-induced aortic regurgitation occurs if the catheter is too low in the aortic root. Similarly, mitral regurgitation occurs with ventricular ectopic beats, or if the catheter interferes with the valve apparatus.

Severe aortic regurgitation is associated with high LVEDP. Severe mitral regurgitation is associated with prominent V waves in the pulmonary capillary wedge pressure trace. This partly depends on left atrial compliance: a large compliant chamber may absorb the regurgitant pressure and damp any V wave.

LEFT-TO-RIGHT SHUNTS

Oxygen saturations taken during cardiac catheterization help quantify left-to-right shunts.

The level at which O_2 saturation steps up (e.g. atrial, ventricular) indicates the level of the shunt, but it can be difficult to distinguish different types of intra-atrial shunt, e.g. atrial septal defect *versus* partial anomalous pulmonary venous drainage. Although sampling from different levels in the IVC may help, TOE, pulmonary angiography or MRI may be required to delineate the anatomy clearly.

Tip: The ratio of pulmonary to systemic flow is given by:

$$\frac{\text{Pulmonary flow}}{\text{Systemic flow}} = \frac{\text{Ao SaO}_2 - \text{mixed venous SaO}_2}{98 - \text{PA SaO}_2}$$

where 98% is the assumed O_2 saturation in the pulmonary veins; mixed venous
saturation $= \dfrac{(3 \times \text{SVC saturation} + \text{IVC saturation})}{4}.$

SYSTEMIC AND PULMONARY VASCULAR RESISTANCE

Vascular resistance is expressed in dyne.s cm^{-5} or Wood units (mmHg l^{-1}
min^{-1}). (80 dyne.s cm^{-5} = 1 Wood unit). Pulmonary and systemic vascular
resistance (PVR, SVR) can be calculated from cardiac output and pressure
measurements – the calculations required are outlined in Chapter 1. PVR is an
important prognostic indicator in patients with valvular heart disease, heart
failure or cor pulmonale. It is especially important in patients who are being
assessed for cardiac transplantation (see Chapter 13).

CABG, PTCA OR MEDICINE?

Angiography is usually performed in patients who are otherwise potential
candidates for revascularization. The indications for revascularization are
complicated and need to be assessed on an individual basis. All interventions
carry potential hazards, including MI and death, so the risk–benefit balance
has to be evaluated and discussed with the patient. Coronary anatomy,
comorbidity and patient preference all have a major bearing on the types of
revascularization used. In young patients revascularization is usually done for
both prognostic and symptomatic reasons. In elderly patients the risks of
interventions increase and symptom control may be the main indication for
therapy.

After documenting coronary anatomy and cardiac function there are four
main options for patients with angina:

- Intensify medical therapy.
- Cardiac rehabilitation (see Chapter 15).
- Catheter-based intervention, e.g. angioplasty (see next section).
- Coronary artery bypass surgery.

CORONARY ANATOMY

Revascularization may not be feasible if coronary artery disease is diffuse or
affects the distal arteries. Favourable anatomical characteristics for PTCA are
described later.

Successful bypass surgery requires good-quality large-calibre distal arteries, although sometimes local areas can be treated with endarterectomy. Bypass grafts are inserted distal to the main flow-limiting stenoses, in the most accessible areas of the heart: usually the distal RCA, mid-LAD, diagonal branches and the obtuse marginal branches of circumflex. The portion of the circumflex artery that runs in the AV groove is usually inaccessible and cannot be grafted. If possible, arterial conduits are used because the long-term patency rate is much better than that of vein grafts.

PATIENT CHARACTERISTICS

The risk of serious complication during CABG is increased by the following:

- Age — 5-fold increased risk if >75 years compared to <55 years
- Chronic renal failure — 5-fold risk
- Previous CABG — 3.5-fold risk
- Peripheral vascular disease — 3-fold risk
- Impaired LV function — 2-fold risk
- Diabetes mellitus — 1.5-fold risk
- Three-vessel disease — 1.5-fold risk.

Patients at greater risk because of three-vessel disease or impaired LV function also have the most potential long-term gain from CABG.

CABG vs PTCA

Culprit lesion PTCA may be appropriate for some patients with multivessel disease who are unsuitable for CABG because of comorbid factors and for palliation in patients with concomitant distal disease which precludes CABG.

CABG improves prognosis (i.e. reduces risk of death) in patients with:

- Left main stem stenosis ≥ 50%
- Three-vessel disease
- Two-vessel disease including significant proximal LAD stenosis.

Particularly if LV function is impaired or stress test strongly positive.

PTCA is a reasonable first-line treatment in patients with limiting angina who have a suitable target lesion and:

- Single-vessel disease
- Two-vessel disease without significant proximal LAD stenosis
- Previous CABG.

INDICATIONS FOR PTCA

Immediate angiographic success is achieved in around 95% of patients who undergo PTCA. This is *usually* accompanied by total or partial relief from angina. Compared with medication alone, PTCA is associated with a reduction in angina symptoms for at least 2 years after the procedure. This reduces the need for antianginal drugs and improves exercise capacity and quality of life. This clinical benefit has to be balanced against a procedure-related risk of death, MI and peripheral vascular complications. Also, restenosis occurs in a significant proportion of patients because of neointimal hyperplasia, resulting in loss of some of the apparent early gain in luminal area. Restenosis affects up to 30% of patients, and may necessitate repeat intervention if symptoms recur.

As yet there is little evidence that PTCA improves prognosis in patients with stable angina, although it does improve symptoms in appropriately selected patients. In many centres PTCA is only considered when medication does not adequately control symptoms. Also, CABG may be more appropriate than PTCA and is preferable in some patients with multivessel disease, as described in the previous section.

INDICATIONS

Stable angina
Patients with limiting angina despite medical therapy with:

- A suitable target lesion, especially if there is objective evidence of ischaemia in the relevant territory on stress testing
- Single-vessel disease, or two-vessel disease without proximal LAD stenosis
- Previous CABG (risk of repeat CABG is high: perioperative mortality 5–10%)
- Multivessel disease not suitable for CABG, but who have a suitable 'culprit lesion'.

Unstable angina and acute MI
See later section.

PTCA – PROCEDURE

PREPROCEDURE CHECKLIST

In addition to the checks described for diagnostic angiography (see earlier), the following should be done:

- Explain the specific risks of PTCA (including death, MI and the possible need for urgent CABG).
- Check blood group and hold serum for potential cross-match.
- Preprocedure ECG (for comparison).
- Antiplatelet therapy: aspirin should be given to all patients for at least 24 h before PTCA. Some centres pretreat with ticlopidine (250 mg bd) or

clopidogrel (300 mg preprocedure, followed by 75 mg d^{-1} afterwards) if stenting is anticipated.
● Review diagnostic angiogram, to anticipate guiding catheter, balloon size, need for elective stent etc.

PROCEDURE

Pharmacological treatment

● **Unfractionated heparin** (70–100 U kg^{-1} IV) bolus prior to instrumentation of the coronary arteries, unless SC heparin/low molecular weight heparin already given, in which case reduce dose).
● Nitrates – some operators give buccal nitrate to prevent coronary spasm. This may exacerbate hypotension associated with PTCA. Intracoronary **GTN** (100–200 µg aliquots) minimizes these systemic effects.
● Analgesia – patients can be pretreated with opiate analgesia (e.g. **morphine** 5–10 mg IV) + antiemetic (e.g. **metoclopramide** 10 mg IV) to minimize discomfort during the procedure.
● IV crystalloid should be available to treat hypotension. Volume depletion is common in patients who take diuretics or who have fasted for a long time.

Arterial access

See earlier section. The femoral route is preferable for PTCA as it is associated with a lower rate of vascular complications.

Equipment selection

The success of PTCA depends on the correct selection of equipment!

Guide catheters

The choice of guide catheter depends upon the artery and the nature and position of the lesion. The following need to be considered:

● Catheter type – such as Judkins, extra back-up, Amplatz
● Catheter size – lumen (6–9 Fr) and length
● Need for side holes.

The size and shape of guide catheters mirror those of diagnostic catheters. Although the 'standard' Judkins right and left guide catheters may be used, interventional guide catheter shapes may provide better back-up.

Back-up refers to the support, or bracing, given to the guidewire and balloon by the guide catheter. A catheter with inadequate back-up will disengage from the coronary ostium when the guidewire or balloon is advanced against a stenosis and may not allow the stenosis to be crossed. Extra back-up is required to traverse complex lesions, tortuous vessels or right-angled bends, or if the risk of procedural complication (e.g. dissection) is high.

These include left coronary extra back-up (e.g. EBU or XB) catheters and the Amplatz right coronary catheter. Very proximal or ostial lesions require catheters with side holes because of the risk of occluding the vessel with the catheter. The RCA is especially prone to catheter-induced spasm, and many operators routinely use side-hole catheters for such interventions.

Guidewires

Wire characteristics need to be considered in the context of the site and type of lesion that needs treatment:

- Stiffness – floppy, intermediate, standard
- Strength – extra support
- Coating - hydrophilic
- Calibre – usually 0.014 in.

Preformed wires are available, but usually the wire tip has to be shaped with a slight bend. This allows the operator to steer the wire into or away from vessel branches and through stenoses. Hydrophilic and stiff wires increase the likelihood of crossing severe, tortuous stenoses, but stiffer wires may traumatize or perforate the vessel. Extra-support wires provide support for the angioplasty balloon, particularly with difficult distal lesions in tortuous vessels. Most balloons operate on a 'monorail' system, where only the distal few centimetres of the balloon catheter ride on the guidewire. 'Over-the-wire' balloons are seldom used and require very long guidewires.

Balloons

Balloon selection depends on lesion length, width and eccentricity. The following need to be considered:

- Balloon length – needs to cover the target diseased segment
- Balloon diameter when inflated to 'nominal' pressure
- Balloon characteristics – compliant or non-compliant; profile when collapsed.

Compliant balloons are most often used for PTCA. This means that as the inflation pressure is increased balloon diameter also increases; a balloon with diameter 3 mm at 'nominal' pressure may increase to 3.5 mm at high pressure. Generally, a larger balloon inflated to low pressure causes less vessel trauma than a smaller balloon at high pressure.

Non-compliant balloons expand relatively little beyond nominal pressure and are useful for hard calcified lesions and localized areas of underexpansion within stents (these situations require high inflation pressure).

Balloon sizing is usually done with reference to an adjacent, non-stenosed vessel segment. Balloon sizing using the angiogram tends to underestimate the true luminal diameter, typically by 0.5 mm. For very tightly stenosed lesions a small-diameter low-profile balloon may be helpful – initial dilation with a small-diameter balloon (predilation) may subsequently allow a larger balloon to cross the lesion.

Basic procedure

After the guide catheter is placed, the coronary guidewire is fed into the catheter through an adjustable haemostatic valve using an introducer needle. The guidewire is threaded into the coronary artery until its tip is positioned as distally as possible in the target vessel. Guidewire placement must be careful to avoid extravasating the wire and to avoid slipping it into side branches. Small contrast injections are usually needed to assist wire positioning. The balloon catheter is then prepared: the central lumen is flushed with heparinized saline and the balloon lumen emptied under negative pressure and replaced with diluted contrast agent. The balloon is fed over the guidewire, without advancing or retracting the wire, and advanced into the artery. Angioplasty balloons have radio-opaque markers to assist positioning over the stenosed segment. When the balloon is correctly positioned it is gradually inflated with diluted contrast agent; screening continues to ensure that the balloon does not slip forwards or backwards. At first the balloon is usually seen to have a 'waist' at the stenosed segment; pressure is increased until either the waist disappears (representing a controlled dissection of the target lesion) or a maximum pressure is reached. Inflation pressures vary according to the balloon used and the compliance of the lesion, but are typically between 4 and 10 atmospheres. The balloon is usually kept inflated for 20–90 s. After deflation the balloon is withdrawn from the artery and an angiogram is done to assess the result.

TROUBLESHOOTING

Unable to engage the guide catheter
See earlier section.

Inability to pass the guidewire
To manipulate the guidewire effectively the guide catheter must be in a stable position. For LAD and circumflex angioplasty, the catheter's angle of entry into the left coronary ostium can be adjusted to point the guidewire towards the target vessel: torsion may help here. Sometimes a sharp bend (e.g. 60°) is needed at the tip of the guidewire to negotiate right-angled bends or tortuous lesions.

Some guidewires have a hydrophilic coating, which helps when crossing tight stenoses. Stiff wires may also help, but risk dissection or vessel perforation. If the lesion cannot be crossed, advancing the balloon up to the lesion sometimes provides the extra support required to prevent the guidewire from kinking or deflecting. Hypotube catheters can also be fed over the guidewire and provide extra support for floppy guidewires, enabling the lesion to be crossed with less risk of trauma.

Unable to introduce the balloon
The balloon should always move freely on the guidewire; it may 'stick' if

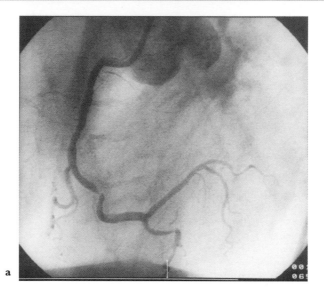

a

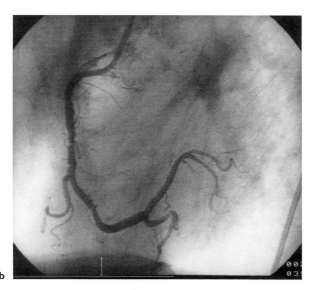

b

Fig. 18.13 (a) Critical RCA stenosis. (b) Angioplasty with suboptimal result (c) necessitated stent insertion to achieve (d) good angiographic result. The crimping of the artery proximal to the lesion (b and d) is an artefact produced by the guidewire.

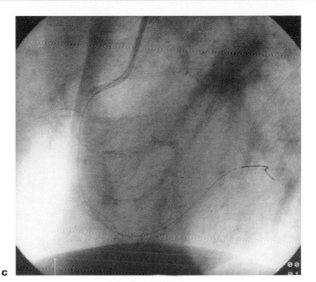

c

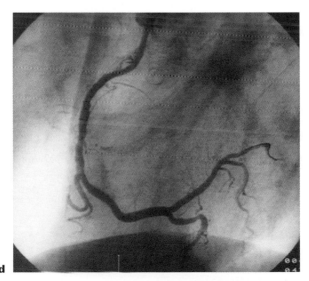

d

Fig. 18.13 (a) Critical RCA stenosis. (b) Angioplasty with suboptimal result (c) necessitated stent insertion to achieve (d) good angiographic result. The crimping of the artery proximal to the lesion (a and d) is an artefact produced by the guidewire.

there is thrombus, contrast medium or debris on the wire. The guidewire should be cleaned regularly with a heparinized saline-soaked sponge to avoid this. The balloon may not cross a stenosis if its diameter (deflated) exceeds that of the stenosis, or if the stenosis is complex or eccentric. If this occurs, the guide catheter will proplase out of the coronary ostium as the balloon braces against the stenosis. If so, try sustained gentle pressure and slight to-and-fro agitation of the balloon catheter, to assist the balloon's passage. If this fails, a smaller-diameter lower-profile balloon may cross the stenosis; once the stenosis is partially opened up, a larger balloon can be used to complete the procedure.

Ostial stenoses

If the stenosis is very proximal, or ostial, the guide catheter often abuts it. Angioplasty is difficult because the guide catheter sits in the proximal part of the stenosis and prevents the balloon from expanding it. In this situation the guide catheter can be prolapsed into the aorta by advancing the guidewire slightly until the balloon is free of the catheter and positioned across the stenosis. This is a tricky technique to master.

Stenosis at bifurcation/side branch

Stenoses often occur at an artery bifurcation, or at the origin of a side branch. Sometimes sacrifice of a small side branch is necessary to preserve a larger artery. When side branches are large and subtend a significant area of myocardium, it is sensible to feed guidewires into both the main artery and the branch. Then, if angioplasty of the main artery compromises the branch artery, the second guidewire permits angioplasty of the branch. Simultaneous inflation of balloons in the two arteries can be tried – the 'kissing balloons' method. This may require the use of a wider-calibre guide catheter and is a difficult technique to perform.

COMPLICATIONS OF INTERVENTION

The likelihood of encountering a major periprocedural complication depends on the clinical situation (higher risk in acute coronary syndromes and in haemodynamically unstable patients), coronary anatomy, LV function and comorbidity. Operator experience and technique also have a major influence.

DETERMINANTS OF RISK

Clinical risk indicators
- Recent or current MI or unstable angina
- LV impairment
- Advanced age
- Female gender

- Smoking
- Diabetes mellitus
- Renal failure.

Anatomical risk indicators
- Long lesion (>20 mm)
- Multivessel disease
- Tortuosity or excessive angulation of target vessel
- Complete occlusion >3 months
- Degenerate vein grafts
- Ostial lesion
- Calcified lesion
- Lesion at bifurcation/major side branch
- Small vessel calibre
- Presence of thrombus.

COMPLICATIONS

Major complications

Coronary stents and contemporary antiplatelet therapy have reduced the incidence of major complications from PTCA. Despite this, there remains a small but significant risk of acute MI (~3%), the need for emergency CABG (~2%) and death (~1%).

Acute vessel compromise/closure

This may occur because of dissection or thrombosis, although sometimes profound coronary artery spasm is the cause. If in doubt, give intracoronary GTN (100–200 µg) or verapamil (250 µg) to exclude spasm. For high-risk complex lesions or acute cases (e.g. unstable angina) pretreatment with a glycoprotein IIb/IIIa receptor antagonist reduces the risk of acute thrombotic vessel closure (see next section).

Coronary dissection. PTCA is a form of controlled dissection. Dissection flaps that partially occlude the lumen or which extend beyond the original lesion may require specific treatment. Dissection most often follows balloon inflation, especially with high inflation pressures in complex or calcified lesions. It can also occur while engaging the guide catheter or manipulating the guidewire. Dissection is the most common cause of acute vessel closure and can usually be treated by placing a stent in the dissected segment. This tacks the dissection flap to the vessel wall and restores flow. Localized dissection, or dissection in a vessel unsuitable for stenting, can be treated with prolonged balloon inflation to 'tack up' the dissection flap. IV abciximab helps prevent secondary thrombosis (see next section). Some dissections require surgical intervention, but this is rare in the era of intracoronary stenting. Where acute vessel closure occurs and catheter-based treatment is unsuccessful, a *perfusion balloon* can be used to provide some distal perfusion prior to emergency CABG.

Thrombotic occlusion is difficult to treat. It is more common if distal run-off is poor (stasis) and in acute coronary syndromes. Mechanical fragmentation of thrombus with an angioplasty balloon can cause distal embolization and *impaired reflow* due to capillary occlusion. Stent implantation may help if thrombus forms at the site of a complex lesion, but may encourage thrombus formation. IV abciximab or intracoronary thrombolysis may help in this situation.

Vessel rupture

This is very rare and occurs if an oversized balloon is inflated at high pressure. Vessels may also perforate because of guidewire extravasation, or with the use of atherectomy devices. Clinical features are chest pain and hypotension. Angiography may show extravasation of contrast – an echo should be performed to exclude tamponade. If the ruptured segment cannot be sealed using a covered intracoronary stent, or if tamponade occurs, emergency surgery is required.

'Minor' complications

Peripheral vascular complications

Anticoagulation and intensive antiplatelet therapy increase the risk of haematoma and pseudoaneurysm formation after coronary intervention (see earlier). These are more likely if larger sheaths are used, especially if the sheath is left in place overnight. Clinically significant vascular complications occur in ~5% of cases. Rarely, distal limb perfusion is compromised. This is more common in patients with peripheral vascular disease and necessitates immediate assessment by the vascular team.

Hypotension

This is common during PTCA, contributed to by fluid depletion (nil by mouth), blood loss (at the access site and via the catheter), myocardial ischaemia and osmotic diuresis due to the contrast agent. IV crystalloid should be given (with care in patients with LV impairment) if this occurs. Hypotension is less common *after* PTCA. It can occur because of arrhythmia, occult haemorrhage, delayed contrast reaction, myocardial ischaemia, or a vasovagal response. The patient should be carefully examined and an ECG performed. Be aware of the risk of GI and retroperitoneal bleeding. The latter is easily missed but is often associated with severe back pain and can be confirmed with CT or ultrasound scanning.

Arrhythmias

PTCA is associated with a low risk of pathological arrhythmia (~2%). As with diagnostic angiography, vigorous contrast injection or catheter damping (especially in RCA) is associated with VF. During PTCA ventricular ectopic beats or non-sustained VT may occur because of myocardial ischaemia.

Bradycardias are common during PTCA to the proximal RCA because of ischaemia of the conus, sinus node and AV node branches. Prophylactic atropine is sometimes used, but may not be effective. Bradycardias are sometimes so readily induced that a temporary pacing wire is required.

Chest pain
This affects up to 50% of patients after PTCA and is usually transient. It may simply result from the trauma of the procedure and is often pericarditic in nature. Ischaemic chest pain may be caused by coronary spasm. If it does not resolve with GTN, or if it is severe, repeat angiography should be performed as soon as possible. Side branch occlusion may result in mild ischaemic chest pain (and sometimes minor ECG abnormalities and elevation of cardiac enzymes).

PTCA – ADJUNCTIVE THERAPY

ANTIPLATELET THERAPY

Aspirin
All patients with known or suspected coronary artery disease should receive antiplatelet therapy, usually **aspirin** 75–300 mg d^{-1}. Prior treatment with aspirin is associated with a 50% reduction in the rate of vessel occlusion after PTCA (4% *vs* 8%).

Thienopyridines
Combination antiplatelet therapy with **ticlopidine** (250 mg bd for 2 weeks: currently not licensed in UK) and aspirin 75–300 mg d^{-1} reduces cardiac events and vascular complications after stent deployment. Ticlopidine causes neutropenia in 1–2% of patients and is likely to be superseded by a related drug, **clopidrogel** (300 mg preprocedure, followed by 75 mg d^{-1} for 2 weeks). This agent is currently being evaluated as an adjunct to PTCA and stenting, but is not yet licensed for this indication.

Glycoprotein (Gp) IIb/IIIa receptor antagonists
These inhibit the final common pathway of platelet aggregation and are potent antiplatelet agents. As such, they are associated with a higher risk of bleeding complications than other antiplatelet agents. **Abciximab** is a monoclonal antibody fragment which blocks the Gp IIb/IIIa receptor and is the most widely used agent. There is a good body of evidence for its efficacy in high-risk coronary interventions, especially in patients with unstable angina. The recommended dose is 0.25 mg kg^{-1} bolus, 10 min preprocedure, then 10 μg min^{-1} for 12–24 hours afterwards. Synthetic oral analogues (e.g. tirofiban, integrilin) are also becoming available and may be useful in the future.

STENT IMPLANTATION

Indications

Stents are usually implanted in one of three situations:

- To 'bail out' if the vessel occludes
- If PTCA achieves a suboptimal result
- Elective (for complex lesions, restenotic lesions, proximal LAD stenosis and vein graft stenosis).

There is no definitive evidence that a policy of elective stenting during all PTCA procedures improves outcome: the modest benefit in terms of reducing symptomatic restenosis is partly offset by the risk of thrombotic occlusion.

Types of stent

Stents come in several designs, including coil, mesh and slotted tube. Most are balloon expandable (i.e. premounted or crimped on to an angioplasty balloon, deployed by inflating the balloon) although some modern stents are self-expanding. Factors which are important in stent selection are:

- Length (should cover entire lesion/dissection)
- Diameter when expanded: most can be expanded within a range of diameters, e.g. 3.5–5.0 mm
- Flexibility (for lesions on a bend, flexible coil stents are useful; coils also useful to preserve side branches)
- Cell density – reflecting the amount of metal in the stent (low density best to preserve side branches)
- Radial strength
- Radio-opacity.

Method of implantation

For elective stenting the target lesion is usually predilated with an angioplasty balloon to give the stent space to straddle the lesion. The balloon and stent are advanced over the stenosis in the same manner as described for the PTCA balloon (see earlier). Be careful not to damage the stent when passing it through haemostatic valve (i.e. open the valve wide!). Stents may not pass easily through tortuous segments or into side branches. Do not force the catheter because the vessel may be traumatized, or the stent deformed or dislodged from the balloon. Always maintain guidewire position, especially if there is a severe dissection or acute vessel closure: it may not be possible to rewire the vessel if the guidewire slips back. The balloon is inflated to a higher pressure during stent implantation than for simple PTCA (typically 10–14 atmospheres) and for a shorter duration (e.g. 10–60 s). The balloon should only be withdrawn after it is completely deflated.

TROUBLESHOOTING

Stent displacement or embolization

Stents can dislodge from the balloon, be incorrectly positioned, or may not cross the target lesion. If the stent remains on the balloon it may be possible to withdraw it back into the guide catheter, but there is a significant risk of displacing the stent off the balloon while attempting this. The stent may embolize down the aorta and cause cerebral, limb, renal or mesenteric ischaemia. For this reason it is often best to withdraw the guide catheter, guidewire and balloon *en masse* into the lower descending aorta before attempting stent retrieval.

The stent may move and become malpositioned during balloon inflation. This can occur if the stent slips in a tapered stenosis, or shortens during deployment. Stent shortening should be anticipated with long stents. The stent **must** be fully deployed: it is dangerous to abort and deflate the balloon with the stent partly expanded. If the lesion or dissection is then not adequately covered, further stenting may be needed.

If the stent displaces from the balloon, **do not pull the guidewire back**. Instead, pull the guide catheter, guidewire, balloon and stent back into the descending aorta, then carefully remove the balloon without withdrawing the guidewire. A retrieval snare can then be used to 'grab' the stent, which should still be on the guidewire. Alternatively, a low-profile balloon (e.g. 1.5 mm) can sometimes be threaded through the stent, inflated distal to it and withdrawn, bringing the stent with it.

An embolized unexpanded stent must be located and retrieved. Fluoroscopy can be used to locate radio-opaque stents. Displaced radiolucent stents are sometimes not located unless they cause vascular compromise. Retrieval snares can be used to extract stents once located. Ask for help from an experienced vascular radiologist before attempting to retrieve lost stents. Surgical retrieval is rarely needed.

ATHERECTOMY

Atherectomy involves the removal or debulking of atheromatous material from a heavily diseased artery segment. It is useful if there is a high plaque load, which may mean successful PTCA is not possible or does not achieve a satisfactory result. There are four main approaches to atherectomy:

● **Directional coronary atherectomy** (DCA). An open chamber is forcibly abutted against the lesion, using a balloon positioned behind the chamber. Tissue invaginated into the chamber is excised using a rotating (2000 rpm) cutting piston. Excised tissue is stored in the distal collecting chamber. DCA is most suitable for bulky lesions in large-diameter (>3 mm) vessels. Restenosis rate is at least as high as with conventional PTCA and DCA is usually reserved for lesions in which PTCA achieves a poor result.

- **Laser atherectomy** destabilizes atheroma by breaking molecular bonds. Thermal laser atherectomy is associated with a high rate of perforation.
- **Rotational atherectomy** involves very rapid rotation (160 000–200 000 rpm) of a diamond-studded abrasive burr, which produces very fine and (supposedly) innocuous 10 μm particles. This technique is useful for treating heavily calcified plaques and in-stent restenosis.
- **Extraction atherectomy** combines atherectomy with suction to extract the excised debris and is useful for diffusely diseased vein grafts.

INTRA-AORTIC BALLOON PUMP

This is useful to stabilize patients before, during or after high-risk PTCA procedures particularly when associated with acute vessel closure, cardiogenic shock or cardiac failure (see Chapter 3).

POSTPROCEDURE MANAGEMENT

After successful PTCA patients should remain supine and be observed in the recovery room and ward. Routine ECG monitoring is not necessary, but heart rate, blood pressure and lower limb pulses and perfusion should be checked regularly for 4 hours.

IMMEDIATE MANAGEMENT

Sheath management
The sheath is usually larger than that used for diagnostic angiography, often 7–8 Fr, and so the risk of arterial trauma is greater. It should be removed when the APTT ratio has fallen below 1.5:1, or immediately if a radial artery approach is used. The APTT should be checked 4 hours after the procedure. After complicated or suboptimal procedures some centres keep patients on IV heparin and nitrate infusions for 12–24 hours. Vascular complications are then more likely to occur during sheath removal and if there is concern about risk of haematoma formation a mechanical clamp (e.g. Femostop) should be available at the time of sheath removal.

Maintaining PTCA patency
Antithrombotic and antiplatelet therapy are discussed in the previous section.

LONG-TERM MANAGEMENT

Patients should be reviewed 2–6 months after PTCA and discharged if appropriate.

Restenosis usually occurs in the first few months after PTCA; around half of cases are symptomatic and patients give a history of initial improvement of angina followed by recurrence. This affects 10–20% of cases and repeat angiography is usually warranted.

> **Tip:** Current evidence is that catheter interventions for stable angina alter symptoms but not long-term prognosis. There is little evidence that stress testing, in the absence of recurrent symptoms, is useful after PTCA, as the main aim of treatment is symptom relief.

PTCA IN UNSTABLE ANGINA AND ACUTE MI

INDICATIONS

Unstable angina
● Persistent symptoms or high-risk features despite treatment with aspirin and heparin (see Chapter 5 for early invasive *vs* early conservative approach).

Myocardial Infarction
● Primary PTCA – most centres reserve primary PTCA for patients with contraindications to thrombolysis, although primary PTCA is valid first-line R_x in centres with experienced operators and 24-hour immediate access to catheterization laboratory.
● 'Rescue' PTCA (for failed thrombolysis) – evidence for efficacy is weak and the benefit is probably confined to patients with haemodynamic instability.
● Persistent postinfarct angina despite aspirin, heparin and β-blockade (treat as unstable angina).

MODIFIED APPROACH TO PTCA

In patients with acute coronary syndromes *in situ* thrombus is common and the complication rate of PTCA greatly exceeds that of elective angioplasty for stable angina. A modified approach is therefore required. In patients with unstable angina allowing an initial 'cooling-off' period with antithrombotic, antiplatelet and anti-ischaemic therapy is a sensible approach. Many centres practise an 'early conservative' approach, in which angiography is only performed in patients who fail to settle with medication or who have persistent high-risk features, or in those whose angina resolves but who have easily inducible ischaemia on predischarge stress testing.

IV abciximab should be given for at least 1 hour before the procedure and for a total of 24 hours. Selective angiography of the artery supplying the unaffected territory (i.e. RCA, if anterior ECG changes) is done first, followed by the suspected culprit artery.

Once the culprit lesion is identified the artery is instrumented in the normal manner. Complete or subtotal occlusions may not be obvious and several views may be needed to identify the site. The guidewire usually passes through quite easily, because fresh thrombus is soft. The potential to create a dissection is still significant because acute coronary syndromes are asssociated with intimal inflammation and rupture.

Arrhythmias commonly occur during reperfusion – this may occur after passing the guidewire, which in itself often restores some blood flow. Flow may be sluggish despite apparently successful angioplasty. This *impaired reflow* phenomenon is the result of many factors, including distal embolization of thrombus, release of vasoconstrictors and spasm. Intracoronary thrombolytics are not usually helpful in this situation.

Stents are usually reserved for severe residual stenoses or dissections that compromise the vessel lumen. Thrombosis should not occur if the stent is fully deployed and IV abciximab is given.

PTCA IN BYPASS GRAFTS

Most patients with saphenous vein grafts have significant graft disease after 8–10 years: 60% of grafts will be occluded. Unstable ischaemic chest pain in patients with previous CABG often requires several days' treatment with IV heparin or SC enoxaparin because impending graft occlusion is often associated with extensive thrombosis in the graft.

Redo CABG carries an operative mortality of around 10% and non-fatal complications are also common. Thus, an initial strategy of PTCA is preferable if possible in patients with previous CABG who develop severe or unstable angina. However, PTCA of venous conduits is itself associated with a high complication rate, which increases procedural risk.

TYPES OF STENOSIS

Graft stenoses which occur soon after surgery at the aortic or coronary anastomotic site usually cause early postoperative symptoms and are sometimes related to surgical technique. Midgraft stenoses which present early are caused by neointimal hyperplasia similar to that produced by coronary intervention. Graft stenoses occurring years after surgery are produced by accelerated atherosclerosis and are very soft and friable. Embolism of lesion material is common during PTCA and distal flow may be poor as a result. Internal mammary graft stenoses are usually anastomotic, but can also occur in the body of the graft. Recurrent symptoms can also occur because of the progression of native vessel disease.

MODIFIED APPROACH TO PTCA

Preprocedure preparation
Because of the high risk of distal embolization of friable vein grafts, patients may need intensive antiplatelet and anticoagulant therapy for several days before PTCA is performed.

Guide catheter
Careful catheter selection is needed to achieve adequate support for the

guidewire and balloon. RCA vein grafts often have a vertical take-off from the aorta; a multipurpose guide catheter may be needed if the Judkins right coronary catheter is unsuitable. Vein grafts to the LAD, circumflex and branches sometimes require a dedicated left coronary artery bypass or Amplatz guide catheter. An internal mammary guide catheter can be used for LIMA or RIMA PTCA, although the brachial or radial approaches are useful alternatives.

Balloon

Vein grafts often need to be dilated with a slightly oversized balloon. High pressure may be required (>10 atmospheres) because vein grafts are often fibrotic. Graft rupture and plaque embolization are potential hazards. A long balloon helps prevent slippage during dilatation: this is especially important during stent deployment. As there is an increased risk of distal embolization of plaque material, extraction atherectomy is sometimes advocated for severely and heavily diseased grafts. Anastomotic and internal mammary artery stenoses require lower (typically 4–10 atmosphere) inflation pressures.

Stent insertion

After PTCA vein graft stenoses are almost always stented to prevent collapse of the graft (which has little exterior support) and restenosis. Self-expanding stents are particularly useful in this situation as they have a large diameter and can cover long diseased segments. Because there is a significant risk of embolism during predilatation, some operators use direct stenting for saphenous vein graft stenoses.

NON-RADIOGRAPHIC EVALUATION

Assessment of coronary artery disease with angiography is sometimes described as 'lumenology', as it only provides information about the artery lumen. Newer technologies allow assessment of the artery wall and the effect of a stenosis on coronary flow. These can help guide decisions about the appropriateness of interventions and are useful for monitoring immediate outcome.

IMAGING MODALITIES

Intravascular ultrasound (IVUS)

IVUS catheters operate at 20–30 MHz, providing excellent spatial resolution. They have either a solid state or a rotating transducer. IVUS catheters are placed in the target vessel over an intracoronary guidewire in the same manner as a PTCA balloon, after giving IV heparin. The catheter can induce spasm, and intracoronary GTN (100–200 µg) should be given before imaging.

Imaging is done while withdrawing the transducer from the distal vessel, across the region of interest. Mechanical 'pullback' devices allow this to be done at a constant speed.

Indications

IVUS is used mainly if there is uncertainty about the angiographic appearance during diagnostic procedures or interventions.

- Clarify anatomy – assessment of suspected left main stem or ostial stenoses, bifurcation disease
- Angiographic 'haziness' – dissection, thrombus and complex stenoses can present this way
- Plaque composition – calcification, fat, fibrous tissue
- Balloon sizing – allows accurate assessment of reference vessel segment and severity of stenosis itself
- Assessment after intervention – IVUS helps assess stent deployment and suspected dissection.

Image interpretation

Landmarks such as pericardial reflections, cardiac veins and side branches are used to orientate the image. The centre of the image represents the catheter itself and the guidewire is also seen as a small acoustic shadow. The artery wall has a three-layered appearance representing the intima, the echolucent media and the adventitia. This appearance is not seen in young subjects because the intima is very thin. Speckling is seen in the lumen, especially when blood flow is sluggish.

Angiographically normal coronary arteries often contain a significant plaque load. This is because of adaptive remodelling, in which the artery expands to accommodate the plaque burden. IVUS helps evaluate plaque composition, ranging from soft fibrofatty plaques, through fibromuscular plaques to calcified hard plaques. Dissections are readily demonstrated using IVUS. Fresh thrombus is sometimes difficult to differentiate from disrupted soft plaque.

Angioscopy

This is a highly specialized approach to directly visualize the coronary arteries; unlike intravascular ultrasound it is available in only a few centres. The imaging catheter is inserted using a monorail system and a proximal occluding cuff is inflated while infusing Ringer's lactate solution to provide a blood-free field for visualization. The central fibreoptic imaging bundle may be advanced or deflected to better image the lesion of interest. This necessitates coronary occlusion and often causes chest pain and ECG abnormalities. Imaging takes 15–30 s and can be repeated if reperfusion is allowed between examinations.

FUNCTIONAL ASSESSMENT OF CORONARY STENOSES

Intravascular Doppler

Intracoronary Doppler wires have been developed that have similar handling characteristics to conventional interventional guidewires, but which have a small piezoelectric cell mounted at the tip to allow assessment of coronary flow velocity.

Coronary flow reserve

The Doppler wire is positioned distal to the diseased segment and a baseline recording of the peak blood flow velocity is made. Hyperaemia is then induced to maximize blood flow, usually with intracoronary adenosine (12–18 µg for RCA and 24–30 µg for LCA). The ratio of basal and maximal peak velocity is determined – this is the *coronary flow reserve* (CFR). A CFR of:

- >2.5 indicates a haemodynamically insignificant stenosis
- <2.0 indicates a haemodynamically significant stenosis
- 2.0–2.5, an intermediate response, can be further assessed by comparing CFR with that of an adjacent artery.

CFR can be used to assess the outcome of PTCA in terms of both increased basal flow (severe critical lesions only) and improvement in CFR.

Pressure wire

These are either solid-state wires or have a simple fluid-filled lumen with multiple distal ports. These wires allow direct measurement of mean intracoronary pressure. Pressure wires have similar handling characteristics to interventional guidewires.

Fractional flow reserve

The wire is positioned at the coronary ostium and the wire transducer calibrated with that of the guide catheter. The wire is moved distal to the diseased segment and simultaneous ostial and intracoronary pressure recordings are made at baseline and after injection of intracoronary adenosine (as for Doppler wire). Myocardial fractional flow reserve, FFR_{MYO}, is the ratio of mean distal coronary artery pressure:mean aortic pressure during hyperaemia. FFR < 0.75 is said to represent a functionally significant stenosis.

RIGHT VENTRICULAR BIOPSY

INDICATIONS

The indications for RV biopsy are limited because there are few situations in which a definitive diagnosis can be made, or in which the biopsy result influences clinical management. Several biopsy specimens should be taken, as many myocarditic processes are patchy. RV biopsy carries a small but significant risk of cardiac rupture and tamponade, especially if the RV free wall is thin (e.g. in dilated cardiomyopathies). Indications are:

- Assessment of rejection in a cardiac transplant recipient
- Assessment of anthracycline toxicity
- Myocarditis: diagnosis and monitoring (unlikely to influence management)
- Diagnosis of secondary cardiomyopathy (e.g. amyloidosis)
- Distinction between restrictive cardiomyopathy and constrictive pericarditis.

COMPLICATIONS

- Tamponade – from free wall perforation
- Septal perforation
- Arrhythmias – usually VPBs or non-sustained VT
- AV conduction defects – usually temporary
- Papillary muscle injury
- Vasovagal syncope
- Embolic complications.

CHAPTER 19

ECHOCARDIOGRAPHY

TRANSTHORACIC 2D AND M-MODE VIEWS

THE FOUR STANDARD VIEWS

The standard probes used for transthoracic echocardiography use 2–5 MHz frequencies and can give high-quality 2D images as well as detailed Doppler signals. Choice of probe frequency is a compromise between image resolution and depth. High-frequency probes provide high-resolution images but have poor tissue penetration. Low-frequency probes can image deeper structures at the cost of resolution. Modern echo machines function across a broad band of frequencies. The recent development of harmonic imaging, in which first-order and harmonics of the transmitted signal are detected, has greatly improved transthoracic image quality.

Parasternal long-axis view

The probe is positioned in the fifth intercostal space at the lower left sternal edge and angled obliquely, with the probe marker pointing to the right shoulder. This provides a longitudinal view of the left ventricle (Fig. 19.1a), with the mitral valve, LA, aortic valve, ascending aorta and RV usually visible.

Parasternal short-axis view

From the long-axis view, rotation of the probe through 90° (marker now pointing towards the left shoulder) brings the ventricles into cross-sectional view. Cranial angulation opens up the aortic valve, with its characteristic 'Mercedez–Benz' appearance of the three cusps. In this plane the tricuspid valve, the atria and interatrial septum, RV and pulmonary valve are seen (Fig. 19.1b). Slow angulation of the probe inferiorly, by pronating the wrist, should bring the mitral annulus and leaflets into view. Leaflet thickening can be detected and planimetry used to estimate mitral valve area. Further inferior angulation opens up the LV at base and at midpapillary muscle level (view used for measuring LV dimensions), and in many cases the apical LV segments.

Apical four-chamber view

With the marker pointing in the direction of the left shoulder, the probe can be slid along the rib space to the cardiac apex. This brings all four chambers of the heart into view (Fig. 19.1c). Further angulation of the probe cranially visualizes the aortic valve and proximal ascending aorta – the five-chamber view.

Apical long-axis and two-chamber views

At the apex, rotation of the probe through 90°, with the marker once more pointing towards the right shoulder, shows the same structures as the parasternal long-axis view, often with a better view of the LV apex because of the imaging angle (Fig. 19.1a). Rotation of the probe through a further 30° produces a two-chamber view of the left ventricle and atrium (the correct

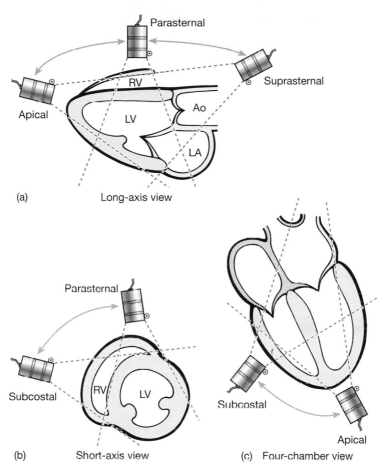

Fig. 19.1 Standard 2D transthoracic echo views. (a) Long axis. (b) Short axis. (c) Four-chamber.

angle is where the aortic valve just disappears from the plane of the image). This view can be difficult to obtain but is very useful for assessing the inferior and anterior LV wall.

TROUBLESHOOTING

No image on screen
Check that the following are appropriately set:

- Probe selection: ensure the probe is plugged in and properly selected on the machine.
- Gain and transmission settings: turn the gain up and you should at least be able to see the gel reflection.
- Depth setting: usually 12–24 cm.

Unable to obtain parasternal views

In some patients, especially the obese or those with a hyperinflated chest, it is impossible to obtain clear images of the heart. Before giving up, try:

- Rolling the patient further towards the left lateral position.
- Change the intercostal position of the probe. High positions visualize the aorta more prominently, whereas low positions tend to give foreshortened apical views. Patients' individual anatomies vary enormously.
- Applying firmer pressure – but note that it is uncomfortable for the patient to have a probe run up and down the ribs with excessive pressure! *Firm* pressure can enhance the image without being uncomfortable to the patient.
- Imaging in held expiration – reduces the amount of lung tissue between probe and heart.
- Apply more gel – there is a tendency to add more and more gel in a vain attempt to improve image quality. Although good contact is essential, copious quantities of gel make the probe less easy to handle and increase the operator's frustration!

Unable to obtain apical views

This is common in obese women, as well as those with lung disease. In addition to the above suggestions, the following manoeuvres may help:

- Lean the patient back towards the supine position.
- Position the probe at the point of maximum apical impulse.
- Angle the probe further cranially.

Unable to obtain any satisfactory standard views

Under these circumstances, consider:

- Alternative views: subcostal and supraclavicular (see next section)
- Transoesophageal echo
- Alternative imaging modalities, depending on the strength of indication for echo, e.g. radionuclide LV ejection fraction in the assessment of LV function (see Chapter 20).

OTHER ECHO VIEWS

These views are used less often as the standard four views are usually able to image the heart satisfactorily. They are useful when imaging is incomplete or technically difficult, as in patients with emphysema or chest wall malformations.

Subcostal views

In addition to the standard views, the subcostal views permit closer examination of the right ventricle and IVC and are particularly useful for assessing the interatrial septum. The subcostal approach is difficult in obese patients.

Long axis

The probe is positioned in the epigastrium, pressed up beneath the left costal border and aimed at the right shoulder with the probe marker pointing to the left hip. This provides a long-axis four-chamber midcavity view that is 60–90° to the apical four-chamber view. The LV apex is not seen well in this view, but the RV, the atria, the tricuspid and mitral valves and the body of the LV are clearly seen.

Short axis

Rotation of the probe anticlockwise through 90° gives a short-axis view 60–90° to the standard parasternal short-axis view. The left ventricle is clearly seen, with the right ventricle in the foreground.

Suprasternal views

This view, if it can be obtained, allows examination of the ascending aorta, the arch and the great vessels. It is often difficult to fit the probe into the suprasternal notch, especially in patients with a hyperinflated chest. This approach is very useful, using a small 'standalone' Doppler probe, for assessing aortic valve flows.

Long axis

The head and neck are slightly extended to permit the probe to sit in the suprasternal notch with the marker pointing posteriorly. This provides a view of the ascending aorta, aortic valve, mitral valve and left ventricle that is 60–90° cranial to the parasternal long-axis view.

Short axis

Usually very difficult – 90° anticlockwise rotation occasionally produces a long-axis view of the ascending and descending aorta as well as the aortic arch and great vessels.

M-MODE IMAGING

M-mode imaging allows the operator to display a graphical representation of the movement of structures throughout the cardiac cycle. A single one-dimensional line is continuously sampled through the heart, displaying tissue depth in the vertical axis and time in the horizontal axis (Fig. 19.2). This produces a 'smeared' image of cardiac motion with time. M-mode images can seem rather daunting and uninterpretable at first, but they are useful and easy

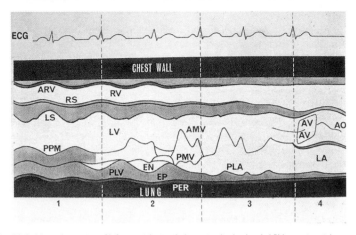

Fig. 19.2 M-mode tracing of left ventricle, just below mitral valve level. ARV, anterior right ventricular wall; RV, right ventricle; RS, right ventricular septum; LV, left ventricle; LS, left ventricular septum; AMV, anterior mitral valve leaflet; PMV, posterior mitral valve leaflet; PPM, posterior papillary muscle; EN, endocardium; EP, epicardium; PLV, posterior left ventricular wall; PLA, posterior left atrial wall; LA, left atrium; AV, aortic valve cusp; PER, pericardium.

to learn. In particular, M-mode imaging allows precise measurement of chamber dimensions.

Standard M-mode tracings

These standard images can be performed in either the long or the short axis of the parasternal view. A clear simultaneous ECG recording is essential to allow timing of structure movement with the cardiac cycle. It helps to make any measurements in both the parasternal short- and long-axis views.

Ventricles and mitral valve

The M-mode cursor line is positioned on screen during 2D imaging. Careful prior alignment of the 2D image is important, since an oblique 'cut' leads to overestimation of chamber dimensions. The cursor is aligned through the tips of the mitral valve, perpendicular to the long axis of LV. The following can be examined:

● LV and RV systolic and diastolic dimensions
● Systolic and diastolic thickness of the interventricular septum and posterior LV wall
● Mitral valve motion – early and late diastolic mitral flow causes the anterior leaflet to describe an 'M'-shape, whereas the posterior leaflet describes a flattened 'W' in sinus rhythm
● Depth of pericardial effusion and any associated RV diastolic collapse (indicates tamponade).

Aortic valve and left atrium

The M-mode cursor line is positioned across the tips of the aortic valve leaflets, enabling measurement of aortic root and left atrial dimensions. The motion of the aortic leaflets can also be assessed and usually describes a 'box' shape. Reduced aortic valve leaflet separation is seen in aortic stenosis and in low-output states.

Measuring cardiac dimensions

Echo software enables precise measurement of cardiac dimensions using on-screen calipers, allowing quantitative assessment of cardiac function and chamber size. LV end-systolic and diastolic diameters, and septal and posterior wall thickness should be measured whenever possible. This allows the estimation of *shortening fraction* (a crude index of LV systolic function) and left ventricular mass.

TABLE 19.1 Adult reference ranges for M-mode assessments

Structure	Parameter	Range	Units
Left ventricle	End-systolic diameter	25–41	mm
	End-diastolic diameter	35–56	mm
	Shortening fraction*	30–40	%
	Ejection fraction*	50–85	%
	Mass*	60–124	g/m^2
Septum	Systolic thickness	9–18	mm
	Diastolic thickness	7–12	mm
Posterior wall	Systolic thickness	9–13	mm
	Diastolic thickness	7–13	mm
Aortic root	Diameter	20–37	mm
	Cusp separation	15–26	mm
Left atrium		19–40	mm
Right ventricle		7–23	mm

* see later section

DOPPLER ECHOCARDIOGRAPHY

Using the Doppler principle blood flow velocity can be measured with ultrasound. There are two complementary approaches to this: colour flow mapping and spectral analysis. Flow velocity is best determined when the direction of flow is parallel to, or within 20° of, the axis of the ultrasound beam. Blood flow velocity estimation becomes very inaccurate when the incident angle exceeds 20° (Fig. 19.3).

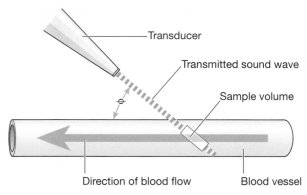

Fig. 19.3 Angle correction for Doppler velocity measurements.

COLOUR FLOW MAPPING (CFM)

This is done during 2D or M-mode imaging. A colour blood flow map is superimposed on the 2D or M-mode image, with blood velocity at any point on the image assigned a colour according to its magnitude and direction. By convention, blood flow towards the probe is usually assigned a red/orange colour, and flow away from the probe is assigned blue/purple. Turbulent blood flow produces a mosaic of colours (because small, high-velocity vortices occur within a turbulent jet) and is easily identified. Some echo systems superimpose a green colour over regions of turbulent flow.

CFM is useful for identifying valve regurgitation and intracardiac shunts, as turbulent, high-velocity flow is often associated with these pathologies. Also, the colour map is often used to guide spectral Doppler sampling during quantitative assessment of valvular blood flow.

SPECTRAL DOPPLER

This produces an on-screen graphical representation of the relationship between blood flow velocity and time. As with M-mode imaging, a clear ECG tracing helps establish temporal relationships during the cardiac cycle. Blood flow is measured using either continuous-wave (CW) mode (where velocities are detected along the entire length of the ultrasound beam) or pulsed-wave (PW) mode (where velocities at a specified tissue depth are detected). The CW cursor line or PW sample box is positioned during 2D imaging.

Continuous-wave Doppler

To record a CW Doppler signal the 2D image ± CFM is used to position the spectral Doppler cursor line along a line of interest (usually across one of the valves). CW Doppler detects velocities all along this line and is useful for recording the maximum flow velocity and the flow pattern through a stenosed valve. Using the modified Bernoulli equation the peak instantaneous valve gradient can be estimated (see next section). Rapid sampling frequency allows high velocities to be detected (up to 8 m s^{-1}).

The density of the signal envelope at a given velocity is determined by the number of red cells travelling at that velocity. When blood flow is laminar, flow velocities all fall within a given velocity range and a band surrounds the Doppler envelope. With turbulent flow, the Doppler signal is more heterogeneous in intensity – this is known as *spectral broadening* (Fig. 19.4).

Pulsed-wave Doppler

Unlike CW, PW Doppler measures blood flow velocity within a small area of the Doppler sample line – this is called the *sample volume*. This is done by sending 'pulses' of ultrasound and measuring the frequency shift of the returning echo to determine blood velocity within the sample volume (Fig. 19.5). PW Doppler is usually limited to a lower velocity range than CW Doppler (maximum 1.5–2.0 m s^{-1}). Measurement of blood flow at a specific depth is useful for detecting acceleration of blood through a stenosed valve. Using PW and CW Doppler, blood flow velocity on both sides of the stenosis can be measured.

VALVE DOPPLER SIGNALS

Aortic and pulmonary valve Doppler signals normally consist of a single

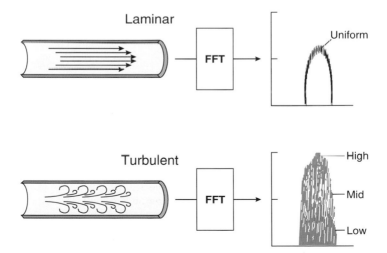

Fig. 19.4 Laminar and turbulent Doppler blood flow signals.

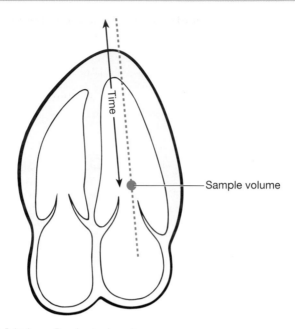

Fig. 19.5 Pulsed-wave Doppler signal sampling.

asymmetric peak of laminar flow. The rate of rise of the Doppler waveform reflects ventricular contractility. The area under the Doppler envelope is termed the *velocity time integral* (VTI); this value can be measured on screen. VTI is directly proportional to blood flow and, in the absence of valve regurgitation, cardiac output (see later).

Tricuspid and mitral valve Doppler signals are double peaked in sinus rhythm because there are two phases to diastolic flow: passive flow in early diastole, followed by 'active' flow due to atrial systole. This gives rise to the 'E' (early) and 'A' (atrial) waves of the Doppler waveform. In healthy individuals, the peak E-wave velocity is greater than that of the A-wave (i.e. *E:A ratio* >1.2:1). The amplitude and duration of the E and A waves give useful information about diastolic function:

● E:A reversal (peak velocity of A wave greater than E wave) occurs with some myocardial pathologies, e.g. in LVH or post-MI (early filling reduced because of ↓ ventricular compliance, atrial 'kick' contributes relatively more to filling).
● E-wave duration prolonged in mitral stenosis (LA and LV pressures take longer to equilibrate).

● Large E wave seen in advanced constrictive pericarditis and restrictive cardiomyopathy (ventricles fill rapidly to maximum capacity in early diastole; atrial kick cannot fill ventricles any further).

The Bernoulli equation

This equation relates pre- and post-valve velocities to the pressure gradient across that valve:

$$\Delta P = 4 \times (V_2^2 - V_1^2)$$

where ΔP = pressure gradient (mmHg), V_1 = pre-valve velocity (m s^{-1}) and V_2 = post-valve velocity (m s^{-1}).

If $V_2 \gg V_1$ then this can be further modified to:

$$\Delta P = 4 \times V_2^2$$

If tricuspid regurgitation is present the Bernoulli equation allows indirect determination of pulmonary artery systolic pressure using the following principles:

● RV and PA systolic pressure are virtually identical in patients who have a normal pulmonary valve.
● RV systolic pressure can be estimated from the tricuspid regurgitant velocity and central venous pressure (CVP):

$$\text{RV or PA systolic pressure (mmHg)} = \frac{4 \times V_{TR}^2 + (CVP + 5)}{1.3}$$

where V_{TR} = tricuspid regurgitant velocity (m s^{-1}). CVP can be estimated by examining the jugular venous pulse.

TROUBLESHOOTING

No Doppler signal

This occurs when the Doppler gain setting is too low, the velocity scale is incorrectly set, the 2D image is poor, or when blood flow is perpendicular to the probe. Increase the gain, check the scale settings or try another view.

Aliasing and the Nyquist limit

Pulsed-wave Doppler produces bursts of signals at a given frequency (pulse repetition frequency) and if the signals fall out of phase *aliasing* occurs. This effect is analogous to the apparent backward rotation of a wheel on a forward-moving stagecoach in an old Western film. Aliasing occurs when the Nyquist limit (half the pulse repetition frequency) is exceeded. On screen, the Doppler signal exceeds the highest (or lowest) point on the velocity scale and 'wraps' around the top or bottom of the display, making it impossible to interpret the tracing. Aliasing is more likely to occur at greater scanning depths and with higher transducer frequencies. It can sometimes be overcome by moving the

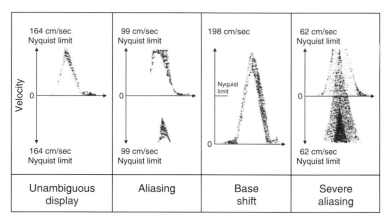

Fig. 19.6 Aliasing and the Nyquist limit.

Doppler baseline to the bottom or top of the display, thereby doubling the Nyquist limit (Fig. 19.6). The pulsed repetition frequency can be increased above the Nyquist limit on some modern echo machines. This allows PW Doppler assessment of higher flow velocities, e.g. in aortic stenosis. Aliasing may also occur when the Doppler velocity scale has been set inappropriately.

Doppler gain
The Doppler gain settings should be adjusted so that there is no background noise while giving a clear Doppler signal envelope. If the gain setting is too high, the background is very noisy and unclear and 'mirroring' below or above the baseline may occur (see Fig. 19.7).

Poor-quality Doppler signal
If the 2D images are poor the Doppler signal usually follows suit. The Doppler signal can be improved using similar methods as with 2D imaging (see next section). However, Doppler measurements are generally limited to certain views, as the transducer axis must be parallel to the line of flow. Some echo machines allow an angle correction factor to be used if the probe cannot be correctly aligned (see Fig. 19.3).

STANDARD TRANSTHORACIC PROTOCOL

The following is a suggested basic echo protocol. Clearly, this can be modified depending on the clinical problem being investigated.

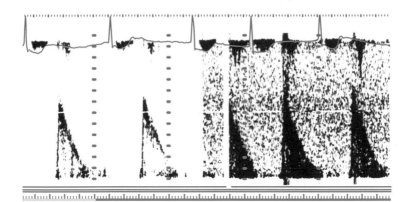

Fig. 19.7 Noise and appropriate gain settings.

TABLE 19.2 Adult reference ranges for spectral Doppler measurements

Measurement	Site	Range	Units
Peak valve velocity	Aortic	0.9–1.8	m s⁻¹
	Mitral	0.6–1.4	m s⁻¹
	Pulmonary	0.5–0.9	m s⁻¹
	Tricuspid	0.4–0.8	m s⁻¹
Mitral valve	Peak early, E	0.5–1.1	m s⁻¹
	Peak late, A	0.2–0.7	m s⁻¹
	E/A ratio	1.2–2.0	

INITIAL PREPARATION

• Make sure you are familiar with the equipment controls and, if not using a digital acquisition system, that the videotape is wound to the correct place (there's nothing worse than recording over someone else's scans!).
• Enter patient details on to system.
• Position patient comfortably and correctly.
• Attach the ECG cable; ensure you have a clear trace – often missed, but essential to time the cardiac cycle.

GETTING IMAGES

Image quality depends on:

• Chest anatomy: patients with emphysema or chest wall deformities are difficult to scan.

- Patient position: rested semirecumbent at 45° and leaning over in the left decubitus position.
- Probe position: place the probe between the ribs and over the pleural window.
- Contact gel.
- Machine settings: ensure correct depth, gain, transmission and processing levels are set.

SUGGESTED ECHOCARDIOGRAM ROUTINE

Parasternal long-axis view
- 2D images
- CFM of mitral and aortic valve
- M-mode of both the mitral and aortic valves. Record aortic root, LA, LV and RV dimensions
- Measure septal and posterior wall thickness in systole and diastole.

Parasternal short-axis view
- 2D images in the following planes:
    aortic valve
    mitral valve
    basal LV
    apical LV
- During above, CFM of tricuspid and pulmonary valve. Also, colour flow mapping of mitral and aortic valves if regurgitation seen in long-axis view.
- CW Doppler of tricuspid and pulmonary flow.
- M-modes: assess mitral and aortic valves. Record LV and aortic dimensions.

Apical four- and five-chamber views
- 2D imaging. Angle probe cranially to obtain five-chamber view.
- CFM of tricuspid, mitral and aortic valves.
- CW and PW Doppler of tricuspid, mitral and aortic valves.

Apical long-axis and two-chamber views
- 2D imaging both in long-axis view (aortic valve/root plane) and two-chamber view (anterior/inferior wall plane)
- CFM of mitral and aortic valves
- CW and PW Doppler of mitral and aortic valves.

ASSESSING LV FUNCTION

LV function can be assessed by echo quantitatively, semiquantitatively and qualitatively. Quantitative methods (which produce indices such as LV ejection fraction) are time-consuming and often inaccurate. Semiquantitative methods, which utilize regional wall motion scores (assessed subjectively by the operator) are easier to apply and are useful for patients with ischaemic heart disease. Qualitative or 'eyeball' assessment is most commonly used, categorizing LV function as normal, or mild, moderate or severe impairment.

2D IMAGING

A systematic approach is needed when assessing LV function, which can be assessed at two levels: global function and regional wall function. *Regional* LV dysfunction suggests an ischaemic aetiology, whereas *global* dysfunction may suggest an underlying cardiomyopathy or LV impairment secondary to valve pathology.

All 2D views need to be examined when assessing LV function. As no single view shows all LV wall segments, reliance on a single view can be misleading. For example, patients with LV dysfunction due to an anterior MI often have an apical wall motion defect with normal function at the base of the heart. Thus, LV function in the parasternal short-axis view will appear normal, but the apical views will show the true extent of LV impairment.

Assessing regional wall motion

The left ventricle can be divided into segments for regional wall motion analysis. Both 9- and 16-segment models can be used; the 9-segment model is quicker and adequate for everyday purposes (Fig. 19.8). The function of each

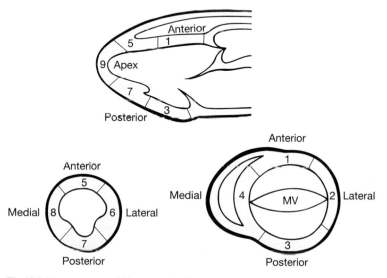

Fig. 19.8 Nine-segment model for regional wall motion assessment.

segment is graded as normal, hypokinetic, akinetic or dyskinetic. To assess segmental function, the following should be examined:

- **Wall thickness** – hypertrophy or thinning (e.g. due to previous MI).
- **Wall motion** – direction and magnitude. This is sometimes difficult to assess because of translational motion of the heart within the chest.
- **Wall contraction** – during systole the myocardium should thicken.

An aggregate wall motion score can be derived from segment analysis, but the main purpose of using a segmental model is to discipline oneself to examine LV function systematically. Wall motion scores themselves are not widely implemented other than as a research tool.

M-MODE IMAGING

This should always be done if image quality allows. Performed correctly, M-mode assessment provides useful additional information about LV function.

LV wall motion

M-mode assessment allows quantitative assessment of LV contraction. However, becuase M-mode assessment is mainly confined to the interventricular septum and posterior wall, it can over- or underestimate cardiac function in patients with *regional* LV dysfunction. In particular, estimation of LV ejection fraction from the M-mode makes the geometric assumption that the LV is conical or ellipsoid in shape and extrapolates global function from the motion of just two segments. Regional wall motion abnormalities render this type of calculation inaccurate.

Valve motion

In low cardiac output states left ventricular ejection time (i.e. duration of aortic valve opening) and leaflet excursion are reduced. Mitral valve diastolic opening time may also be reduced because of high LV end-diastolic pressure.

DOPPLER ASSESSMENT

The aortic valve CW Doppler signal can be used to estimate cardiac output, as follows:

- The area subtended by the CW signal envelope (i.e. velocity–time integral (VTI); see earlier) is directly proportional to cardiac output. VTI is measured in cm.
- The area through which blood flows, i.e. the aortic root, can be estimated by measuring the aortic root diameter. Aortic root area is measured in cm^2.
- VTI $\times$ aortic root area = stroke volume, measured in ml.
- Stroke volume $\times$ heart rate = cardiac output, measured in ml min^{-1}.

Using the M-mode recording in both parasternal views at the mitral valve tips, left ventricular end-systolic (LVESD) and diastolic diameters (LVEDD) and septal (IVSWT) and posterior wall thickness (PWT) should be measured and averaged. These measures are made at the end of diastole, coincident with the R wave of the QRS complex. The end-systolic dimension is measured at peak of contraction. The shortening fraction is defined as:

$$\text{Shortening fraction, SF} = \frac{100 \times (\text{LVEDD} - \text{LVESD})}{\text{LVEDD}}$$

The ejection fraction can be estimated by the simple cube (Teicholz) method:

$$\text{Ejection fraction, EF} = \frac{100 \times (\text{LVEDD}^3 - \text{LVESD}^3)}{\text{LVEDD}^3}$$

The modified Simpson's rule provides a more accurate assessment of ejection fraction but requires two measurements of left ventricular end-systolic and diastolic diameters equidistant along the ventricle – usually at the tips of the mitral valve and at the level of the papillary muscles – and determination of left ventricular length.

The Penn convention calculates left ventricular mass as follows:

$$\text{Left ventricular mass (g)} = 1.05 \times [(\text{LVEDD} + \text{IVSWT} + \text{PWT})^3 - \text{LVEDD}^3]$$

TABLE 19.3 Estimating global LV function. Limitations are described above

LV function	Shortening fraction(%)	Ejection fraction (%)
Normal	>25	>45
Mild	18–25	36–45
Moderate	10–17	28–35
Severe	<10	<28

$$\text{Cardiac output, CO (ml min}^{-1}\text{)} = \frac{\text{VTI}_{ao} \times \text{HR} \times \pi \times D_{ao}^2}{4}$$

where HR = heart rate (min^{-1}).

This assumes the absence of significant aortic valve disease and, crudely, cardiac output can be gauged by the magnitude of the aortic outflow velocity. Thus, low-output states have low Doppler velocities and high-output hyperdynamic states have high velocities.

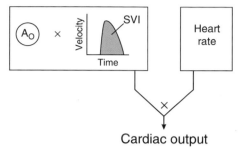

Fig. 19.9 Doppler determination of cardiac output.

The accuracy of cardiac output estimation depends upon the accurate measurement of aortic root diameter and on the correct alignment of the ultrasound beam in the direction of aortic blood flow.

Diastolic LV function

The mitral valve PW Doppler signal can provide an indication of left ventricular diastolic function. The two main Doppler indices are the E:A ratio (see earlier and below) and isovolumic relaxation time, but they are highly load and heart rate dependent. The isovolumic relaxation time (normal range 48–65 ms) is the time taken from the closure of the aortic valve to the onset of diastolic filling, and equates to the period between the second heart sound and the onset of the E wave of the mitral valve Doppler signal. This measurement therefore necessitates the simultaneous recording of the phonocardiogram.

Acoustic quantification will potentially provide a more useful method of assessing left ventricular diastolic dysfunction. Here, the endocardial border is continuously mapped to produce a volume/time curve. This requires the appropriate computer software, and border detection is facilitated by the use of echogenic contrast agents.

TABLE 19.4 Echo indices of diastolic dysfunction. IVRT = isovolumic relaxation time, i.e. the interval between aortic valve closure and mitral valve opening

	<30 years	30–50 years	>50 years
E:A ratio	<1.0	<1.0	<0.5
E-wave deceleration time (ms)	>220	>220	>280
IVRT (ms)	>92	>100	>105

LEFT-SIDED VALVE DISEASE

MITRAL STENOSIS (Fig. 19.10)

The severity of mitral stenosis is assessed by the valve's appearance on the 2D image and by Doppler assessment of the mitral valve pressure gradient. Additional supporting information is obtained by measuring left atrial size and by estimating PA pressure using the Bernoulli equation (see earlier).

2D imaging

In mitral stenosis leaflet movement is restricted, giving them the characteristic 'hockey stick' appearance in the long-axis and four-chamber views; the commissures fail to separate and leaflet tissue bows into the left ventricle. In the short-axis view planimetry of the mitral valve orifice can provide an accurate assessment of valve area, provided measurements are made precisely at the leaflet tips. Left atrial enlargement is seen with moderate or severe mitral stenosis and, when associated with low cardiac output, spontaneous echo contrast is seen owing to sluggish blood flow, rouleau formation and eddy currents. Dystrophic calcification is often seen within the mitral annulus and subvalvular apparatus.

M-mode imaging

Mitral leaflet separation is restricted and the normal M-W pattern is replaced by an orthogonal box. Left atrial diameter may be increased.

Doppler assessment

The colour flow map usually shows accelerated turbulent diastolic flow at the valve orifice and may show associated mitral regurgitation. CW Doppler shows prolongation of the E wave (because it takes longer for LA and LV pressures to equilibrate in diastole) and spectral broadening. The peak diastolic velocity is related to the peak pressure gradient across the valve (Bernoulli equation, see earlier). Mitral valve area and the mean pressure gradient can be calculated from the diastolic flow envelope.

MITRAL REGURGITATION

Mitral regurgitation is easy to detect using modern echo technology; very mild degrees of mitral (and tricuspid) regurgitation are nowadays regarded as a normal finding. However, although it is easy to detect, it is less easy to quantify without resorting to complicated and potentially error-prone methods.

2D imaging

This helps identify the aetiology of mitral regurgitation. The mitral valve and supporting apparatus should be examined systematically:

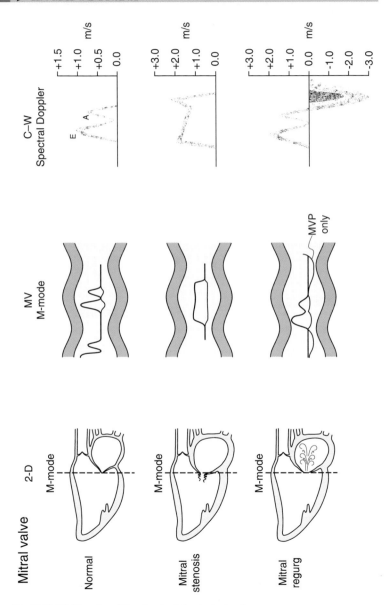

Fig. 19.10 2D, M-mode and Doppler signals in mitral valve disease.

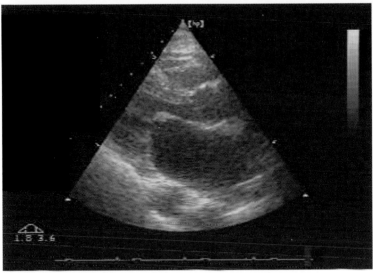

Fig. 19.11 2D views of stenosed mitral valve.

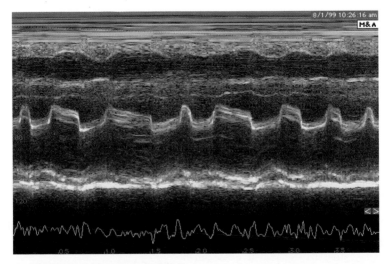

Fig. 19.12 M-mode of stenosed mitral valve.

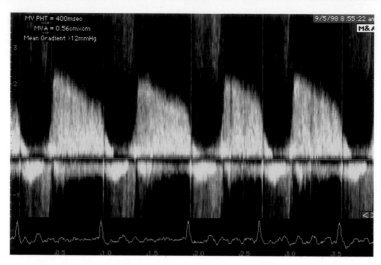

Fig. 19.13 Spectral Doppler signal in mitral stenosis.

● Mitral leaflet shape: calcified / rheumatic leaflets (rheumatic mitral regurgitation), vegetations
● Mitral leaflet motion: do leaflets fail to meet (e.g. annular dilatation), or does one leaflet prolapse behind the other?
● Chordae: any sign of chordal calcification (may restrict leaflet motion) or rupture?
● Papillary muscle function: any wall motion abnormality in segments associated with papillary muscles (i.e. posterior wall and septum)?
● Left ventricle: is it dilated? (This is the most common cause – *functional* mitral regurgitation due to LV dilatation.)

> **Tip:** Severe mitral regurgitation with a normal-sized left atrium suggests an acute aetiology. Look carefully for signs of chordal or papillary muscle rupture.

M-mode imaging
M-mode imaging provides additional supportive information:

● Leaflet motion – displacement and separation of the mitral leaflets seen in late systole
● Left atrial size – quantitative assessment
● Left ventricular dimensions.

Pressure half-time (PHT) is the time taken for the pressure gradient to fall to half its initial value. As there is a squared relationship between pressure and velocity, this translates into the time taken for the velocity to fall by ~30%. Mitral valve area (MVA) can be estimated as follows:

$$MVA \ (cm^2) = \frac{220}{PHT \ (ms)}$$

These measurements are made from the mitral CW Doppler envelope, by tracing around it. PHT is calculated from the rate of fall of flow from the peak of the E wave. In patients with atrial fibrillation measurements from several cardiac cycles should be averaged. Aortic incompetence can also prevent accurate estimation of MVA by distorting the CW envelope and by inducing functional mitral stenosis. In the absence of significant mitral regurgitation, the continuity equation provides an alternative method of calculating mitral valve area:

$$MVA \ (cm^2) = \frac{SV}{VTI_{mv}}$$

where SV = stroke volume $\frac{(VTI_{ao} \times \pi \times D_{ao}^2)}{4}$; and VTI_{mv} = velocity time integral of the mitral flow.

TABLE 19.5 Severity of mitral stenosis assessed using spectral Doppler measurements

Severity	Valve area (cm²)	Mean gradient (mmHg)	Pressure half-time (ms)
Normal	4.0–6.0	–	<60
Mild	2.2–1.6	<5	100–149
Moderate	1.5–1.0	5–10	150–220
Severe	<1.0	>10	>220

Doppler assessment

Colour flow mapping (Fig. 19.14)

This usually reveals a jet of regurgitant flow into the left atrium. Examination of the colour jet helps identify the cause of the valve leak. A central jet is associated with annular dilatation and functional mitral regurgitation. An eccentric jet is often associated with rheumatic disease and mitral valve prolapse and can be easy to miss as only a small part of the jet may appear in any one imaging plane.

Semiquantitative assessment of mitral regurgitation can be made from the colour flow map:

● Jet length mapping: the jet is graded from + to ++++ as follows:
    +   trivial regurgitation seen behind leaflets

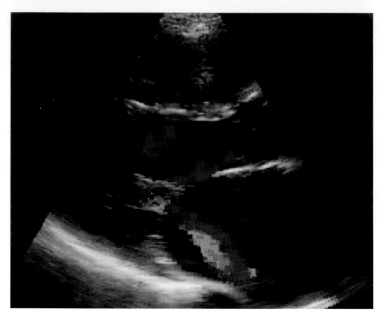

Fig. 19.14 Colour flow mapping of mitral regurgitation.

++   jet extends 1/3 way back into left atrium
+++   jet extends 2/3 way back into left atrium
++++   jet extends to back wall of left atrium.

Jet length mapping is error-prone and dependent on Doppler gain settings, velocity scale and left atrial size.

● Planimetry of colour jet: time-consuming and gain-dependent, inaccurate with eccentric or wall jets.

● Proximal isovelocity surface area (PISA) method: the most accurate method but time-consuming. Involves examining the colour flow map on the *ventricular* aspect of the mitral valve. Using a low-velocity scale setting a cone shape is seen on the colour map, centred on the leaflet tips. This represents blood accelerating into the regurgitant orifice. The volume of the cone is proportional to the regurgitant volume.

Spectral Doppler
Spectral Doppler gives limited information about the type and severity of mitral regurgitation. CW Doppler is sensitive at detecting small jets, but these are usually clinically unimportant. The regurgitant jet is usually of high velocity (>4 m s^{-1}), reflecting LV systolic pressure.

● Jet density mapping is used as a crude index of severity of regurgitation, based on the assumption that a denser CW envelope indicates more blood cells regurgitating.

● The onset of mitral regurgitation in late systole indicates mitral valve prolapse.

● If the pulmonary veins can be seen on the 2D image, PW Doppler can be used to examine pulmonary vein flow. In severe mitral regurgitation pulmonary vein flow reverses in systole as a result of increased left atrial pressure.

ASSESSING PROSTHETIC MITRAL VALVES

Metallic valve prostheses generate large acoustic shadows, making structural assessment very difficult. Mitral prostheses are often aligned in an anteriorly rotated position. This should be borne in mind during Doppler assessment, as the outflow jet is often eccentric. Forward flow can be readily measured from a transthoracic approach, but prosthetic mitral regurgitation is much more difficult to detect because the prosthesis' acoustic shadow masks the left atrium. Transoesophageal echo largely overcomes this limitation and should be used if the clinical index of suspicion is high. Despite the limitations, transthoracic echo does provide useful information:

● **Peak diastolic velocity** – if increased above reference range for the particular model of prosthesis (Table 19.6), may indicate paraprosthetic regurgitation or, less commonly, restriction of opening of the prosthesis.

● **LV function** – hyperdynamic LV contraction often accompanies severe prosthetic or paraprosthetic regurgitation.

Mitral valve prostheses usually have a slightly stenotic flow profile on Doppler assessment, which relates to aperture size.

TABLE 19.6 Normal values (± standard deviation) for selected prosthetic valves in the mitral position. These values are affected by valve size (smaller valves relatively more obstructed)

	Peak velocity (ms)	Peak gradient (mmHg)	Pressure half-time (ms)	Valve area (cm²)
Mechanical				
Starr–Edwards	1.97 ± 0.42	15.5 ± 5.8	113 ± 29	1.95 ± 0.50
St Jude	1.56 ± 0.29	10.0 ± 3.6	77 ± 17	2.88 ± 0.64
Bjork–Shiley	1.62 ± 0.30	10.7 ± 2.7	90 ± 27	2.40 ± 0.62
Tissue				
Carpentier–Edwards	1.76 ± 0.74	12.5 ± 3.6	90 ± 25	2.45 ± 0.74
Hancock	1.54 ± 0.26	9.2 ± 3.2	129 ± 31	1.71 ± 0.41
Ionescu–Shiley	1.46 ± 0.27	8.5 ± 2.9	93 ± 25	2.36 ± 0.75

AORTIC STENOSIS (Fig. 19.15)

2D imaging

Aortic valve morphology is often distorted in aortic stenosis because of fibrosis and calcification. The parasternal views are the most helpful for assessing valve structure and associated abnormalities:

● Leaflet separation. If leaflets are not clearly seen to separate, aortic stenosis is likely to be severe.
● Leaflet closure line (long-axis view) – if off-centre relative to the aortic annulus, the aortic valve may be bicuspid. Confirm in short-axis view and M-mode.
● Proximal aorta (long-axis view) – look for poststenotic dilatation.
● LV wall thickness – LVH accompanies moderate or severe aortic stenosis.
● LV function – dilated and impaired if decompensation occurs.

M-mode imaging

Look for:

● Thickening of leaflets and loss of normal 'box' appearance
● Reduced leaflet excursion due to cusp fusion
● Eccentric closure line in bicuspid aortic valve
● Increased LV wall thickness ± dilatation.

Doppler assessment

Colour flow mapping shows a turbulent jet in the aortic root. A regurgitant jet is often seen in association with aortic stenosis. CFM is not useful for assessing the severity of aortic stenosis: this is done using spectral Doppler as follows:

● In the apical five-chamber view, align the LV outflow tract with the Doppler cursor line.
● Position the PW sample volume in the LV outflow tract, just under the aortic valve and measure the peak systolic velocity. This is the peak 'pre-valve' velocity.
● In the same alignment, use CW Doppler to measure the peak systolic velocity through the aortic valve. Fine adjustments in probe position are usually needed to 'catch' a clean flow envelope. This gives the peak 'post-valve' velocity.
● Repeat the 'post-valve' measurement using a 'stand-alone' Doppler probe from the upper right sternal border and suprasternal notch and use the highest recorded post-valve velocity for calculations.
● The ratio of pre-valve:post-valve velocity is used to estimate the peak systolic gradient across the valve, using the Bernoulli equation. A pre:post-valve ratio ≥ 1:4 is associated with severe aortic stenosis.
● Do not rely on post-valve velocity to assess the severity of aortic stenosis: it

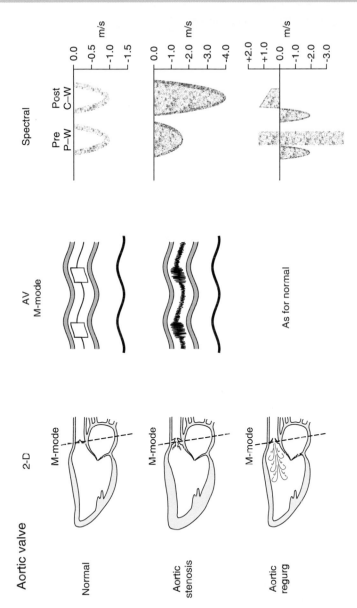

Fig. 19.15 2D, M-mode and Doppler signals in aortic valve disease.

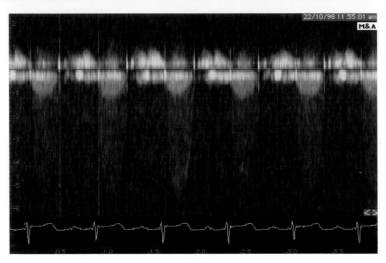

Fig. 19.16 Spectral Doppler signal of aortic stenosis.

can be increased by other factors, e.g. anaemia or sepsis and reduced if LV function is impaired. The pre:post-valve velocity ratio is the most reliable index.

TABLE 19.7 Severity of aortic stenosis using spectral Doppler measurements

Severity	Valve area (cm²)	Peak velocity (m/s)	Peak gradient (mmHg)	Mean gradient (mmHg)
Normal	2.5–3.5	0.9–1.8	–	–
Mild	1.0–1.5	≤ 2.5	<25	<15
Moderate	0.5–1.0	2.6–3.9	25–64	15–50
Severe	<0.5	≥ 4.0	>64	>50

AORTIC REGURGITATION

2D imaging

The valve may appear structurally normal, but look for the following:

- Aortic root dilatation
- Calcified/rheumatic cusps
- Vegetations

- LV dilatation/rapid diastolic filling/systolic impairment in severe aortic regurgitation
- Fluttering of anterior mitral leaflet due to impingement of the regurgitant jet.

M-mode imaging
- Failure of cusp apposition (rarely seen)
- Fluttering of anterior mitral leaflet, early closure due to high LVEDP in severe aortic regurgitation
- LV dilatation ± hypertrophy.

Doppler assessment
As with mitral regurgitation, the severity of aortic incompetence is difficult to assess. Using colour flow mapping the width the regurgitant jet and the distance it travels into LV are indicators of severity. If the jet fills the entire width of the LV outflow tract, this suggests severe regurgitation. Spectral Doppler provides additional information:

- Increased systolic flow in LV outflow tract (>1.5 m s^{-1}) may indicate a large regurgitant volume.

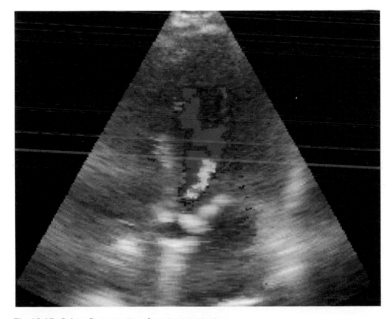

Fig. 19.17 Colour flow mapping of aortic regurgitation.

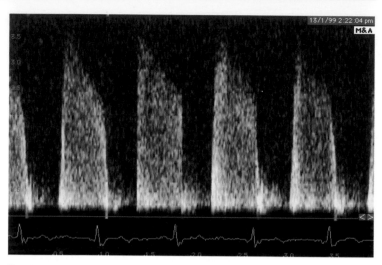

Fig. 19.18 Spectral Doppler signal of aortic regurgitation.

● The shape of the regurgitant flow envelope indicates how rapidly aortic and LV pressures equilibrate in diastole. A flat diastolic flow envelope indicates mild regurgitation; a rapid deceleration in diastolic flow velocity indicates severe regurgitation.

ASSESSING PROSTHETIC AORTIC VALVES

Although aortic prostheses also generate large acoustic shadows, their alignment allows for easier assessment of function than with mitral valve prostheses. Paraprosthetic leaks and systolic flow velocities can be readily assessed using the apical views. Most aortic prostheses produce a mildly stenotic flow profile on Doppler assessment, with higher postvalve velocities generated by small diameter valves. Very small prostheses (e.g. 17 mm) can produce a peak systolic pressure gradient of around 50 mmHg.

RIGHT-SIDED VALVE DISEASE

The pulmonary and tricuspid valves are assessed in a similar way to the aortic and mitral valves, but they are less easily imaged and a modified approach is needed.

PULMONARY VALVE DISEASE

The pulmonary valve is often difficult to image from the standard

TABLE 19.8 Normal values (± standard deviation) for selected prosthetic valves in the aortic position. These values are affected by valve size (smaller valves relatively obstructed)

	Peak velocity (ms)	Peak gradient (mmHg)	Mean gradient (mmHg)
Mechanical			
Starr–Edwards	3.10 ± 0.47	38.6 ± 11.7	24.0 ± 4.0
St Jude	2.37 ± 0.27	25.5 ± 5.1	12.5 ± 6.4
Bjork–Shiley	2.62 ± 0.42	23.8 ± 8.8	14.3 ± 5.3
Tissue			
Carpentier–Edwards	2.37 ± 0.46	23.2 ± 8.7	14.4 ± 5.7
Hancock	2.38 ± 0.35	23.0 ± 6.7	11.0 ± 3.3
Ionescu–Shiley	2.49 ± 1.71	24.7 ± 7.7	14.0 ± 4.3

transthoracic windows. It is best seen in the parasternal short-axis view, in the plane of the aortic valve. Complete visualization is unusual and often only the posterior cusp is seen.

Colour flow mapping may show pulmonary regurgitation, a common finding in pulmonary hypertension (see Chapter 13). CW Doppler is used to measure regurgitant velocity, which allows estimation of PA diastolic pressure using the Bernoulli equation (see earlier). PW and CW Doppler are used to measure pre- and postvalve systolic flow, in a similar manner as for aortic stenosis. Pulmonary systolic flow velocity may be increased (>1.5 m s^{-1}) in any of the following situations:

- Increased cardiac output (see earlier)
- Pulmonary regurgitation
- Left-to-right shunt (e.g. VSD).

TRICUSPID VALVE DISEASE

The tricuspid valve is best imaged in the short-axis and four-chamber views, but it is not usually possible to distinguish the three cusps in these views. The four-chamber view allows assessment of the leaflet attachments (displaced towards the apex in Ebstein's anomaly – see Chapter 13). Tricuspid regurgitation is a very common finding and its presence allows the assessment of PA systolic pressure by assessing pulmonary pressures and hypertension (see earlier).

The formula given above for estimating mitral valve area does not apply to the tricuspid valve. Tricuspid stenosis can be detected by other means:

- Tethering or 'doming' of the tricuspid leaflets
- Increased diastolic flow velocity, turbulence
- Right atrial enlargement.

Note that severe tricuspid stenosis is often associated with a very small pressure gradient.

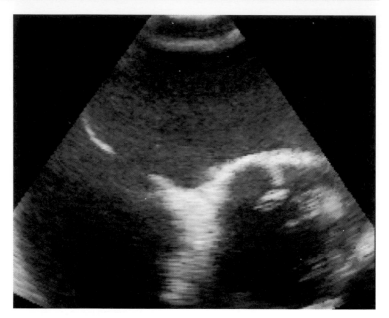

Fig. 19.19 Atrial septal defect.

INTRACARDIAC SHUNTS

ATRIAL SEPTAL DEFECT (Fig. 19.19)

Detection of ASDs using transthoracic echo can be difficult. Careful selection of views and interpretation of images is essential. Of the 'standard' transthoracic views, two provide a window on the interatrial septum – the four-chamber view and the short-axis view in the aortic valve plane. Both are prone to artefact, called 'echo dropout', in which a 'hole' is seen in the interatrial septum at its thinnest part because it is aligned along the ultrasound beam.

2D imaging

If an ASD is suspected the subcostal views provide the best window. Echo dropout is less likely and the structure of the interatrial septum and associated abnormalities can be examined:

- Discontinuity of septum
- Atrial septal aneurysm (associated with multiple small ASDs – fenestrated septum)

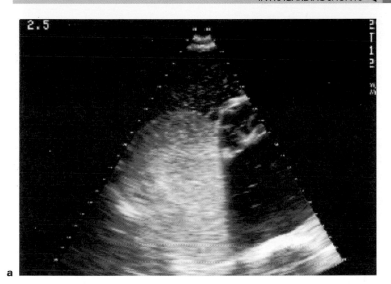

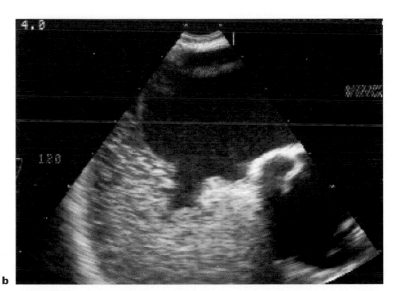

Fig. 19.20 Atrial septal defect imaged with echo contrast.

- Right-sided chamber dilatation
- Endocardial cushion defects (e.g. mitral valve prolapse, VSD).

Doppler assessment

- CFM of the interatrial septum (take care not to interpret tricuspid regurgitation, caval or coronary sinus flow as an ASD).
- Compare left and right ventricular outflow velocities; increased RVOT flow (>1.5 m s^{-1}) in left-to-right shunt. As pulmonary hypertension develops the shunt may lessen.
- Long-standing moderate or large ASD associated with pulmonary hypertension: assess pulmonary and tricuspid regurgitant flows to estimate PA pressure (see previous section).

Contrast echocardiography

If there is uncertainty about the diagnosis of ASD, contrast echocardiography is helpful. Agitated saline is the most widely used contrast agent, but commercial agents are now available which may be more sensitive at detecting intracardiac shunts. Agitated saline contains microbubbles which are very echo-reflective and are easily seen filling the right-sided chambers following IV injection. Microbubbles do not normally pass into the left side of the heart and are trapped in the pulmonary capillary bed before being absorbed into the bloodstream. Great care should be taken during agitated saline injection if a right-to-left shunt is suspected, as there is a risk of systemic air embolism.

How to do an agitated saline contrast echo

- Obtain peripheral IV access.
- Attach three-way tap and two 10 ml syringes to the IV cannula.
- 10 ml of saline is rapidly pumped to-and-fro between the two syringes to induce microbubble formation. No air should be present.
- Inject the agitated saline rapidly into cannula.
- In the subcostal or four-chamber view, agitated saline contrast is easily seen as it opacifies the right atrium and ventricle.
- A right-to-left shunt is indicated by the passage of microbubbles into the left-sided chambers.
- A left-to-right shunt is indicated by the presence of a contrast-free jet within the opacified right atrium.

VENTRICULAR SEPTAL DEFECT

Congenital VSDs most often occur in the membranous part of the interventricular septum, adjacent to the aortic valve (see Chapter 14). VSDs are best detected using colour flow mapping in the parasternal and apical views. CW Doppler often detects a high-velocity jet, although this may be absent if there is pulmonary hypertension or if Eisenmenger syndrome has developed. The severity of the shunt is in part related to the size of the jet, but left and right ventricular outflow velocities should be compared to estimate shunt size.

Acquired VSDs due to acute MI more often occur in the mid or apical septum. Multiple jets, or a fenestrated appearance, may be seen because of the serpiginous nature of postinfarct VSDs. RV dilatation may be seen; this is an ominous prognostic sign.

RUPTURED SINUS OF VALSALVA

Aortic root abscesses, particularly those associated with valve prostheses, can cause rupture of the sinus of Valsalva. Colour flow mapping shows a turbulent jet extending from the aortic root into the right atrium, or less frequently the left atrium. The jet tends to run along the superior aspect of the AV valve leaflets. CW Doppler may demonstrate a high-velocity jet. Vegetations and aortic regurgitation are common associations (see Chapter 4).

INTRACARDIAC MASSES

Intracardiac masses are usually spotted when an echo is ordered in one of the following clinical situations:

- Embolic events (e.g. TIA or peripheral embolism)
- Suspected endocarditis
- Incidental finding – echo ordered for unrelated indication.

It is often difficult to tell what the mass is, using echo criteria alone: images have to be interpreted in the context of the clinical picture. Although there are features that suggest, for example, tumour or thrombus, these features are not definitive. 2D imaging is the most useful modality; M-mode and Doppler add little information. When a mass lesion is identified, examine it systematically as follows:

- Number of lesions
- Lesion size (use on-screen callipers to measure in at least two axes)
- Echogenicity (relative to normal myocardium)
- Site (attached to valve, adherent to chamber wall, partly intramural?)
- Attachment (e.g. attached by stalk, or fixed over larger area?)
- Mobility (is lesion likely to embolize?).

Failure to identify thrombus or vegetations does not exclude their presence, and if clinical suspicion is high transoesophageal echo is indicated.

THROMBUS

Fresh thrombus is not particularly echogenic, but as it becomes organized it becomes more echogenic and produces a brighter signal than the surrounding myocardium. Thrombus is seen in one of three sites: adherent to the ventricular walls (mural thrombus), in the atrial appendages and, rarely, in transit through the heart.

> **Tip:** Acoustic artefact is often misdiagnosed as mural thrombus, especially at the LV apex. Try to confirm its presence in at least two views.
>
> *In situ* thrombus formation almost never occurs in patients with a normal ECG and CXR, except when associated with cardiac tumours.

Mural thrombus

Mural thrombus is most often seen in the LV, becoming visible as early as 48 hours after acute MI. It is most common after anterior transmural MI, is seen in up to 30% patients and is especially common at the LV apex or overlying large akinetic, dyskinetic or aneurysmal segments. It is very rare to see mural thrombus over a segment of myocardium that contracts normally. Mural thrombus also occurs with dilated cardiomyopathy, especially after viral myocarditis. Embolization is likely if the thrombus is frondlike, sessile or very mobile.

Atrial thrombus

Thrombus tends to form in the atrial appendages of patients who have mitral or tricuspid valve disease associated with atrial fibrillation. Patients with gross atrial enlargement often have 'spontaneous contrast' in the atria – a smokelike appearance caused by swirling of microaggregates which form as a result of stasis. Unfortunately the atrial appendages cannot be seen using transthoracic echo. Left atrial thrombus should be suspected in any patient with a recent history of an embolic event and atrial fibrillation, especially if there is evidence of mitral valve disease.

Pulmonary embolism/thrombus in transit

Long strands of mobile thrombus are occasionally seen in the right-sided chambers of patients who present with pulmonary embolism: this is thrombus 'in transit' from the leg or pelvic veins to the lungs. This appearance is exceptional, but serves to confirm the diagnosis. More often the echo is normal or shows signs of RV strain – RV dilatation, impaired systolic function, flattening of the interventricular septum in the short-axis view and tricuspid and/or pulmonary regurgitation.

VEGETATIONS

Thickening of valve leaflets is common in the elderly and in patients with rheumatic heart disease. It can be difficult to distinguish this from organized vegetations. The following features are suggestive of vegetations:

- Mobile
- Multiple lesions
- Shimmery; has a sessile, friable or variegated appearance
- Site:
    on the low-pressure side of the valve or defect
    opposite a jet lesion (e.g. VSD, aortic incompetence jet)
- Low density relative to rest of valve.

TUMOURS

These are discussed in depth in Chapter 13; the echo characteristics of the two most common primary cardiac tumours are discussed here.

Atrial myxoma

Atrial myxoma has a characteristic bright, gelatinous loculated appearance (Fig. 19.21). The myxoma is usually attached by a pedicle to the interatrial septum and may prolapse through the mitral valve. CW Doppler may confirm interruption of late diastolic flow. Right atrial myxomas also occur, but less commonly (5:1, left:right).

Papillary fibroelastoma

These small tumours usually arise from the papillary muscle or adjacent valve

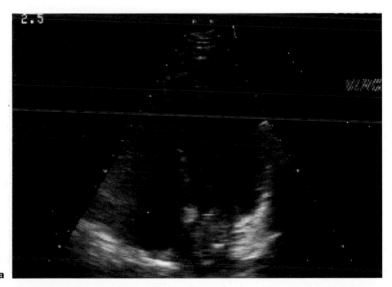

a

Fig. 19.21 a, 2D image of an atrial myxoma.

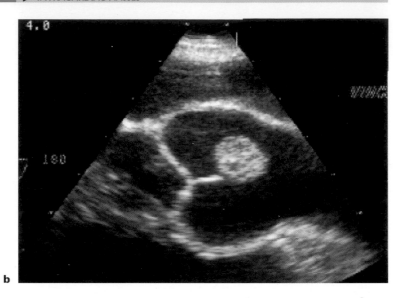

b

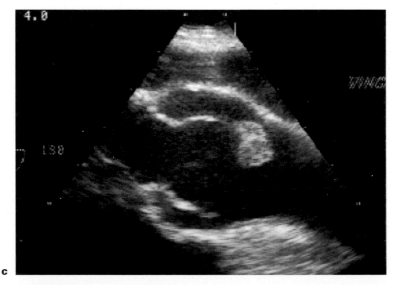

c

Fig. 19.21 b and **c**, aortic valve fibroelastoma.

structures. They are often small, of similar echo density to myocardium, mobile, well circumscribed, clinically silent and often present as an incidental finding. The most common associated symptoms are those associated with systemic embolization.

MYOCARDIAL AND PERICARDIAL DISEASE

HYPERTROPHIC CARDIOMYOPATHY

The clinical features of hypertrophic cardiomyopathy are discussed in Chapter 13. This condition can be difficult to detect in its early stages; evidence of impaired diastolic function may precede overt LVH.

2D imaging

● LVH	– symmetrical (concentric LVH)
	– asymmetric septal hypertrophy (ASH), leading to outflow obstruction
	– apical hypertrophy
● LV cavity obliteration	– reduced cavity size, banana shape in four-chamber view
● LA enlargement	– due to ↓ LV compliance
● RV hypertrophy	– occasionally accompanies LVH.

M-mode imaging

The assumptions used to estimate LV mass only apply when the LVH is concentric (see earlier). The following features may be seen:

- Asymmetric septal hypertrophy (ASH) = septal:posterior wall thickness >1.3:1
- Reduced LV end-systolic dimension
- Systolic anterior motion of mitral valve (SAM) due to outflow obstruction
- Increased LA diameter.

Doppler assessment

LV outflow obstruction

PW Doppler is helpful to determine flow velocity at different levels in the LV cavity. If there is significant acceleration of flow between midcavity and the LV outflow tract, with a high outflow velocity (>1.5 m s^{-1}), outflow obstruction is likely. CW Doppler helps identify the peak systolic velocity in the outflow tract, an index of the severity of obstruction. Outflow obstruction is accentuated by exercise, GTN or the Valsalva manoeuvre. The shape of the PW Doppler trace is often asymmetrical, or 'scalloped', with relatively slow flow early in systole, accelerating rapidly to a peak late in systole as outflow obstruction occurs.

Diastolic dysfunction
Decreased LV compliance may lead to diastolic dysfunction; see Table 19.4 for indices.

DILATED CARDIOMYOPATHIES

Echo is used to assess the severity, complications, progression and prognosis of dilated cardiomyopathy. The main echo finding is a dilated, impaired left ventricle (see earlier section). Serial echo studies can be used to monitor disease progression:

- LV systolic and diastolic dimensions
- LV systolic function
- Assessment of aetiology: regional *vs* global dysfunction
- Functional mitral and tricuspid regurgitation (due to dilatation of valve annuli)
- PA pressure from tricuspid and pulmonary flow (secondary pulmonary hypertension).

RESTRICTIVE CARDIOMYOPATHY

Restrictive cardiomyopathy is caused by infiltration of the myocardium with abnormal material, e.g. amyloid protein. This impairs the ability of the ventricles to relax, increases wall stiffness and in advanced cases compromises systolic function. The ventricular walls may appear thickened and of abnormal echogenicity and left and right atrial pressures increase, causing these chambers to dilate. It is extremely difficult to distinguish restrictive cardiomyopathy from constrictive pericarditis using echo, as the effects on diastolic function are similar.

2D imaging
- LVH appearance, with abnormally bright 'ground-glass' myocardial signal
- Dilatation of LA and RA
- Impaired LV systolic function
- (Sometimes) thickening of valve leaflets and interatrial septum.

M-Mode imaging
- Increased LV wall thickness
- Normal or reduced LV cavity size
- Impaired LV systolic function.

Doppler assessment
- (Early) – E:A reversal due to diastolic impairment
- (Late) – high-velocity E wave with sharp deceleration, small A wave due to severe restriction (ventricles fill to maximum capacity early diastole, atrial kick contributes little to filling). A wave may be lost due to atrial fibrillation

- Little variation of right-sided Doppler flows with respiration (more marked variation seen in constrictive pericarditis).

PERICARDIAL EFFUSION

Echo is very sensitive at diagnosing pericardial effusion (Table 19.9). It is very common to see a thin rim of pericardial fluid during echo studies and this can be regarded as normal. Echo gives information about the location, size, aetiology and composition of a pericardial effusion.

- Location   – circumferential, regional (e.g. posterior) or loculated
- Size   – can be estimated approximately from thickness of fluid on echo
- Aetiology   – myocardial rupture (thin-walled, echolucent, akinetic segment)
                  – aortic dissection (aortic incompetence, dissection flap in aortic root)
- Composition   – fibrinous fronds are seen in inflammatory and haemorrhagic pericardial effusions.

The distribution of pericardial fluid helps decide whether a subxiphoid or an apical approach is preferable if the effusion needs to be drained. Tamponade is a clinical diagnosis and supportive information may be given by echo:

- RV collapse early in diastole (use M-mode from parasternal long-axis view for timing)
- RA collapse (four-chamber view)
- LA and LV collapse (uncommon)
- Respiratory variation in tricuspid and mitral flow (↑ tricuspid and ↓ mitral flow on inspiration).

TABLE 19.9 Estimating volume of pericardial effusion from echo

Severity	Depth of effusion (cm)	Approximate volume (ml)
Mild	0.5	300
Moderate	1.0	500
Severe	2.0	700

Tip: After cardiac surgery the RA and RV may adhere to the pericardium. Any pericardial effusion may be localized to the posterior LV wall, compressing it and compromising LV function. The characteristic RV and RA collapse of tamponade may not be seen.

Differential diagnosis

The following may be mistaken for pericardial effusions:

- Pleural effusions
- Pericardial fat pad
- Pericardial cysts or tumours.

AORTIC DISSECTION

See Chapter 4 for clinical presentation.

Transthoracic echo is not a good imaging modality for diagnosing aortic dissection, but does provide useful supportive information in these cases. It cannot exclude dissection because only the aortic root and proximal ascending aorta can be imaged clearly. The following should be sought:

- Intra-aortic flap: may be seen in long-axis and suprasternal views in proximal type A dissection
- Aortic root dilatation and aortic incompetence
- Pericardial effusion due to rupture into pericardial space
- Regional wall motion abnormality due to coronary artery dissection (most commonly RCA – inferior wall)
- LVH – evidence of long-standing hypertension, predisposes to dissection.

> **Tip:** Acoustic artefact in the long-axis parasternal view often gives the appearance of a dissection flap in the ascending aorta.

Confirmation of the diagnosis and assessment of the extent of dissection requires one of the following: spiral CT scan, MRI scan or transoesophageal echo.

STRESS ECHOCARDIOGRAPHY

Stress echo is an evolving technique which assesses myocardial function during pharmacological or physiological stress. By examining the response of wall segments to stress it is possible to derive information about myocardial viability and regional perfusion. Stress echo has two main applications: risk assessment in patients with suspected IHD and assessment of myocardial viability in patients known to have IHD. The following principles are applied when interpreting stress echo:

- During stress, reduction of wall motion (in a segment which contracts when patient is at rest) implies that the segment is subtended by one or more flow-limiting coronary stenoses.
- During low-dose pharmacological stress, improvement of function in an

impaired segment implies that the segment is viable (either **'stunned'** after a period of ischaemia/reperfusion, or **'hibernating'**, i.e. subtended by a critically stenosed vessel).

The diagnostic accuracy of stress echo is highly dependent on the training and experience of the operator. Operators skilled in conventional echo require hands-on training from an experienced operator before undertaking stress echo studies.

INDICATIONS

Risk assessment in patients with suspected IHD
Some patients with suspected IHD cannot be reliably assessed using exercise ECG. Alternative, non-invasive approaches such as stress echo and stress myocardial perfusion scanning (see Chapter 20) are helpful in these cases. (In experienced hands stress echo has superior sensitivity and specificity for diagnosing underlying CAD than exercise ECG.) Indications are:

- Resting ECG abnormality which precludes interpretation (e.g. LBBB, LVH with ST segment depression)
- Inconclusive exercise ECG
- Inability to reach target heart rate/time during exercise ECG (e.g. due to immobility, coexisting lung disorder) – pharmacological stress echo
- Coronary stenosis of uncertain functional significance at angiography.

Detection of large/multiple hypokinetic or akinetic segments during stress suggests a flow-limiting stenosis of a major vessel, or multivessel disease. In cases where such prognostically important disease is suspected, angiography may be indicated with a view to revascularization.

Assessment of patients after MI
Stress echo can help identify myocardial segments which are prone to ischaemia and identify regions of viable but impaired myocardium after MI. Dobutamine stress echo (DSE) is reasonably safe when performed at least 5 days after MI. Stress echo can be useful after MI in the following groups of patients:

- When exercise ECG cannot be completed or result is inconclusive
- Significantly impaired LV function, to assess myocardial viability and likely improvement of LV function when angioplasty or CABG is being considered
- Suspected ischaemic LV dysfunction (e.g. exertional dyspnoea disproportionate to degree of resting LV impairment).

Assessment of myocardial viability
A low-dose IV infusion of a positive inotrope, usually dobutamine, can be used to stimulate the heart during stress echo. This is sometimes sufficient to

improve the function of segments that do not contract well at rest but which are viable. Three possible responses to DSE are seen in wall segments with impaired motion at rest:

- **Improvement with low-dose dobutamine.** Reperfused *stunned* (non-functioning at rest) myocardium may respond to low-dose dobutamine. These segments, which are hypokinetic or akinetic at rest and which improve during stress, often recover function after several weeks or months. Further improvement of segmental function with higher doses of dobutamine implies lack of critical stenosis in the infarct-related artery.
- **Improvement with low-dose dobutamine and deterioration with higher-dose dobutamine (biphasic response).** This implies a stunned segment subtended by a critical stenosis (i.e. ischaemia induced by high-dose dobutamine results in wall motion impairment). The term 'hibernating myocardium' is used to describe these segments, which may recover function after revascularization.
- **No improvement with dobutamine.** These segments tend not to recover in the long term and are probably infarcted.

STRESS PROTOCOLS

Exercise stress

LV function is assessed using the standard echo views at rest and immediately after a symptom-limited exercise test. A standard treadmill protocol, such as the Bruce protocol, is most often used (see Chapter 16). Because regional dysfunction can improve quickly after stopping exercise, a limited time window is available in which to obtain postexercise views. This can be partly avoided by using a supine bicycle rather than a treadmill, as long as adequate views are obtained in the exercise position. Exercise stress is further limited by respiratory artefact caused by hyperventilation, but is the most physiological of the stressors used.

Pharmacological stress

Although drugs do not produce identical physiological responses to exercise, the stressor can be given with the patient in an optimal position for imaging. The advantages in terms of image quality, the ability to image during rather than after stress and utility in patients who cannot exercise, make pharmacological stress very useful. The main stressors used are **dobutamine** and **arbutamine**. Adjuvant agents such as atropine and dipyridamole can be used to augment the heart rate response during stress. The protocols given for dobutamine stress are widely used (see Box), although many variations exist.

Recently, computerized infusion devices have been developed that monitor heart rate response to a challenge dose of inotrope. The device calculates a stress protocol adapted to the patient's evoked heart rate response, which helps prevent overshoot of the target heart rate.

Dobutamine stress protocols

Normal dose protocol – detection of inducible ischaemia
- Rest scan, then scan during **dobutamine IVI** for 3 min using the following incremental doses: 5, 10, 20, 30, 40 µg kg^{-1} min^{-1}.
- IVI is not increased to next increment if heart rate reaches target (85% of age-predicted maximum – see Chapter 16) or if significant chest discomfort develops.
- **Atropine 0.25 mg** aliquots can be given, to maximum of 1 mg, if adequate chronotropic response to dobutamine does not occur.

Low-dose protocol – assessment of myocardial viability
- Rest scan, then scan during **dobutamine IVI** for 3 min using the following incremental doses: 2.5, 5, 7.5, 10, 20 µg kg^{-1} min^{-1}.
- IVI is not increased to next increment if heart rate reaches target (85% of age-predicted maximum – see Chapter 16) or if significant chest discomfort develops.

Atrial pacing

This involves siting an oesophageal electrode or transvenous atrial pacing wire and incremental atrial pacing to stress the heart. This is a less 'physiological' stressor as little positive inotropic effect or peripheral vasodilatation occurs and is less sensitive at detecting inducible ischaemia than the methods outlined above. It is also uncomfortable for the patient and is little used.

IMAGE INTERPRETATION

Stress echo images are best stored on an ECG-gated digital image acquisition system. This allows side-by-side synchronized comparison of resting and stress images. A methodical approach maximizes diagnostic sensitivity. Regional wall motion analysis is performed using either a 9- or a 16-segment scoring system, as described earlier. The following are examined during each increment of the test:

- **Segmental appearance**: previously infarcted segments may appear thinned or abnormally bright at rest (recently infarcted segments may appear dark or echolucent).
- **Segmental wall motion**: net inward systolic motion of the segment.
- **Segmental wall thickening**: wall motion alone can mislead, since an akinetic segment may appear to move inwards when adjacent to a hyperdynamic segment. Contracting myocardium thickens during systole.
- **Left ventricular outflow velocity–time integral** (optional): this marker of cardiac output may remain static or decrease with stress if there is marked ischaemic LV dysfunction.
- **Mitral valve Doppler assessment** (optional): papillary muscle ischaemia may cause mitral regurgitation and can be detected using CFM and CW

Doppler. This should be done if there is an inducible septal or posterior wall motion defect, or if exertional breathlessness is a prominent symptom.

COMPLICATIONS OF PHARMACOLOGICAL STRESS

Stress echo is a safe procedure. The complications described below were noted in a published experience of over 2800 pharmacological stress studies; major complications occurred in 9 (< 0.5 %) patients. In that series there were no deaths (Secknus M A, Marwick T H. Evolution of dobutamine echocardiography protocols and indications: safety and side effects in 3,011 studies over 5 years. J Am Coll Cardiol 1997; 29:1234–1240).

Minor complications
- Flushing, dizziness
- Transient chest discomfort (an end-point of the test)
- Breathlessness
- Extrasystoles, transient SVTs
- Anticholinergic side effects (blurred vision, dry mouth) with atropine.

Major complications
- Sustained VT requiring intervention
- Myocardial infarction
- Sustained SVT requiring intervention
- Hypotension.

TRANSOESOPHAGEAL ECHOCARDIOGRAPHY (TOE)

TTE is simple, non-invasive and easy to perform. However, it has its limitations and in approximately 10% of cases satisfactory images cannot be obtained because of the patient's chest wall anatomy or build. TOE has many advantages over the transthoracic method. The ultrasound probe is positioned closer to the heart and uses a higher frequency, which provides better resolution. The signal-to-noise ratio is superior, providing better image contrast.

INDICATIONS

TOE is indicated in the diagnosis and evaluation of the following:

- Aortic dissection and thoracic aneurysms
- Infective endocarditis
- Prosthetic valve function (especially mitral)
- Congenital heart defects
- Aortic coarctation
- Assessment of mitral valve for repair or valvuloplasty
- Intraoperative assessment of valve repair or replacement
- Detection of thrombus in LA appendage.

CONTRAINDICATIONS

- Oesophageal disease or dysphagia (especially oesophageal strictures, pouches or varices)
- Respiratory compromise and hypoxaemia, such as with severe respiratory or left ventricular failure
- Cervical spine pathology (especially rheumatoid arthritis) – risk with neck flexion or hyperextension.

PREPROCEDURE CHECKLIST

The TOE procedure has a very small but quantifiable mortality risk which relates partly to the acute illness of some patients undergoing the procedure, e.g. aortic dissection. When TOE is performed carefully it is a relatively simple and safe technique.

- Check equipment.
- Explain procedure and risks.
- Obtain written consent *before* administering sedation.
- Check allergies.
- Remove dentures.
- Ensure patient fasted for at least 4 h.
- Topical local anaesthetic spray to oropharynx – very bitter! (e.g. 10% lignocaine pump spray (2–3 'shots' = 20–30 mg)).
- Attach ECG, blood pressure cuff and pulse oximeter.
- (Optional): sedation, usually short-acting benzodiazepine, e.g. **midazolam** 2.5–10 mg in small aliquots by slow IVI.

Warning: Rapid reversal of benzodiazepines can be achieved using flumazenil 0.2–0.5 mg, slow IVI, if patient becomes hypoxic or hypotensive during the procedure.

TRANSOESOPHAGEAL ECHO PROCEDURE

Before doing a TOE procedure for the first time it is strongly recommended that trainees obtain experience with oesophageal intubation alone. It is best to intubate 20–30 patients under the supervision of a trained gastroenterologist during an elective upper GI endoscopy list.

OESOPHAGEAL INTUBATION

After the preprocedure checklist has been completed the patient is rolled on to their left side. A mouth guard is inserted and the probe lubricated.

With the head flexed, the probe is advanced through the mouth guard and over the top of the tongue. When the patient reacts to the probe at the back of the mouth, the probe is temporarily angulated down to deflect it towards the oesophagus and gently advanced with continuous pressure. The probe is allowed to straighten and the patient is instructed to swallow. The probe should slide into the oesophagus with minimal resistance.

TROUBLESHOOTING

Agitation
Oesophageal instrumentation is uncomfortable and additional sedation may be needed. If the patient gags or retches, the oropharynx may not be adequately anaesthetized. Oversedation puts the patient at risk of hypoxia and arrhythmias, so use small aliquots (e.g. IV **midazolam** 2 mg). Ask the patient to concentrate on their breathing and to take slow, deep breaths. Even with heavy sedation some patients find the procedure intolerable and general anaesthesia or an alternative diagnostic modality may be needed.

Failed intubation
Maintain head flexion to ensure that the probe angles towards the oesophagus. Head extension, or passage of the probe along the hard palate, pushes the probe towards the trachea. Excessive angulation of the probe during intubation risks pharyngeal or oesophageal trauma. The probe may double back on itself, making oesophageal instrumentation impossible. Again, ensure that the patient is appropriately sedated.

Resistance to the probe
Never use excessive force with the probe, as laryngeal and oesophageal trauma may ensue. Consider anatomical abnormalities such as oesophageal pouches or strictures. If doubt remains, fibreoptic endoscopy may be necessary to identify any obstruction.

No image
- Check probe plugged in and selected.
- Check depth and gain settings.
- Ensure probe is correctly sited (left atrial level = 30–40 cm).
- Rotate probe and/or angulation it to improve contact with oesophageal wall.

COMPLICATIONS

These are uncommon but include:

- Bradycardias – usually vagally mediated and include AV block. IV **atropine** 500 µg may be required if patient compromised
- SVT
- Bronchospasm and respiratory depression

- Tracheal intubation, laryngeal trauma
- Aspiration due to vomiting
- Pharyngeal trauma
- Oesophageal tear or rupture.

TRANSOESOPHAGEAL VIEWS AND INTERPRETATION

TOE images are usually much clearer than transthoracic images, for reasons explained earlier. The standard TOE views are obtained as the probe passes down the oesophagus and into the stomach. A systematic approach helps ensure a complete and thorough examination. TOE probes have depth markers to help orientate the operator during the procedure.

Multiplane probes (which allow any imaging angle, from sagittal to transverse) allow selection of the best imaging plane, particularly when the alignment of the heart is unusual. In this section the standard biplane (transverse and sagittal) views are described. You will need to start thinking upside-down – these views appear inverted compared with their transthoracic equivalents! (Fig. 19.22).

STANDARD VIEWS

Transverse views

- **Ascending aorta** (25–30 cm) – reveals the ascending aorta, the left and right atria and their appendages and the right ventricular outflow tract.
- **Pulmonary valve** – as with the transthoracic short-axis views, the pulmonary valve is not always clearly seen. It comes into view as the probe is advanced to aortic valve level.
- **Aortic valve** (30–35 cm) – similar to the transthoracic short-axis view, shows left and right atria and interatrial septum (near field), aortic and tricuspid valve and right ventricle and its outflow tract (far field). The origin of the left main coronary artery is often visualized in this view. To see the aortic valve in true cross-section requires a multiplane probe with the beam angled to 20°.
- **Four-chamber view** (35–45 cm) – gives an oblique view of all four chambers, with the ventricles foreshortened. The mitral and tricuspid valves, left ventricular outflow tract, interatrial septum and atria are seen. Depending on the position of the heart relative to the oesophagus, the LV may be seen more along its long axis. This can also be produced using angulation of the beam with a multiplane probe.
- **Short-axis gastric view** (45–50 cm) – as the probe enters the stomach the liver is readily seen in this view and a true cross-sectional view of the ventricles is obtained.

Longitudinal views

With the probe at the level of the four-chamber transverse view (35–40 cm),

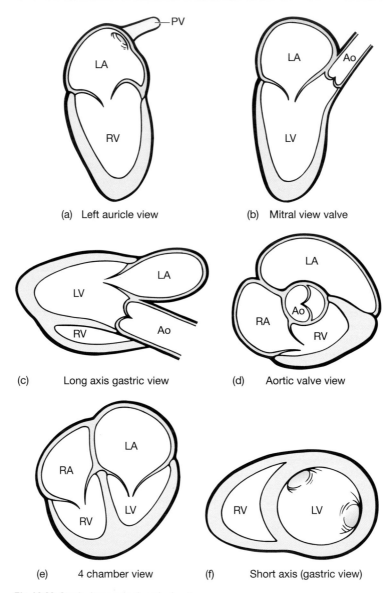

(a) Left auricle view

(b) Mitral view valve

(c) Long axis gastric view

(d) Aortic valve view

(e) 4 chamber view

(f) Short axis (gastric view)

Fig. 19.22 Standard transoesophageal echo views.

the longitudinal plane is used with a biplane probe or the beam is rotated to 90° with a multiplane probe. Longitudinal views are obtained by rotating the entire probe from left to right.

● **Left auricle view** – the probe is rotated to the left to image the left atrium and appendage, mitral valve and left ventricle. The left pulmonary artery is seen in cross-section and slight rotation brings the pulmonary veins into view.

● **Mitral valve** – subsequent rotation to the right gives a longitudinal two-chamber view of the left atrium and ventricle. The aortic valve and LV outflow tract may also be seen in this view.

● **Pulmonary valve** – further rotation to the right gives an excellent view of RV, RVOT, pulmonary valve and main PA. The left atrium, mitral valve and a small section of LV are seen between the probe and the right ventricle.

● **Superior vena cava** – further rotation to the right, with slight cranial tilt, gives a view of the right atrium and appendage, interatrial septum and superior vena cava. Lateral angulation brings the ascending aorta (left) and aortic valve (right) into view.

● **Gastric views** – passage of the probe into the stomach, and cranial angulation, allows imaging of the heart from the gastric fundus. The longitudinal view allows closer examination of the LV apex. Transverse views are similar to those obtained using the short-axis views from the lower oesophagus.

Aortic views

These views are very important for the assessment of aortic dissection (see Chapter 4). Transverse views of the aortic arch and ascending aorta are obtained from around 25 cm. Anticlockwise rotation through 120° brings the descending aorta into view. Passage of the probe further into the oesophagus permits examination of the entire descending thoracic aorta. The aortic valve and ascending aorta can be inspected using the superior vena cava view, above.

IMAGE INTERPRETATION

The approach to the assessment of cardiac and valvular function with TOE is the same as for transthoracic echo. As orientation of the cardiac structures is inverted compared to transthoracic echo, images may appear quite confusing at first. Some conditions lend themselves to assessment with TOE and are described below.

Atrial septal defect

The transverse aortic valve and four-chamber views are used to assess the interatrial septum. ASDs are identified using colour flow mapping and spectral Doppler. Occasionally, contrast injection with agitated saline is required (see earlier). With larger left-to-right shunts a dilated RV may be seen. Tricuspid and pulmonary regurgitant flows can be used to estimate pulmonary artery pressure. Filamentous and highly mobile structures may be seen in the enlarged RA – the Chiari network.

Percutaneous closure of ASDs requires prior assessment with TOE. This allows the operator to see whether there is enough free margin around the ASD to secure a closure device and also allows correct sizing of the device.

Atrial thrombus

The atrial appendages are a common site for thrombus formation in patients with atrial fibrillation, although trabeculae within the appendages may give a false impression of thrombus. The left atrial appendage is best assessed using the ascending aorta transverse and left auricle longitudinal views. CFM should be used to confirm that flow is present within the auricle. TOE is far more sensitive than transthoracic echo at detecting spontaneous contrast and atrial thrombus.

Assessment for mitral valvuloplasty or mitral valve repair

Careful patient selection is required for percutaneous balloon mitral valvuloplasty, as severe mitral regurgitation (requiring urgent valve replacement) can complicate the procedure. Features that predict a poor outcome or suboptimal result are:

- Leaflet rigidity

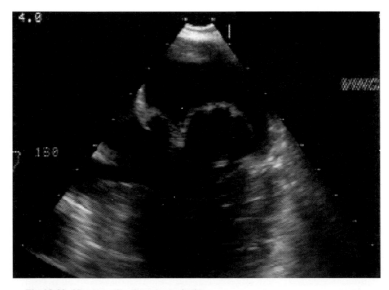

Fig. 19.23 2D image of prolapsing mitral valve.

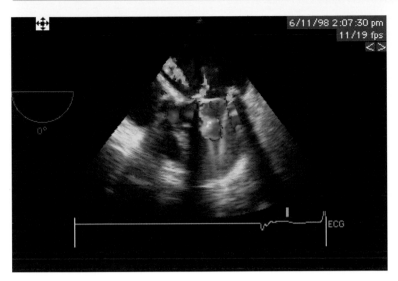

Fig. 19.24 2D image of prosthetic mitral valve with paraprosthetic regurgitation.

- Leaflet thickening
- Valvular calcification
- Subvalvular disease.

These four features may be scored on a 0–4 scale and an overall total above 8 indicates an unfavourable outcome.

Reconstruction or repair of the mitral valve may be possible in patients with non-calcific mitral regurgitation, pliable mitral valves, ruptured posterior mitral valve chordae, mitral valve prolapse (Fig. 19.23) or mitral valve annular dilatation. Adverse features are similar to those described for mitral valvuloplasty.

Mitral valve prostheses

The transverse aortic valve and four-chamber views give good views of the left atrium and of mitral prostheses. Regurgitant jets can be identified in these views, but the left ventricle may be obscured by acoustic shadow. The gastric views give a less obstructed view of the left ventricle.

Aortic dissection

The probe should be positioned at the level of the aortic valve in the transverse view. Retraction of the probe reveals the ascending aorta. Intimal tears are apparent as the flap traverses the lumen. Occasionally, involvement of the coronary artery ostia can be detected with TOE. The longitudinal mitral valve view can be used to examine the aortic valve and proximal ascending aorta – CFM should reveal any aortic regurgitation. Rotation of the probe through 180° shows the descending aorta, which can be examined in transverse and longitudinal views.

CHAPTER 20

NUCLEAR CARDIOLOGY

NUCLEAR CARDIOLOGY AND RADIOPHARMACEUTICALS

Nuclear cardiology encompasses a range of imaging techniques, both qualitative and quantitative, which use radiopharmaceuticals as a photon source. As such, they represent emission rather than transmission techniques and have constraints owing to the random vectors of radionuclide photons and the physical properties of the detector (γ-camera). Thus, they have poorer spatial resolution than conventional X-ray techniques such as angiography. However, they readily lend themselves to functional (e.g. myocardial perfusion imaging) and quantitative (e.g. ventriculography) cardiac assessment.

The generic term *radiopharmaceutical* describes a γ-ray or positron emitting radionuclide bound to one of several molecules used specially to target an area of interest. The term is used to describe γ-ray emitters such as technetium (^{99m}Tc) and thallium (^{201}Tl) chloride, and positron emitters such as ^{18}F fluoro-2-deoxyglucose (^{18}FDG). ^{99m}Tc photons (140 keV) are suited to the optimal energy range of γ-cameras (100–200 keV) and have a half-life of 6 hours. In contrast, ^{201}Tl (a $^+$K analogue) has relatively low energy (60–80 keV) and a biological half-life of 58 hours.

Dosimetry

- The average dose equivalent for a single ^{201}Tl scan is 18 mSv. This is equal to approximately three thoracic CT scans, or almost two coronary angiograms.
- A 2-day protocol ^{99m}Tc -tetrofosmin perfusion scan imparts a total of 6 mSv.
- An equilibrium ^{99m}Tc RBC ventriculogram imparts 7 mSv.

The following summarizes these radiopharmaceuticals according to their nuclear cardiology applications.

Radiopharmaceutical agents

^{99m}Tc (technetium)-labelled agents

- ^{99m}Tc-labelled red cells   – blood pool studies
                                         – ventriculography
- ^{99m}Tc tetrofosmin *or* ^{99m}Tc MIBI – myocardial perfusion imaging
- ^{99m}Tc pyrophosphate   – infarct scanning

^{111}In (indium)-labelled agents

- ^{111}In antimyosin antibodies   – infarct scanning

^{201}Tl (thallium)-labelled agents

- ^{201}Tl chloride   – myocardial perfusion imaging.

Positron emitters

- Usually cyclotron produced – high energy, short half-life (<2 h)

- Expensive and not widely available
- Gold standard for detecting hibernating myocardium
- ^{18}F fluoro-2-deoxyglucose (^{18}FDG) – hibernating myocardium
- ^{13}N ammonia – myocardial perfusion imaging
- ^{15}O – oxygen utilization.

IMAGING TECHNIQUES

SINGLE-PHOTON EMISSION COMPUTED TOMOGRAPHY (SPECT)

In addition to conventional static planar projections for ventriculography, SPECT is now routinely used for myocardial perfusion imaging. This employs a rotating γ-camera head which moves around the thorax acquiring multiple projections, from which a three-dimensional image is generated. Multiple detector heads (two or three) give superior resolution and shorter acquisition times.

POSITRON EMISSION TOMOGRAPHY (PET)

This uses the two high-energy photons (511 keV cf. 140 keV for ^{99m}Tc) that are emitted when a positron encounters an electron and annihilation ensues. Unlike the random vectors of single photons, these travel at 180° to each other, allowing paired detectors (usually a ring of 1500 small detectors) to register photon pairs by coincidence counting. PET therefore offers a higher spatial resolution than SPECT. The available short-lived emitters, e.g. ^{11}C, ^{13}N and ^{15}O, allow substitution in biologically active compounds, allowing observation and quantification of biochemical and metabolic processes. Despite these advantages, the routine clinical use of PET is constrained by limited availability and high cost.

RADIONUCLIDE VENTRICULOGRAPHY

Radionuclide ventriculography is one of several imaging modalities used to assess and quantify LV function. Echo is the most commonly used, is inexpensive, quick, and adequate for most applications, such as post-MI assessment. For accurate quantitative LV assessment, however, echo is limited by geometric constraints, interobserver variability and patient echogenicity. X-ray angiography also suffers from geometric limitations and is invasive. Radionuclide ventriculography is one of the most accurate and reproducible methods for LV assessment, with an interstudy variability of less than 5% and an interobserver variability (for ejection fraction estimation) as low as 2%, compared to up to 11% for echo. LV assessment can be made either by equilibrium ventriculography or by a first-pass technique, providing both global and regional information.

EQUILIBRIUM VENTRICULOGRAPHY

This is the most common technique and uses a sample of the patient's blood labelled with ^{99m}Tc to produce a blood pool acquisition of several hundred summated beats, gated to the QRS complex. These are acquired in a 45° left anterior oblique projection. Atrial fibrillation and extrasystoles may cause significant underestimation of ejection fraction and should be taken into consideration when interpreting the study.

FIRST-PASS VENTRICULOGRAPHY

This involves tracking a high-energy radionuclide bolus with a fast γ-camera. It is now possible to perform a ventriculogram at the same time as a perfusion scan using ^{99m}Tc-labelled agents such as tetrofosmin. The first-pass technique can also be used to detect and quantify intracardiac shunts using a pulmonary time–activity curve.

Indications for radionuclide ventriculography

- Management and prognosis post myocardial infarction (exercise LVEF gives information about ischaemic LV dysfunction)
- Prior to treatment with ACE inhibitors
- Risk assessment prior to major surgery, e.g. abdominal aneurysm
- Prior to cardiotoxic drugs, e.g. doxorubicin (baseline LVEF should not be <30%)
- Shunt detection and quantification
- Cardiac transplantation
- Assessment of cardiomyopathies
- Identification of LV aneurysms and diagnosis of coronary disease – rarely used.

Global ejection fraction is a good prognostic indicator post MI: an LVEF of <30% is associated with an annual mortality of 22% after a first MI, compared to 1% for those with LVEF >30%. LVEF <40% is also associated with a poorer outcome from elective abdominal aortic aneurysm surgery.

> **Tip:** The calculation of LVEF will vary depending on technique, and it is important to be familiar with the normal range (usually more than 50–65%) for your centre.

MYOCARDIAL PERFUSION IMAGING

Myocardial perfusion imaging allows the estimation of regional myocardial blood flow capacity by examining the relative distribution of a radiopharmaceutical after stress and at rest. During stress, territories subtended by a flow-limiting coronary stenosis will receive relatively less blood (and emitter) than territories with normal perfusion. [201]Tl is commonly used; tomographic imaging is performed immediately following a single injection of ^{201}Tl at the point of maximal exercise. This is followed by redistribution imaging at 3–4 hours.

[201]Tl has been the main perfusion agent used over the last 20 years, but has been superseded in many centres by [99m]Tc -labelled compounds such as *sestamibi* or, more recently, *tetrofosmin*. These agents provide higher resolution using a lower radiation dose than [201]Tl. The higher photon flux of ^{99m}Tc agents also makes it possible to acquire gated data for perfusion and LV function simultaneously. Unlike ^{99m}Tc, ^{201}Tl does redistribute and is therefore theoretically able to demonstrate hibernating myocardium on the delayed images. The relative merits of the two agents are summarized below:

---

[201]Tl vs ^{99m}Tc compounds

Thallium
- Single injection, so 1-day protocol with redistribution scan after 3–4 h
- Less expensive than ^{99m}Tc agents
- Theoretical advantage in demonstrating hibernating myocardium (reinjection)
- Less hepatobiliary uptake, so may image inferior wall better

Technetium compounds
- Higher photon energy, so better spatial resolution and diagnostic quality
- Up to one-third lower radiation dose than [201]Tl
- Tracer 'fixed' in myocardium, so no need to image immediately. This means that the treadmill need not be next door to the γ-camera
- Gated studies possible – LV function and perfusion simultaneously
- 2-day protocol preferable – resting scan can be avoided if stress normal

---

Stressors

Stressors used for myocardial perfusion imaging are exercise, dipyridamole, adenosine, dobutamine and arbutamine. Pharmacological stress is indicated for patients who cannot exercise. Although exercise (if possible) is the stressor of choice, drug stress is used preferentially in some centres for ease of scheduling.

- **Adenosine** or **dipyridamole** are preferable for patients with LBBB – tachycardia exacerbates poor diastolic septal blood flow.
- **Dobutamine** or **arbutamine** are preferable for asthmatics who cannot exercise (adenosine and dipyridamole can cause bronchospasm).
- **Exercise** should be the first-choice stressor for patients with good effort tolerance, even if prior exercise ECG is non-diagnostic.

Indications for stress myocardial perfusion imaging

Myocardial perfusion imaging is indicated in situations in which clarification of the presence, distribution or threshold of inducible myocardial ischaemia is required:

- High clinical suspicion with negative exercise test
- Low clinical suspicion with positive exercise test
- Borderline or uninterpretable exercise test
- Resting ECG precludes stress ECG test (e.g. LBBB, LVH with 'strain' pattern)
- Culprit vessel identification in multivessel disease
- Assessment post CABG or PTCA
- Identify hibernating myocardium (aids decision making when considering revascularization)
- Work-up for cardiac transplantation (to help exclude coronary revascularization as an option)
- Risk stratification prior to major non-cardiac surgery (e.g. vascular surgery).

Interpreting results

A photon-deficient area which remains unchanged on both phases of the study (*fixed defect*) may represent an area of infarction (Fig. 20.1). A defect on

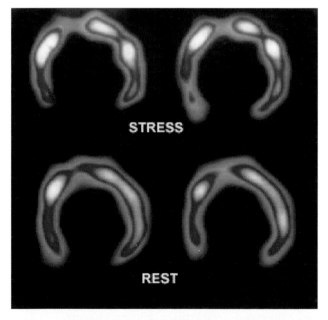

Fig. 20.1 ^{99m}Tc tetrofosmin scan with pharmacological stress, short-axis view. Stress images show dilated LV, an irreversible inferior defect and thinning of the anteroseptal segment. There is some reversibility in the lateral wall on the resting study. Severe three-vessel disease was found at angiography.

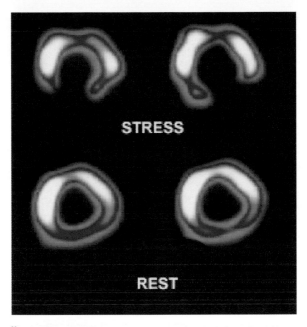

Fig. 20.2 ^{99m}Tc tetrofosmin scan with exercise stress, short-axis view. Stress images show a well defined inferior defect which reverses on the resting study. Minor anterior thinning. A severe PDA stenosis was found at angiography.

the post-stress scan which subsequently completely or partially normalizes (*reversible defect*) usually represents reversible ischaemia (Fig. 20.2). Perfusion defects may not be due solely to angiographically demonstrable coronary artery disease.

Prognostic assessment

In stable angina myocardial perfusion imaging is superior to stress ECG testing for detecting flow-limiting coronary stenoses, with a sensitivity of 90% and a specificity of 95%. The risk of cardiac death or MI is <1% in patients with angina and a negative perfusion scan. Cardiac events are extremely unlikely in patients with a positive exercise ECG and a negative perfusion scan. Single small defects are also associated with a good prognosis. In patients with positive perfusion scans the risk is related to the number and size of the perfusion defects (left main stem disease is more often associated with multiple, rather than single, large defects) and to the presence of *high lung uptake*, which is a marker of severe disease and poor prognosis.

Causes of perfusion defects other than macrovascular disease

Normal variants
- 'Patchy' low count scans – low injected activity or attenuation due to obesity
- Some inferior wall attenuation is common in men
- High diaphragm in obese patients also attenuates inferior wall
- Large or dense breasts attenuate anterior wall
- Apical thinning is a frequent normal finding
- Basal septum is membranous – may appear attenuated

(Most of these will show similar defects on both phases of the study)

Pathological
- Small vessel disease, e.g. in diabetes mellitus
- Cardiomyopathies
- Infiltration, e.g. amyloidosis, sarcoidosis
- Coronary artery spasm
- LBBB (may be pathological – can be difficult to interpret)

Identifying hibernating myocardium

Conventional ^{201}Tl perfusion imaging will significantly underestimate the amount of viable myocardium. ^{201}Tl reinjection techniques have shown that up to 50% of apparently fixed defects improve on delayed imaging. ^{201}Tl is better than ^{99m}Tc agents for this purpose and is almost as sensitive as PET scanning, in which ^{18}FDG is the gold standard.

IMAGING OF MYOCARDIAL INFARCTION

Myocardial infarction is normally diagnosed from the clinical history, electrocardiogram and cardiac enzyme estimation. In the presence of a non-diagnostic ECG or borderline enzyme elevation the diagnosis may be in doubt. In these situations, ^{99m}Tc pyrophosphate scanning can be used to identify recently infarcted myocardium.

Indications for infarct zone imaging
- Late presentation with normal cardiac enzymes
- Non-diagnostic ECG, e.g. LBBB
- Detection of peri-infarct MI after CABG.

Infarct zones are detected either using a 'hot spot' technique, which uses infarct-avid tracers (e.g. pyrophosphate), or 'cold spot' scanning, which uses a perfusion agent.

^{99m}Tc pyrophosphate (developed as a bone scanning agent) is taken up in Ca^{2+} deposits in necrotic myocardium >10–12 h post infarct. Peak uptake is at 48–72 h. Some uptake remains at 5 days, returns to normal within 10 days. SPECT imaging improves sensitivity (Fig. 20.3). ^{111}In antimyosin antibodies (murine monoclonal antibodies to myosin) are highly sensitive and specific

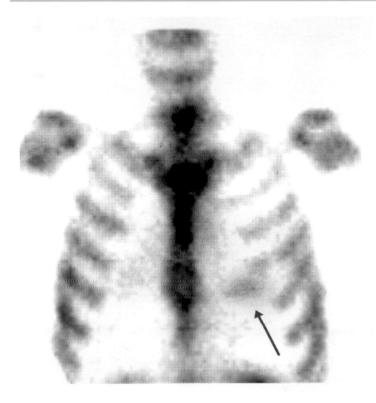

Fig. 20.3 ^{99m}Tc pyrophosphate scan showing a patch of abnormal increased uptake in the inferior wall (arrow). Recent suspected inferior MI with equivocal cardiac enzyme result.

for infarcted myocardium, but their high cost and the increased radiation dose currently preclude routine clinical use.

Causes of false positive ^{99m}Tc pyrophosphate scan

- Recent myocardial injury – contusion, myocarditis, pericarditis
- LV aneurysm, mural thrombus
- Calcified heart valves
- Amyloidosis
- Extracardiac abnormalities – rib/costal cartilage trauma, breast/lung tumours, surgical drains, defibrillator burns

INDEX

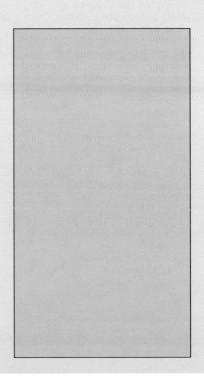